THE

INDISPENSABLE

CANCER

HANDBOOK

THE INDISPENSABLE CANCER HANDBOOK

A Comprehensive, Authoritative
Guide to the Latest and Best
in Diagnosis, Treatment, Care,
and Supporting Services

KATHRYN H. SALSBURY
ELEANOR LIEBMAN JOHNSON

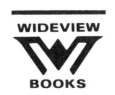

WIDEVIEW

BOOKS

Manufactured in the United States of America.
Second Printing
Wideview Books/A Division of PEI Books, Inc.

Line drawings by Eleanor Liebman Johnson.

Grateful acknowledgment is given for permission to reprint previously published material:
"The Patient's Bill of Rights" is reprinted with the permission of the American Hospital Association, copyright © 1972.
"The Dying Person's Bill of Rights," copyright © 1975, American Journal of Nursing Company, is reproduced, with permission, from *American Journal of Nursing*, Vol. 75, No. 1.

Library of Congress Cataloging in Publication Data

Salsbury, Kathryn H.
        The indispensable cancer handbook.

        Includes bibliographies.
            1.   Cancer—Handbooks, manuals, etc.   I.   Johnson, Eleanor Liebman.   II.   Title.
RC263.S24   1981b   616.99′4   81-50337
ISBN 0-87223-729-X (pbk.)   AACR2

Acknowledgments

We would like to thank the twenty oncologists and oncology nurses at the National Cancer Institute who helped check the accuracy, timeliness and quality of information in this volume. Despite their eighteen-hour-a-day schedules, they devoted many extra hours to insure that this was the kind of book we all felt should be written. Conflict-of-interest problems prevent us from thanking them by name, but we are forever in their debt—not only for the help they gave us, but also for setting the standard for the highest quality care to which we feel every cancer patient ought to be entitled.

Table of Contents

PART I

Understanding Cancer

Chapter Five: DIAGNOSTIC PROCEDURES AND TESTS— WHAT, WHY, AND HOW

Table of Contents

PART II

Specific Cancers

Table of Contents

PART III

Appendices

Introduction

One out of every four people gets cancer. There are 1,230,000 new cases diagnosed each year. Clearly then, cancer is not an isolated experience—especially when one considers that not only the patient but the patient's family, friends, employer, and neighbors will all be affected. If only twenty people are concerned with each patient (and that estimate is considered low), then over twenty million Americans become involved with cancer each year.

There seem to be two kinds of fear that people face. First, there is fear of death. A very quick look at the statistics—that over forty million of us are, right now, walking around with cancer, but only 400,000 of us will die from it this year—makes it obvious that having cancer is not an immediate death sentence. The real problem is living and dealing with cancer, not dying from it. And that leads us to the second kind of fear, which concerns the "unknowns" of cancer, and the complex world of cancer diagnosis and treatment.

The only way to deal with this welter of complicated, fear-laden treatment information is by self-education. The new knowledge required—specific, complete, and understandable—is presented from the patient's perspective in this book.

The traditional roles played by cancer patients, doctors, and other health professionals were based on two assumptions: that "cancer" always meant a painful, terminal illness; and that only the doctors had the ability to decide what patients should know. In the last ten years, both of these assumptions have been discarded. Tremendous advances have been made in the treatment of many kinds of cancer, and revolutionary changes have taken place in the treatment of pain and in the treatment of patients who are dying.

The biggest change is attributable to the rise of the consumer health movement, which contends that health is not a subject that can be left only to the professionals. They advocate that every member of society be responsible for his or her own good health, and that laymen cannot maintain their responsibility without being fully informed.

Until 1972, the amount of information provided to the patient was decided solely by his physician. The test of what was a "reasonable" amount of information was whether or not other "reasonable practitioners" would have given the same information in a similar situation. Since most doctors felt that medical decisions should be left to professionals, and that the more information a patient had, the more fearful he would become (an attitude particularly prevalent when dealing with cancer patients), patients were told very little. But, in *Canterbury* v. *Spence* (1972) the courts declared that doctors were legally obligated to conform to a standard of "informed consent," which the court defined as follows:

Doctors must disclose everything that, on the basis of medical training and prior experience, they would expect the average, reasonable patient to consider material to a decision to undergo the proposed treatment. This includes items such as the diagnosis, nature and proposed treatment plus its probability of success and its attendant risks and consequences, similar information concerning alternative treatment possibilities, and the prognosis if no treatment is received. An item of information is "material" if, by itself or in combination with other applicable information, it would cause the patient to refuse the recommended treatment.*

This right of full disclosure was not just a judicial whim that disregarded what was psychologically best for the patient. Studies of the relationship between doctors and cancer patients found that, contrary to doctors' beliefs, patients do want to know what is going on. Rather than increasing patient anxiety, information gives the patient a sense of control over his life, allowing him to become a partner in the healing process. This new definition of "adequate information" has been strongly supported by those health professionals whose main job it is to deal with people, not disease: the nurses and social workers.

The first step in becoming knowledgeable on the subject of cancer and its treatment is understanding that "cancer" is an umbrella word that covers over a hundred different disorders of cell growth. Because it centers around cells and how they work, both alone and in relation to other cells in the body, you must understand something of cell biology (the structure, function, and biochemistry of cells) and the human immune system to understand cancer. A glance at the Table of Contents will give you an idea of the diverse areas to be covered in acquiring an understanding of cancer.

During the preparation of this book, over a dozen cancer specialists checked the accuracy and timeliness of the information, insuring that

---

* Arnold J. Rosoff, "Informed Consent: A Developing Subfield of Medical Jurisprudence," in *The Cancer Patient: Social and Medical Aspects of Care,* ed. Barrie R. Cassileth (Philadelphia: Lea and Febiger, 1979), p. 81.

the procedures described reflect "best current practice." In addition to their specific input, many felt compelled to voice general concerns. Their points, as follow, are important to keep in mind when seeking and undergoing treatment for cancer:

Diagnosis and Treatment. Patients should make sure that they are dealing with doctors and hospitals that are expert in the diagnosis of cancer and in the planning and administration of potentially curable modes of therapy for their form of cancer.

Monitoring. All patients should adhere religiously to their schedule of checkups once treatment is finished.

Statistics. Physicians would prefer that statistics relating to prognosis not appear at all. One explained the problem this way: "Professionals find interpretation of claims in the literature about cure rates difficult. Individual patients have features that could make their outcomes much better or much worse than those in the literature. I think it is more useful to explain treatment in terms of 'likely to produce long-term complete remission and possibly cure' or 'unlikely to cure,' etc."

Epidemiology and the High-Risk Patient. Epidemiologists voiced concern that more space was not devoted to the preventability of the vast majority of cancer deaths. (See part III.) Clinical oncologists, however, were concerned that too much of certain types of epidemiological data had been included.

The Informed Patient. The reader should bear in mind that this book is a bridge to medical knowledge and not an end in itself. A partially informed patient can be very dangerous to his own care if he attempts to manage his own treatment. Specific treatments and diagnostic work-ups change rapidly in many instances, so patients must maintain flexibility in their expectations of physicians.

How to Use This Book

The *Handbook* was written to cover every kind of cancer. At the same time, we realized that most readers would have an immediate interest in understanding only one kind of cancer. Therefore, in organizing a book of this kind, a balance had to be struck between the fact that each type of cancer is unique and the fact that many aspects of diagnosis and treatment are common to a number of cancers.

Part I, "Understanding Cancer," includes subjects that relate to all or most cancer patients. Here you will find explanations of the biology of cancer: detailed explanations of the diagnostic process, diagnostic procedures, treatments, and support services; and directions for finding the best help available.

Part II deals with specific cancers. They have been arranged here alphabetically by primary site (bone, breast, etc.). Systemic cancers like leukemias and lymphomas are treated as sites and are listed with the others. If you are not sure of the primary site, or know the cancer by another name (such as "Wilms's tumor"), look it up in the index. This book covers every kind of cancer.

As a rule of thumb, in part II we discuss in detail only those things that relate specifically to a given type of cancer. All concepts and procedures involved in the diagnosis and treatment of one cancer, but which relate to many kinds of cancers, are listed in **boldface letters.** You can find the explanations for these in part I. Under site listings, you may also be referred to detailed information in the appendices, and to explanations appearing in other site discussions.

Each of these site discussions includes the following information:

Introduction. This gives a general description of the particular type of cancer, where it is located (you will want to refer to the drawings and diagrams in Appendix A), and its idiosyncrasies and epidemiology.

Symptoms. All symptoms for a given type of cancer are listed. (See also chapter 4, "Diagnosis," for general information on symptoms.)

Diagnosis and Staging. Diagnosis refers to that part of the process where the cancer is identified. Staging involves tests and procedures that pinpoint how far the cancer has spread from the primary site. All procedures and tests are listed, but only those that are unique to a given type of cancer are described in detail. Chapter 5 gives detailed descriptions of all procedures and tests that appear in boldface. Occasionally you may be referred to another site discussion for a description of a procedure. Chapter 4, "Diagnosis," contains a detailed discussion of the diagnostic process (including what is involved in a medical history and physical examination) and an overview of the various types of hospital tests.

Types of Cancer. This section identifies the specific cell types of cancer that affect particular parts of the body.

Treatments. This section briefly summarizes the standard treatments for each type of cancer. Treatment forms are described in detail in the chapters on surgery, radiation, chemotherapy, and lesser-known treatments, and supportive treatments. As a rule, the only comprehensive explanations you will find in this section are specific surgical procedures. (Note: Drugs currently being used in chemotherapy, hormone therapy, and immunotherapy are listed in part III.)

Experimental Treatments. What they are and how one becomes involved in them are discussed in chapter 6, "How to Find Help." In this section, therefore, we briefly list the types of experimental programs being conducted, with appropriate comments. The section ends with a list of initials, acronyms for the clinical cooperative groups working on each type of cancer. You can find names and addresses of the people to contact in these groups in Appendix H. (Note: Not all experimental programs will accept all patients.)

Doctors Who May Be Involved in Treatment. Several specialists can be involved in the "average" case of cancer. At least two of the specialists listed should be involved either directly or as consultants for confirming diagnosis and designing the treatment plan. This list is provided as a starting point in your search for appropriate treatment.

Resources and Further Reading. In this section we have included support programs and additional information written for the layman, if available.

A word about prognosis. Everyone is extremely interested in knowing his "chances." However, with the exception of those cancers where standard treatments are providing excellent results, we have not given statistical information on prognosis in the site chapters. The "odds" in any individual case are almost impossible to predict, and the available statistics are based on old information that may not be relevant to newer treatments. In the site chapters we do indicate whether certain standard treatments have had better response or survival rates than others, and whether certain experimental programs—which are incomplete but far enough along to give preliminary data—show significantly better results at this point than the standard treatments. Patients may want to make an extra effort to become involved in these experiments.

The appendices constitute part III. Here you will find four types of information referred to elsewhere in the book: anatomical drawings and diagrams; cancer statistics; technical information, including a list of all drugs used in standard and experimental treatments; and treatment information and resources. The latter includes phone numbers and addresses of diagnostic, treatment, and informational resources, organized alphabetically by state, as well as descriptions of National Cancer Institute programs and where to contact the Clinical Cooperative Groups, who administer experimental programs.

We suggest that you begin by reading through the table of contents and by skimming the site section in part II that describes the type of cancer in which you are interested. At this point there will be a great deal that you will not understand, but a fast read will let you know which chapters in the first section are particularly important for you. Later, you can reread the site discussion.

PART I

Understanding Cancer

Chapter One

CELLS AND TUMORS

Introduction

Cancer is a disorder of cell growth. Normal cells grow, divide, and band together into organized groups of organs and tissues. Although there are different types of cells, each is a part of a team whose sole reason for being is the creation and maintenance of the human body. Cancer cells also grow, divided, and band together, but their existence serves no useful purpose, and their behavior can cause great harm.

Until very recently, this limited explanation of cancer—the "cells gone mad" story—was the only one available to the general public. We now know that we need far more information to decide where to go for diagnosis and treatment.

We will begin by exploring the subjects of cell biology (the growth and function of both normal and abnormal cells), and epidemiology (why certain groups of people are particularly susceptible to specific types of cancer). We will discuss the numbers and words used to describe prognosis (what your chances are) and responses to cancer treatment. Armed with this information, you will be prepared for a fuller understanding of why "cancer" is presently considered to be over a hundred different diseases, why the diagnostic process has to be so thorough, and why different treatments have been developed and how they work. We will also explain why various lines of research are being pursued (or rejected), why each patient must be considered a unique case, and why the questions that you ask your cancer specialists—even those who are the best in their fields—cannot be answered with the degree of certainty, simplicity, and exactness that you would like.

The Normal Cell

Our body is made up of between five billion and one trillion cells. Each cell has a function in the body and its own special life cycle. Cell activities are controlled by the genetic programming contained in the strands of DNA found in the nucleus of each cell.

The cells in our body are constantly reproducing themselves. Every minute of our life, three million cells die and are instantly replaced. Yet different kinds of cells replace themselves at different rates: Nerve cells in the brain only replace themselves if they become damaged; while our white blood cells, which act as the main strike force for the immune system, completely replace themselves every six hours. If damage occurs anywhere, the cells responsible for making repairs will rush to the rescue, begin dividing very rapidly until the damage is repaired, and then return to their normal rate of growth.

Each part of a cell's life cycle is essential for it to accurately reproduce itself by dividing into two daughter cells. The life cycle of a cell is usually described as a five-phase process. G_0 is a resting phase, where no activity has yet been observed. It is followed by the G_1 phase, in which the cell prepares itself for the synthesis (production) of DNA. This leads directly to the S (synthesis) phase, in which the DNA reproduces to make an exact copy of the original chromosome blueprint. The cell then enters another preparation phase, G_2, when it readies itself for actual division. The final phase is the M (mitosis) phase, where the cell actually divides itself in two. These two daughter cells immediately go into the G_0 phase, and the cycle begins again. Each different type of cell has its own time clock that regulates how long this process takes. Not only do they differ in the length of time involved in completing the whole cycle, but different types of cells may stay in any one of the five phases for varying amounts of time.

In a healthy cell, the growth process functions in a very specific way that insures the continued health of the body as a whole. Each cell's growth is not only governed by the genetic master plan locked in the DNA, but also responds to signals indicating that the body has specific immediate needs. Cells are able to do this because they are differentiated. That means that the mature cells have very special and identifiable forms and functions. Differentiation can be seen not only in the role that each type of cell plays in maintaining the health and functioning of the body, but in the very complex jobs that each part of each cell must perform in order for the cell to remain that type of cell and carry out its proper function.

Although there are many kinds of cells in the human body, they have certain things in common. Each cell is surrounded by a membrane, which serves as a sentinel, protecting the cell and deciding which substances may go in and out of the cell. The membrane also identifies what kind of cell it is to other cells, and insures that the cell grows only so far and does not interfere with neighboring cells or invade their territory. This particular type of restriction on cell growth is called "contact inhibition."

Inside the membrane are the cytoplasm and protoplasm—made up of water, fats, sugars, and proteins. Living in this sticky stuff are the mitochondria and lysosomes. The mitochondria are not really a part of the cell, but are microscopic creatures that live there in a mutually advantageous situation: They provide energy and breathe for the cell, and the cell provides them with proteins to eat and a place to live. The lysosomes are powerful enzymes that also break down proteins. Lysosomes can be so powerful that they can cause the cell to self-destruct if it is placed under conditions of extreme stress. Besides having mitochondria and lysosomes for destroying proteins, cells also have two parts for protein production, called the endoplasmic reticulum and the Golgi apparatus.

Directing all this activity is the single nucleus, the control center for each cell. Inside the nucleus is the DNA (deoxyribonucleic acid). DNA is a protein that looks like two strands of ribbon wound around each other. On each strand are twenty-three genes, which carry the blueprint for our whole body and for the identity and functioning of each cell therein.

The DNA also sets limits, preventing cells from doing what normal cells do not do. One thing normal cells don't do is reproduce themselves beyond a certain point. Cells "know" when the organ of which they are a part has reached the right size, and how many and what kind of specialized types of cells are needed in order for the organ to function properly. If damage should occur to certain cells, only those damaged cells are replaced. Normal cells also know their place; they do not travel around the body searching for new and interesting places to grow.

In addition to the limits on growth set by the DNA and maintained by mechanisms like contact inhibition, growth is also regulated by chemicals called "hormones," which are produced by various glands throughout the body. Hormones can be thought of as the body's chemical communicators. They usually flow through our body, keeping the various systems fine-tuned to our immediate biological needs, and they also play a crucial role in emergency situations. When the body

5

is put in a physically or psychologically stressful situation, our hormone balance changes, sending a chemical message to all parts of the body to shift priorities. The so-called stress reaction is a very basic adaptive mechanism for reacting to situations of immediate physical danger which were a common part of life for primitive man. It prepares one for fight or flight by diverting energy from the normal cell activities (reproduction and warding off infectious diseases) and focusing the body's resources on physical strength. Obviously the body does not have to worry about producing children or even getting sick if it is about to be eaten by a bear.

In short, normal cells have a regular, predictable shape (which varies depending on what kinds of cells they are) and a certain number of parts, which have specific functions to perform. Normal cells follow the rules regarding growth and behavior which are set down by the genetic programming found in the DNA, and are fine-tuned to meet immediate needs of the body by correctly responding to messages conveyed by chemical communicators.

Cancer Cells

Cancer cells are cells that don't play by the rules. They are human cells and they do grow and multiply by division, but the daughter cells display the same abnormal characteristics as the parent cell. The word "abnormal" covers a wide range of traits and behaviors: Some abnormal cells will have no effect on the body at all; others can be fatal. Because of the tremendous range of variation to be found in abnormal cells, scientists have classified them on the basis of several factors: their physiology (what they look like and how their biochemistry works); their growth rate; their ability to spread (metastasize); and the extent to which they can perform the jobs necessary for normal functioning.

Physiology, the first major classification, distinguishes between non-malignant (benign) and malignant (cancer) cells. We will discuss benign cells in the next section. In this section we will describe the range of characteristics that define malignant cells and lead to the further subclassifications of those cells into the hundred-plus different kinds of cancer.

Physiology. Cancer cells don't look like normal cells, but there is a great variety in their appearance. Some look very much like the healthy cells around them (which makes the diagnostic process difficult), while other cells are truly bizarre: They can display such strange membranes that it is difficult to distinguish between where one cell stops and another begins; or have too many nuclei, or none at all; or too few chromosomes, or too many. Even the biochemistry of a cancer cell is different from that of a normal cell.

Growth rate. Cancer cells divide and multiply faster than the normal cells in the surrounding tissue. But since normal cells differ so greatly in their rate of growth (from rarely dividing once the body reaches adulthood, to reproducing every few hours), we see the same variety in cancer cells. Many cancers are slow-growing and do not produce symptoms for years; others have such rapid growth rates that they can reach lethal proportions within weeks. The average life-span of an active cancer cell is from one to ten days (that's the time between the birth of a cell and cell division). Determining the rate of growth of cancer cells is vital to correct diagnosis and treatment.

Metastasis. When doctors talk about metastasis, they are referring to the way in which the cancer spreads. Cancer cells do not respond to the normal limits placed on cell growth by contact inhibition or signals given off by hormones. Cancer cells grow right over other cells and invade healthy tissue—beginning as one abnormal cell in healthy tissue and spreading to other parts of the body as well. By using the blood and lymph systems as a form of transport, cancer can metastasize to distant parts of the body. Cancer cells also have the ability to fool the immune system, so that the normal forces that the body musters to fight off anything harmful are not called into play.

Differentiation. The range of differentiation to be found in various kinds of cancer cells is a factor in the types of treatment it responds to and how well it will respond. (See "Stages and Grades of Cancer" in chapter 2 for a more detailed discussion.) Scientists call all damaged cells "cancer" cells, or neoplasms. These include the nonmalignant cells found in warts, scar tissue, and benign tumors, as well as those malignant cells that most people think of as cancer. In this book we will use "cancer" in the usual sense—that is, to describe a malignancy.

The abnormal cell does not begin to cause problems for the body until it has reproduced itself enough times to be considered a mass. This mass of abnormal cells is called a "tumor." There are two types of tumors: malignant and benign. Malignant tumors are the main subject of this book, but it is also important for you to have some knowledge of benign tumors and their relationship to cancer.

Benign Tumors

Tumors not usually considered life-threatening are called benign. It may be easiest to think of benign tumors as collections of healthy cells

7

that are behaving in some respects like cancer cells. Though comparatively slow-growing, they do grow more rapidly than normal cells, producing an abnormal mass of tissue. They stay where they are, however; they do not spread to surrounding tissue, and they do not invade different parts of the body far from the original site.

Which is not to say that benign tumors are necessarily harmless. While they do not harm the body in the same way as a malignant tumor (by spreading and invading healthy tissue and cells), they may be dangerous in other ways, depending on where they are located. For example, benign tumors of the liver (which affect only the liver) can cause massive bleeding and death. If a benign tumor occurs at an important body site—such as in the intestinal tract, the windpipe, the brain, or the spinal cord—the obstruction the tumor creates can be life-threatening.

Some benign tumors are always benign; some have the potential to become malignant; and some types can be either benign or malignant—and still be called the same thing. (See "Benign Tumors" in part III for a list of which tumors belong in what category.)

The diagnostic process is the same for both malignant and benign tumors. Treatment depends on diagnosis: If the tumor is completely benign, it may be surgically removed along with some of the surrounding healthy tissue; radiation or chemotherapy is not used unless the tumor is one of the borderline types that may become malignant.

Since benign tumors do not come back and do not spread, once they are removed the patient is generally considered cured.

Chapter Two

MALIGNANT
TUMORS

Introduction

Malignant tumors respect no limits on growth or territory. They invade and take over vital organs and tissues in the body, but they cannot assume the functions of these now-damaged organs. They have no capacity for fighting infection, yet they can survive alone, cut off from their points of origin, and travel freely through the blood and lymph systems to new locations in the body. When doctors term a tumor "malignant," or "aggressive," they are describing primarily the ability of that tumor to grow and spread. In addition, doctors are concerned with the actual physiology of the tumor: what kinds of tissues gave rise to the tumor, and how the cancer cells look and function. All of this information goes into building a system of tumor classification that constitutes a basis for finding and using effective treatments.

Tumor Growth: The Doubling Rate

The doubling rate is the amount of time it takes a tumor to double in size. We have already talked about the doubling rate for individual cancer cells. Although all tumors begin as just one abnormal cell, as the tumor grows not all the cells continue to double at the same time. While the average doubling time for cancer cells is between one and ten days, doubling rates for tumors range between ten and four hundred days.

A benchmark of tumor size is the number of doublings one cell must go through before becoming 1 centimeter in diameter (a little less than a half-inch across). A tumor of 1 centimeter has reached its thirtieth doubling. This is usually the earliest that a tumor located deep inside the body can be felt. By the time a tumor has doubled for the fortieth time, it is often untreatable. And if by the fortieth doubling the tumor has reached a diameter of 10 centimeters (about the size of a man's fist), fatal complications may be present.

As mentioned above, there is a tremendous range of variation in the amount of time it takes for a doubling to take place. For example, a tumor with a 100-day doubling cycle will take eight years to grow from a single cell to a tumor 1 centimeter in diameter, while a tumor with a doubling cycle of six days will take only six months to reach 1 centimeter. The doubling rate of the tumor must be calculated on a case-by-case basis, comparing the time the first symptoms appeared with the size of the tumor when diagnosis is made. This rough guess at doubling rate is improved upon as doctors observe the tumor grow further, and as certain key tests are repeated.

Even with one kind of cancer, the variation in doubling rates can be enormous. In breast cancer, for example, the doubling rate can be anywhere between 6 and 540 days. The doubling phenomenon makes it extremely urgent to get a complete diagnosis and start treatment as quickly as possible. Even a fast-growing cancer can take months to produce a tumor large enough to feel, but once it reaches that size, the visible growth rate is explosive: A tumor that has taken almost a year to grow to the size of a large pea will take only another six weeks to grow to the size of a baseball if the doubling rate is ten days.

To complicate the situation even further, some cancers grow at very uneven rates. They may grow quickly for a while, and then, for some reason, appear to take a rest (which may last months or even years) before resuming their growth.

Because there is such a wide range of growth behavior in different cancers, and because treatment for all kinds of cancer is most effective in the early stages of growth, it is obviously best to find and treat any cancer as soon as possible.

Major Groups of Malignant Tumors

Doctors use some general terms to describe how tumors look. A **solid** or **true tumor** is what we generally think of when we imagine a tumor: a ball-like mass of cancer cells. **Disseminated tumors** are those in which the growth of abnormal cells is not confined to one area of the body. The term "disseminated" actually can refer to two slightly different conditions: a cancer, like leukemia, that never forms a solid tumor but is noted for abnormal cells distributed throughout the body; and cancers that may form masses but can appear in many places, due to the tendency to split off and travel from the primary site. Doctors informally refer to these two groups of tumors as "lumpers" and "splitters."

You may also hear the words "primary" and "secondary" (or "secondary-primary") and "double-primaries." The primary tumor is where the cancer first began, and is usually (but not always) the first cancer to be discovered. The presence of both primary and secondary tumors does not mean a cancer has spread (metastasized) to a different site; it means there are two different cancers that started separately. Double-primaries are two tumors of the same type that develop in different parts of the same tissue. For example, some patients with a specific type of cancer in one breast may develop it in the other breast. Some patients with colon cancer may develop it in another part of the colon. The chances of a second primary cancer developing varies according to the location of the first primary, genetic factors, cancer-causing properties of the treatment, and problems with the patient's own immune system. For more information, see chapter 3.

Solid tumors may or may not form in the kinds of cancers that originate in the blood and lymphatic systems (leukemias, lymphomas, myelomas). For these cancers you will hear descriptions of the "tumor" based on the characteristics of the cells involved: differentiated, undifferentiated, nodular, diffuse, lymphocytic, histiocytic, hyperplastic, anaplastic, etc. See the site sections for these types of cancers for a complete definition of these terms.

In the laboratory, cancers may be classified in as many as 1000 separate categories, depending on their histological characteristics. Histology is the study of the tiny structures of cells, tissues, and organs in relation to their function. For the layman, the most important classifications are the six major divisions created by identifying cancer cells according to the type of tissue in which the cancer began:

CARCINOMAS.   Eighty-five to ninety percent of all malignant tumors are carcinomas. Carcinomas start in the epithelial tissue. This is the tissue that covers all the parts of our body: the skin, the lining of the stomach, colon, the surfaces of the nerves, glands, genital system, etc. Carcinomas may be found in the esophagus, breast, lung, stomach, uterus, colon, kidney, etc.

SARCOMAS.   These are the rarest of all malignant tumors, but they may be the most virulent. About 2% of malignant tumors are sarcomas—solid

11

tumors that originate in connective tissue found in muscle, bone, lymphatic, nerve, and fat tissue.

MIXED TUMORS. These are solid tumors composed of both epithelial cells and connective tissue. In other words, within the same tumor mass, you will find cells that are identifiable as sarcoma and other cells that are identifiable as carcinoma. Treatment must be planned to take into account that one is dealing with these two different types of cells.

LEUKEMIAS. Four percent of all cancers are leukemias. These are not solid tumors but are characterized by an abnormal number of white blood cells produced by the bone marrow.

LYMPHOMAS. These account for 5% of all cancers, and are cancers of the lymphatic system. Like leukemias, they are characterized by an abnormal number of white blood cells, but these white blood cells are produced by the lymph nodes and the spleen. Although a cancer of the lymph system, lymphomas may produce solid tumors nearly anywhere in the body.

MYELOMAS. These start in the plasma cells produced in the bone marrow. They are very rare.

Carcinomas, sarcomas, and mixed tumors may be found anywhere in the body, and are more specifically identified according to their primary site (where they began). Pinpointing the primary site is important because, just as the subtypes of normal tissue have different characteristics (for example, the skin and the lining of the stomach are both epithelial tissues, but their characteristics and functions are quite different), their abnormal counterparts are equally different. This has implications both for the course of the cancer itself and its response to the various possible types of treatment. Although lymphomas may produce solid tumors, the location of these tumors is not as important as the specific cell type of lymphoma. Leukemias and myelomas remain confined to the tissues in which they began—leukemias to the blood cells, and myelomas to the plasma and bone cells.

How Cancer Spreads

Tumors are called "malignant" because they have the capacity to invade and infiltrate normal tissues (replacing healthy cells with cancer cells) and to metastasize (spread) to other parts of the body. Death from cancer often comes not from the primary site (where the cancer first began) but from the metastases. For example, a patient with stomach cancer may actually die from liver failure after the cancer has spread to that organ.

Metastasis takes place in many ways: through the lymphatic system, the bloodstream, invasive spread, or through implantation.

The most common way for cancer to spread is through the lymphatic system, and is called "embolization." The lymph system has its own channels that circulate throughout the body (see the diagram in Appendix A), similar to the veins and arteries of the bloodstream. These channels are very small and carry a fluid called lymph throughout the body. Lymph glands or nodes are located at various points along the system. They filter impurities in the body and are a part of our immune system. The lymph glands most people know best are those located in the sides of our neck and under our armpits—the "swollen glands" we get when we have certain types of infection. Although a system unto itself, the lymphatic system does join up with the bloodstream.

When cancer spreads via embolization, cells from the original solid tumor break off and start traveling through the lymphatic system. Carcinomas spread through the lymphatic system more quickly than sarcomas. Lymphomas are cancers that start in this system, and therefore they can spread very rapidly. Often when a solid tumor is removed by surgery, the surgeon will remove not only the tumor but the neighboring lymph glands, even though there is no visible sign of cancer in those glands. This is done as a precautionary measure, because if even one cell has broken away from the tumor and lodged in the lymphatic system, the cancer could continue growing and metastasizing.

Cancer can also metastasize through the bloodstream. Cancer cells, like healthy cells, must have a blood supply in order to live, so all cancer cells have access to the bloodstream. Malignant cells can break off from the tumor and travel through the bloodstream until they find a suitable place to start forming a new tumor. (Tumors almost always metastasize through the veins rather than through the arteries.) Sarcomas spread through the bloodstream, as do certain types of carcinomas, like carcinoma of the kidneys, testicular carcinoma, and Wilms's tumor.

Some cancers have a tendency to "switch-hit": They can spread through either the lymphatic system or the bloodstream. Lung and breast cancers, for example, are switch-hitters.

When a certain type of cancer spreads to another part of the body, it does not change its classification. For example, if a person with lymphoma develops a tumor in the lung through metastasis, he does not have lymphoma and lung cancer; he still only has lymphoma. The treatments for lymphoma and lung cancers are very different. The only treatment that will be effective against this particular lung tumor will be the treatment for lymphoma. This, again, is why doctors go to great lengths to establish the primary site of any cancer. (How this is done will be discussed more fully in chapter 4, "Diagnosis.")

Cancers can also spread by local invasion—that is, by intruding on the healthy tissue that surrounds the tumor. Cancers that spread this

13

way usually do not venture very far from the original site. An example of this type of cancer is basal-cell carcinoma of the skin. When this kind of cancer is removed by surgery and a wide area of healthy tissue surrounding it is also removed, it is usually "cured" immediately. Unless it has spread to the lymph system, it is very unlikely that it will recur. (However, it is possible that the same kind of cancer may start to grow at a later time at a completely different site—although the new growth has nothing to do with the first.)

A very rare type of metastasis is caused by implantation or inoculation. This can happen accidentally when a biopsy is done or when cancer surgery is performed. In this case malignant cells may actually drip from a needle or an instrument (this is also called a "spill"). Because of this danger, however remote, certain conditions suspected of being early portents of cancer are never explored surgically. For example, ulcers of the stomach are rarely biopsied for cancer involvement.

Isolated factors also may cause the spread of cancer—such as injury to a bone, tumor cells growing in an old scar, or a lung scarred from inactive tuberculosis.

Cancers do not spread in a completely random fashion—some parts of the body are more vulnerable to becoming metastatic sites than others. Cancers almost never spread to the skin, but they often spread to the liver and lungs. Since each type of cancer has its own predictable pattern for metastasis, see the individual site discussions in part II for information about where any particular cancer is likely to spread.

Growth Patterns of Tumors

There is a progression that cells go through from the first sign of abnormality to the final stage of widespread metastasis. Since carcinomas are the most common kind of cancer, we will describe the steps involved in the growth of carcinomas. Although the pattern described below is generally true, cancers have a very annoying tendency to be highly individualistic; some cancers may actually skip a stage, while others will remain in one stage and go no further.

Step 1: Precancerous Lesions or Dysplasia

The word "lesion" is usually used to mean a wound or injury. When applied to cancer, however, it refers simply to a change in the pathology of the cell. Changes that can be observed under a microscope in the size, shape, and organization of the adult cells in healthy tissue are

14

termed "lesions." Certain lesions are known to be the first changes in cell structure that can lead to cancer (which is why they are termed "precancerous"). It is difficult to predict which lesions will turn into cancer and which will just go away. Research has shown that certain lesions, especially those that occur in people who are particularly susceptible to cancer (see chapter 3), and/or those that appear in certain body parts, have a great probability of becoming cancerous. If a doctor is able to detect and treat a precancerous lesion, it is likely that cancer itself will never develop. For example, cancer of the cervix can be recognized in this stage and treated effectively—hence the importance of women having regular Pap swears.

Step 2:   In-situ or Preinvasive Cancer

At this point cancer has developed, but is located in one place and involves only the outer covering (epithelium) that surrounds an organ. This is the least serious type of localized cancer.

Step 3:   Invasion

In this stage the tumor spreads out from the original surface location and infiltrates and actively destroys the surrounding tissue. Invasive cancer is another form of localized cancer, although more serious than *in-situ* cancers.

Step 4:   Metastatic Cancer

In this final step, tumor cells have broken off from the original tumor and have spread throughout the body. This is the most serious form of cancer. Successful treatment depends on the type of cancer, how much and how far the cancer has spread, and whether the metastases have interfered with vital organs.

The time required for the cells to progress from the dysplasia stage to the *in-situ* stage may be as much as ten or twenty years. Some cancers may never go past the *in-situ* stage. See part II for details on the particular cancer you are concerned with.

Stages and Grades of Cancer

Systems of grading and staging tumors enable a medical staff to concisely communicate a great deal of information about any one case of cancer. Unfortunately, although the concept of grading and staging is widely accepted, different classification systems are being used (which is why in the site discussions—where we outline specifically what is meant by each stage of cancer at that site—we list which classification system we are using. Your doctor may be using a different system).

Grading and staging a tumor are different processes, but they are both based on how the tumor grows and spreads and what it looks like.

Grading Cancer

Grading is based on how the cells look under the microscope. A pathologist examines the tissues and cells under the microscope and determines the kind of cancer by looking at how differentiated the cells are. This differentiation is a function of how mature the cells are.

The differentiation of normal cells is that process by which cells become specialized to serve a useful function in the body. Differentiation in cancer cells means that they still act like the normal cells from which they grew. Only mature cells are specialized. Some cancer cells never reach full maturity, which means they do not differentiate. If they are completely undifferentiated, they are called "anaplastic." Anaplastic cells have no relation to the primary tissue in which they arose, and their organization is so chaotic that the cells actually pile on top of each other in a jumble and cannot carry out the job normally assigned to them. For example, in the blood cells called "leukocytes," malignant leukocytes cannot do the job of fighting disease and infection that healthy leukocytes can. The pathologist may also note other changes in the cells, like hyperplasia, a condition where the cancer cells cause the organ to become enlarged.

There are usually four grades assigned to any particular type of cancer:

Grade I   well-differentiated tumors
Grade II   moderately or poorly differentiated tumors
Grade III   similar to Grade II but less differentiated
Grade IV   undifferentiated (or dedifferentiated) tumors

As a rule of thumb, the higher the grade, the poorer the prognosis (chances for long-term remission). For example, in the case of epidermoid cancer of the tongue, the five-year survival (cure) rate is 75% if it is detected and treated in Grade I, but only 15% if it is detected and treated in Grade IV.

Staging Cancer

Staging is a way of describing how much cancer is in the body and the extent of metastases. The specific criteria used for defining each stage varies from cancer to cancer (see the site discussions for staging of particular cancers), but the criteria do form a general pattern. The most important criteria used in staging are how deeply the cancer has invaded healthy tissues and how malignant (how fast-growing and -spreading) it is. Generally four stages are defined, although many types of cancer are divided into substages of each level.

Stage I   The tumor is limited to the organ where it began. Generally these patients have the best chance of survival (70–90%).

Stage II   There has been local spread to surrounding tissues and lymph nodes. These patients have a good chance for survival (50+%).

Stage III There has been extensive growth of the primary tumor and possible involvement of other organs, such as bone and lymph nodes. These patients have some chance of survival (20+%).

Stage IV   In this stage, the cancer has spread far into the body and generally chances for survival are not good.

Obviously, it is best to find and treat cancers in Stages I and II. However, for several types of cancer that are fast-growing and hard to detect in the early stages, there have been excellent results using chemotherapy—even in Stage IV. The percentages used above are general figures that are a composite of all types of cancer. Do not use them to judge your particular type of cancer. Besides using the site discussions as a source of statistics for particular cancers, please read chapter 7 very carefully. The numbers used to describe the prognosis for cancer types and effectiveness of various treatments are often misleading and confusing.

Another set of classifications was developed by the International Union Against Cancer and the American Joint Committee for Cancer Staging and End Result Reporting. This is called the TNM classification. "T" stands for tumor, "N" stands for node (as in lymph node), and "M" stands for metastasis. Numbers after each letter (on a scale from 0 to 4) indicate the size of the original tumor, how much involvement of the lymph system has taken place, and whether or not the cancer has spread widely throughout the body. For example, $T^0N^0M^0$ means that the cancer is *in-situ*—there is no spread to the nodes and there are no distant metastases. In contrast, $T^4N^4M^4$ means that the original tumor is very large and has invaded the original organ, there is widespread involvement of the lymph nodes, and the cancer has metastasized to many sites.

17

The staging process is done on two levels, which are called "clinical staging" and "pathological staging." Clinical staging is done on the basis of clinical evidence—tests and examinations that do not involve removal of cell and tissue samples to look at under a microscope. It includes the direct physical evidence your doctor can see with his eyes and feel with his hands, as well as the pictures provided through X rays, scans, etc.

Pathological staging uses all this evidence but takes it one step further and examines the cells and tissues microscopically. Pathological staging is the most accurate and constitutes the only way of being completely certain of exactly what type of cancer a person has. Although cancer specialists would always prefer to have any cancer staged pathologically, certain cancers—because of their location—cannot be staged this way, and treatment must be designed on the basis of clinical staging.

The actual staging process will be discussed fully in chapter 4 on diagnosis.

Further Reading

Laurie Garrett, "The Biology of Cancer," in *Understanding Cancer*, eds. Mark Renneker and Steven Leib (Palo Alto: Bull Publishing, 1979). This is an excellent detailed explanation of cells and tumors and how they work and behave. ($12.95 paperback.)

Chapter Three

EPIDEMIOLOGY— FACTORS THAT MAKE "HIGH-RISK" PATIENTS

Epidemiology is the study of how disease affects groups of people. Epidemiologists try to discover why certain groups of people are more susceptible to some diseases—including cancer. This information eventually leads to suggested methods for preventing and curing cancer. Epidemiologists compile statistics on cancer, outlining the morbidity (who gets it) and mortality (who dies from it) rates, and the effectiveness of various kinds of treatment for various groups of cancer patients.

Epidemiologists have found that certain factors are closely linked to the development of cancer: geography; heredity; carcinogens (cancer-causing substances) found in the environment; viruses; and stress. If one or more of these factors is present in a person's life, he has a greater risk of developing certain types of cancer: He is a so-called high-risk patient.

Geographic Factors

Factors present in certain locations and societies make various types of cancer more likely to appear. These factors range from improper diet, to exposure to carcinogens, to genetic susceptibilities found in the population as a whole. For example, cancer of the liver is most common among men in Asia, appearing rarely in the United States and Europe. On the other hand, lymphatic leukemia is common in the United States and Europe, but rare in Asia. Even within the United States you can see definite geographic differences in the incidence of different types of cancer: There is, for example, a higher rate of bladder cancer in Pittsburgh than in Atlanta. Some of these differences can be clearly traced to carcinogens known to be present in certain regions. Other differences are not clearly understood and form the basis for further research into the causes of cancer.

Sex, Age, Race

Different types of cancer are more common among various age groups, more common to men or to women, or appear more commonly among certain racial groups. Table 1 lists the types of cancers that affect men and women most frequently in the United States.

TABLE 1
Most-Common Cancers in U.S.

Men	Women
lung (22%)	breast (27%)
prostate (17%)	colon and rectum (15%)
colon and rectum (14%)	uterus (13%)
urinary (10%)	lung (8%)
leukemias and lymphomas (8%)	leukemias and lymphomas (7%)
oral cancers (5%)	ovary (4%)
pancreas (3%)	urinary (4%)
skin (2%)	pancreas (3%)
	oral and melanomas (2% each)

Some of the gender differences in susceptibility to certain cancers are due to the actual physiological characteristics of men and women. Others reflect dissimilarities in life-style that our society imposes on the sexes. For example, since women have begun to enter traditionally masculine career fields in greater numbers and begun to smoke more heavily, the incidence of lung cancers in women has increased.

In childhood, for both sexes, the leading types of cancer are leukemia, cancers of the brain and nervous system, and cancers of the kidney, bone, and connective tissue. In addition, genetic links to cancer appear to play a much more important role than in any other age group.

The susceptibility of certain U.S. racial groups to certain cancers may also be genetic (see "Heredity" below). Other explanations stress coincidental circumstances: Some racial groups, for example, are located in geographic areas that expose them to cancer-causing agents, and also to conditions of poverty. There are odd constellations of high-risk groups: Breast cancer affects black women more frequently in Pittsburgh than anywhere else in the U.S., but it affects white women more often in Minneapolis-Saint Paul. Both black and white women show an equally great tendency to develop breast cancer in San Francisco.

Heredity

People whose parents have had certain types of cancers have a greater risk of developing cancer themselves. A strong family history of cancer (meaning that several members of the family have had cancer, however diverse the types of cancer) also increases the risk. It is important to understand that increased risk is not certainty; it means only that the possibility of cancer is higher.

Why some families are cancer-prone and others cancer-resistant has not been clearly established. It is possible that some families lack certain enzymes, have different hormone patterns, or have some problem with the function of the immune system. This is an area still under close study.

Certain types of cancer are known to be strongly linked to hereditary factors. These are: retinoblastomas (childhood tumors of the eye), some melanomas, breast cancer, Wilms's tumors, leukemias, and cancer of the tongue.

Carcinogens

Carcinogens are substances that cause or promote the development of cancer. They can be found in ray form (X rays, solar rays, or radioactive elements), in heavy metals (zinc, mercury, etc.), or in various chemicals—some which occur naturally and some of which are man-made. Epidemiologists now estimate that more than 80% of all cancers are the result of exposure to carcinogens.

In large doses, carcinogens kill cells. In small doses, carcinogens cause cells to mutate. Mutation is a permanent physical change in a cell, usually involving the genes. Because mutation is locked into the genes, all the daughter cells of the mutated cell will exhibit the same abnormal characteristics. Often the cancer that develops may result from exposure to more than one carcinogen, and this combination of factors may destroy the body's natural defense system.

Some substances are known to cause cancer in animals when given in large doses, but when used by humans in small amounts have a negligible effect. Other chemical substances (additives used in food, chemicals in cigarette smoke, etc.) have been shown to produce cancer in humans exposed to moderate amounts.

All of us are exposed to varying amounts of carcinogens throughout our environment—in what we eat, breathe, and come in contact with physically. Not everyone exposed to a carcinogen will develop cancer; it depends largely on which organ is affected and how the carcinogen is distributed in the body.

Occupational Factors

The National Cancer Institute is conducting research on the relationship between jobs, exposure to carcinogenic substances (agents), and the development of specific cancers. Some of the relationships already identified are shown in table 2.

Drug Use

Another area being investigated is the link between drug use and the development of cancer. Nonprescription drugs such as tobacco and alcohol are implicated. Tobacco can cause cancers of the lung, mouth, and throat, and smoking unfiltered cigarettes can lead to bladder cancer. When a person combines tobacco and alcohol use, the risk is considerably greater for cancers of the tongue, esophagus, and lung.

Some evidence suggests strongly that certain prescription drugs may also cause cancer. The use of DES (diethylstilbestrol) by expectant mothers may cause vaginal cancer in their female offspring. Studies are now under way to determine whether there is a link between mothers who took DES and male children who develop testicular cancers. Links have already been established between various hormones and cancer, and the use of coal-tar ointments and skin cancer.

22

TABLE 2
Job-Related Cancers and Their Causative Agents

Site	Agent	Occupation
Liver	Arsenic	Tanners, smelters
	Vinyl chloride	Plastic workers
Nasal cavity	Chromium	Glass, pottery
& sinuses	Nickel	Battery workers, electrolysis workers
	Wood & leather dust	Wood, leather, shoe workers
Lung	Arsenic, asbestos, chromium, coal dust, mustard gas, nickel, ionizing radiations	Miners, asbestos workers, glass & pottery workers, coal-tar and pitch workers, iron foundry workers, radiologists, chemical workers
Bladder	Coal products	Asphalt, coal-tar workers
	Aromatic amines	Dyestuff users, rubber workers, leather workers, shoemakers, paint manufacturers
Bone	Ionizing radiations	Radium-dial painters
Bone marrow	Benzene, ionizing radiations	Benzene workers, dye users, painters, radiologists
Skin	Coal tar, ultraviolet rays, arsenic, ionizing radiations	Stokers, pitch workers, miners, outdoor workers, radiologists

Two medical treatments—drug therapy and radiation—are known to be carcinogenic, but both are employed (with the patient's knowledge) because the risk to the patient of not using these treatments is often greater than the risk presented by using them. Several of the anticancer drugs (see chapter 10 on chemotherapy) are known to be carcinogenic, and the drugs used to prevent rejection of a transplanted kidney may produce cancer.

Viruses and Contagion

At this time, scientists have direct evidence of a link between viruses and cancers only in animals, not in humans. They continue to explore this area because there are aspects of virus behavior and cancer that support a possible link. For example, viruses can change the genetic properties of a cell and cause chromosome breaks, and the damage to chromosomes may cause cancer. It has yet to be proved that viruses alone cause cancer in man, but it is estimated that there may be a viral element in approximately 5% of tumors. There are also specific instances in which a virus is suspect: For example, patients who have had hepatitis virus B infections seem more prone to liver cancer.

As of this date, all evidence indicates that cancer is not contagious. Talk about contagion (the spread of disease from one human to another through contact) usually increases when the media report "epidemics" of cancer in one geographic area, such as ten cases of Hodgkin's disease in one small town, or a hundred cases of bladder cancer reported in one area of New Jersey. Studies have shown that such phenomena are either the result of freak mathematical distributions or that people in a certain region have been exposed to high levels of carcinogens.

The only type of cancer for which the contagion theory is still being explored as a possibility is cancer of the cervix. Studies show that cervical cancer is almost nonexistent in nuns, but has a high rate of incidence among prostitutes and sexually promiscuous females. As of now, nothing has been proved.

Stress

An area under increasing professional scrutiny is the role that stress plays in both the development of cancer and the effective management of the disease.

There are many illnesses in which we know stress to play an important part: high blood pressure, cardiac accidents, gastric ulcers, and mental disturbances. Cancer has been added to the list of stress-related illnesses.

Stress, as scientists use the term, is a general, nonspecific, physiological response by the body to any demand. The stress itself may be psychological, physical, or chemical. What distinguishes the stress response (also called the General Adaptation Syndrome, or GAS) is that it makes no difference what the specific cause, for the body's reaction is the same: The adrenaline level shoots up, the hormone balance changes, the immune system stops working normally, the reproductive system is put on hold. Nature designed the response to be an adaptive one (as explained in chapter 1), and only temporary— allowing the body to react effectively to extreme conditions, survive, and then return to normal. But if the stress agent is too severe, if situations arise that keep the stress response activated for too long a time, the chemical changes in the body—particularly the effect on the immune system—set the body up for the development of diseases.

What specific disease develops depends on the "weak link" in any

24

individual. Because each of us is different—with different genes, different life-styles, different environments—individual reactions to stress vary enormously.

Nutrition

Attempting to define the role of nutrition in the development of cancer poses some very perplexing problems. It is extremely difficult to study the role of nutrition in a way that leads to clear, scientifically valid conclusions. To work up a case, we must consider the whole field of human biochemistry (and knowledge about that area is very incomplete) and study everything that a person eats and drinks—a huge task that has only just been undertaken.

We know that we ingest certain carcinogens along with our food and beverages. Carcinogens enter our food through pollution, particularly of our water supply, and also by means of chemicals used in producing our food (pesticides, chemicals fed to animals to enhance their growth rate), chemicals used in processing and preserving our food, and chemicals added to food for no other purpose than to enhance flavor and appearance. The Food and Drug Administration is constantly testing chemicals to determine safety.

Identifying known carcinogens in the diet is but the first task in identifying nutritional factors leading to cancer. The great unknowns include substances we eat that are not carcinogens in their natural form but can be converted by the body's own chemistry into carcinogens; what types of diets may set the stage for cancer development (in the same way that a sugary diet sets the stage for tooth decay); and what constitutes an "unbalanced" or "deficient" diet, engendering the lowering of a body's resistance to cancer. For only a few types of cancer do we have direct links between diet and the cancer itself: For example, a lack of fiber and roughage in the diet may help set the stage for cancer of the colon.

The High-Risk Patient

The knowledge gained from the study of epidemiology is used in every area of cancer research, prevention, and treatment. From the patient's point of view, the most important use of this information is in aiding the diagnostic process.

As we have said, it is important to diagnose cancer as early as

25

possible. But the earliest signs of cancer are so often ambiguous and general that they could be signs of much less serious diseases and conditions. In the normal, competent practice of medicine, these less serious possible causes will be thoroughly checked out before one even thinks about the possibility of cancer and the much more complicated diagnostic process that goes along with it. However, if one does have cancer, much valuable time can be lost ruling out these other possibilities. Therefore, the first stage in the diagnosis of any disease is an examination of your medical history. By asking questions not only about the illnesses you have had but also about your family's medical history, where you work and live, your life-style, and the possibility of stresses in your life, the doctor will know immediately whether you should be considered a high-risk patient.

For example, if you have had minor problems with urination but you are a 50-year-old man who has worked for thirty years in a chemical plant, the doctor will immediately schedule tests to rule out cancer of the urinary tract, particularly the bladder.

Further Reading

There has been an enormous amount written about the epidemiology of cancer—both professional literature and lay publications. The books listed below are only meant to serve as a starting point for the interested reader. They all offer bibliographies that can guide the reader to information of greater detail.

Overviews and General Information

Joseph F. Fraumeni, *Persons at High Risk of Cancer* (New York: Academic Press, 1975).
   This professional outline of epidemiology was written by the head of the Epidemiology Branch of the National Cancer Institute.
Mark Renneker and Steven Leib, eds., *Understanding Cancer*, Part III: "Etiologies of Cancer" (Palo Alto: Bull Publishing, 1979).
Cancer Facts and Figures (New York: American Cancer Society, 1979).

Geographic Factors

General information about geographic factors can be found in the books listed above. For a very detailed analysis (complete with maps) of the geographic distributions of different kinds of cancer in the United States, see the *Atlas of Cancer Mortality for U.S. Counties*, by Thomas J. Mason, Frank W. McKay, Robert Hoover, William J. Blot, and Joseph F. Fraumeni. Published by the Department of Health, Education, and Welfare, HEW Publication Number (NIH) 75–780.

Age, Sex, Race

See books cited above.

Heredity

See books cited above.

Carcinogens and Occupational Factors

Larry Agran, *The Cancer Connection—And What We Can Do About It* (Boston: Houghton Mifflin, 1977).

A comprehensive study of chemical carcinogens and jobs, written for the layman.

Samuel S. Epstein, *The Politics of Cancer* (San Francisco: Sierra Club Books, 1978).

This is a study of environmental carcinogens.

Donald Hunter, *The Diseases of Occupations,* 6th ed. (Boston: Little, Brown, 1978).

See also "Occupational Cancer" by Phyllis Lehmann, and "Cancer: Detecting the Chemical Culprits" by Roger Lewin, in *Understanding Cancer* (cited above). At the end of this book is a comprehensive chart, "Industrial Agents Associated with Cancer," which lists forty-four carcinogens and summarizes the exposure occupations.

Stress

Jean Tache, Hans Selye, and Stacey B. Dan, eds., *Cancer, Stress and Death* (New York: Plenum, 1979).

Part of the Sloan-Kettering Cancer Institute Series, this book is fairly technical, but most of it is very readable. The presentations by cancer specialists, pathologists, researchers, epidemiologists, psychiatrists, sociologists, pain specialists, and stress specialists show why the interdisciplinary approach has been developed, why very different fields have independently found studying the stress phenomena to be important, and suggest lines of future research.

O. Carl Simonton, Stephanie Matthews-Simonton, and James L. Creighton, *Getting Well Again* (Los Angeles: J. P. Tarcher, 1978).

Chapters 3 ("The Search for the Causes of Cancer"), 4 ("The Link Between Stress and Illness"), and 5 ("Personality, Stress and Cancer") are highly recommended. There is also a very extensive bibliography, listing over 250 books and articles.

Nutrition

See the books cited above under "Overviews" and also the "Further Readings" at the end of chapter 15.

Chapter Four

DIAGNOSIS

A complete and accurate diagnosis is the first and most important step in effectively dealing with cancer. In order to plan treatment, the cancer specialist must know five things:

1.   the *primary site* (where the cancer began)
2.   the specific *cell type* of cancer
3.   the extent of *metastasis* (how far it has spread, the *stage* it is in)
4.   how *malignant* it is (the rate of growth)
5.   the patient's general state of health, including the medical history as well as his present physical condition.

For the patient, the diagnostic process is a bewildering one. Symptoms are often confusing, confounding even the best doctors. There are numerous tests involved, some administered in hospital departments with ominous-sounding names like Nuclear Medicine. Frequently the highly sophisticated equipment looks frightening. There are also endless waiting periods: waiting for tests to be scheduled, waiting for your body to be ready for a test (not eating or drinking for a period of time, waiting for dyes to flow through your system), waiting for the results of specific tests to confirm something that looked "suspicious," and so forth. The whole process can create a great deal of anxiety; not only is there fear of what the test results will be, there is the often greater fear caused by not understanding what is happening to you.

In this chapter we will explain what needs to be done to formulate a diagnosis, why these things need to be done, and provide you with an overview of the most common procedures. In the next chapter, sixty-five procedures will be explained in detail. No one patient will undergo all of what is explained here; check under the appropriate site discussion of a specific cancer to see what diagnostic procedures are routine for the kind of cancer that concerns you. Note that we are covering only the most routine procedures here. In any one case, doctors may want other tests done, or may find that they do not need to perform the full range of possible tests.

Symptoms

Some cancer symptoms are exactly the same as those found in less serious illnesses: fatigue, a shift in weight, vague stomach distress, and so on. A competent doctor will first rule out the most usual causes of these problems.

Moreover, different types of cancer, and even benign tumors, may produce similar symptoms, or, in their early stages, none at all. Many cancers are detected during routine physical examinations, before the patient is even aware of any symptoms. This is particularly important in the case of deep tumors, which will only produce symptoms after they have reached an advanced stage.

The American Cancer Society has widely publicized the seven warning signs of cancer: change in bowel or bladder habits; a sore throat that does not heal; unusual bleeding or discharge; a thickening or lump in the breast or elsewhere; chronic indigestion or difficulty in swallowing; obvious changes in a wart or mole; and a nagging cough or hoarseness. But even these do not definitely indicate the presence of cancer; they just indicate that something is going on that ought to be checked immediately. See the site discussions of specific cancers for the symptoms associated with each one.

Doctors Involved in the Diagnostic Process

Once cancer is suspected, a carefully planned series of tests and diagnostic procedures is scheduled by your doctor. During the diagnostic process, patients often become confused about who "their doctor" is.

Until this time, your doctor was probably the family physician, internist, or some other specialist who first suspected cancer. For example, if the first symptoms appeared in your stomach, you may have gone to a gastroenterologist (stomach specialist). If signs of cervical cancer turned up in a Pap smear during a regular pelvic exam, your doctor would be the gynecologist who did the test. Your doctor may call in a cancer specialist to consult on the design of the diagnostic process, and to help interpret results. Certain tests may be done by cancer specialists or be performed in a major cancer center, but the cancer specialist, or cancer team, will not become your doctor(s) until the diagnosis is complete. Until that time, all test results will be reported to your original physician.

The diagnostic process requires a large number of tests by many different highly trained specialists: doctors, nurses, and technicians. Hospitals often have teams that specialize in certain types of procedures. Four types of physicians are commonly included on the diagnostic team:

Surgeons: to collect tissue samples for some biopsies and perform surgical diagnostic procedures
Pathologists: to look at the tissue, fluid, and cell samples under a microscope and make the definitive diagnosis
Diagnostic radiologists: to perform and interpret radiological tests
Nuclear-medicine specialists: to perform and interpret scans

In addition, doctors who specialize in diagnostic work on particular parts of the body will be called in as needed.

The Diagnostic Process

The diagnostic process is structured in such a way that each step is dependent on the step before it. Certain base-line information will be obtained for all cancers: a medical history; a general physical examination; samples of blood, urine, and feces for routine laboratory tests; and a sample of the suspected tissue (if it is possible to get such a sample). Beyond that, tests are scheduled according to what type of cancer is suspected and what previous tests have shown. Some test results will tell the doctor that there is no reason to go on with a line of diagnostic questioning; other test results will suggest that he needs to know more, so he will schedule more tests.

Physicians rely very heavily on their sight and sense of touch in making diagnostic judgments. Cancer can be easily seen when it forms on the skin, lips, mouth, tongue, vulva, and penis. More information can be collected by feeling (palpating) suspected tumors: Benign tumors tend to be soft; cancers tend to be hard and painless; and abscesses tend to be hot and painful. Palpable tumors are found only in the breasts, rectum, prostate, ovaries, bone, testes, and peripheral lymph nodes (those in the groin, neck, and under the arm), and even in these places the cancers must be relatively large and advanced before they can be felt.

Medicine has developed a range of technologies to help doctors extend their powers of vision into parts of the body that fifty years ago would only have been accessible by surgery. By using tubes containing a light source and viewing lens, it is possible to go in through natural openings in the body to examine the gastrointestinal tract, the female reproductive system, and the urinary system (see "Endoscopy" on page 56). Other areas can be examined by X-rays, scans, and ultrasound.

Some of the most crucial diagnostic information is obtained by using a microscope to examine the biopsy (a sample of the suspected tumor and adjacent normal tissue), blood, urine, feces, and other natural secretions.

Medical personnel often describe diagnostic procedures by placing them in one of two categories: invasive and noninvasive. An "invasive" procedure involves going into (invading) the body. Procedures like biopsies, which require cutting out tissue, are considered invasive. All surgical procedures and most of the endoscopies are invasive. Tests like X rays, where the doctor does not have to physically go into the body, are called noninvasive.

It may be more useful to think of the different procedures in terms of whether they take place in the doctor's office or in the hospital. Hospital procedures can be divided into two groups: those that must be done on an inpatient basis (you must check into the hospital and stay overnight) and those that can be done on an outpatient basis (you must have the tests done at the hospital, but there is no need to stay overnight).

In the Doctor's Office

A great deal of diagnostic information will be obtained in your doctor's office. Here he will take down your medical history; give you a physical examination; collect samples of blood, urine, feces, and secretions (like those used for a Pap smear) for examination in a laboratory; and, if necessary, perform more-specialized physical exams, like an eye examination, etc. Some biopsies can also be done in the office (if the suspected tissue is easily accessible and would require

31

only local or no anesthetic), as can minor surgical procedures (like the removal of a wart or mole) and some endoscopies.

Medical History

One of the most important procedures done in your doctor's office is taking down your complete medical history. You will be asked about any past illnesses, when the symptoms first began that brought you to the doctor, and whether you have had similar problems in the past. The answers to these questions will help the doctor determine the probable location of the primary site of the cancer, when it began, and will help in selecting the kind of treatment that will be best for you. In addition, they will provide information that will help to anticipate very specific problems that may arise from the cancer itself and from the proposed treatment.

You will also be asked about your life-style and about the medical histories of other people in your family. Your answers will help the doctor to determine if you are a high-risk patient—someone who is more likely to develop cancer than the average person (see chapter 3). At this stage, this information gives the doctor a context in which to interpret signs and symptoms of disease. Because many of the symptoms associated with cancer are ambiguous, any indication that you may be a high-risk patient will alert the doctor to check out symptoms that otherwise might be ignored.

Physical Examination

A general physical examination consists of listening to the patient's heart and lungs; measuring weight, height, and blood pressure; looking at the mouth, throat, ears, and eyes; and collecting samples of blood (a tubeful taken from a vein in your arm with a needle, as well as a finger prick which is immediately smeared on a slide), urine, and feces (you provide the samples in a sterile container). When cancer is suspected, the doctor will also palpate the site as well as examining the groin, the neck, and the area under the arm for signs of metastasis in those lymph nodes. The physical usually does not hurt, although palpation may cause some temporary soreness and tenderness. Specialized physical examinations, like those of the eye and rectum, are described in the individual site discussions.

In the Hospital

Most diagnostic tests take place in the hospital. They consist of highly sophisticated procedures that require special equipment and material, and must be done by highly trained doctors, nurses, and technicians. Some procedures, although possible to do in a doctor's office, are safer and more comfortable for the patient when done in the hospital.

Certain procedures must be done on an inpatient basis; others may be done either as an inpatient or as an outpatient. How it will be handled in your case depends on the series of tests scheduled for you (for example, if one inpatient procedure must be done, other procedures may be scheduled while you are in the hospital) and on other factors, which your doctor will discuss with you.

Types of Tests

The individual tests and procedures (described in the next chapter) may be easier to understand if they are divided into six groups:

Surgical procedures: These include biopsies and laparotomy. Surgery also may be a part of other procedures: For example, the insertion of a catheter may require minor surgery. The different kinds of biopsies are listed by name under "Biopsy" in chapter 5. Their names derive from the types of instruments used to get the tissue sample, or the part of the body from which the biopsy was taken.

Endoscopies: An endoscope is a tube, either rigid or flexible, which is inserted through the mouth, rectum, vagina, or urethra. This allows the doctor to look at and collect cell and tissue samples from various internal organs. With the creation of the flexible tube, and the advances made in filament optics and miniaturization, it is now possible to thread through a narrow tube a light source and a lens (both for direct viewing and for relay to a TV screen and videotape) and even tiny instruments for cutting, brushing, and washing (to get cell samples). All the tests in this group end with "-oscopy." See "Endoscopy" in chapter 5 for a full list of these tests. The start of each name indicates the part of the body being examined.

Radiological films: These can be subdivided into three types:

33

1. Plain films. No special preparation of the patient is needed. Plain films are used for X-rays, mammography, tomography, and xerography.
2. Contrast films. A substance—either air, chemical dye, or a radioactive material—is introduced into the body in order to make the area under examination stand out clearly in the picture. These tests include arteriograms, upper and lower GI, encephalography, gallbladder series, lymphangiogram, aortography, and venacavography.
3. Fluoroscopies (flow studies). These also make use of a contrast material, but, using a machine called a fluoroscope, the doctor can actually observe the material as it moves through a system and take pictures of it. Fluoroscopies include IVP's and renal blood flow studies and might be used in conjunction with any of the contrast film procedures listed above.

Scans: Scans provide an overall picture, or map, of an organ or section of the body. Different organs pick up different isotopes (radioactive forms of certain elements). When these are injected into the body, they enable the doctor to tell which tissues are normal and which are cancerous. Some isotopes are only picked up by healthy tissues, so that any part of the organ that does not pick up the element (these show up as dark, or cold, spots) is suspect. Other isotopes are only picked up by abnormal tissue, so on these scans the suspect areas show up as light, or hot, spots.

The radiation given off by the isotopes is detected by special crystals that convert the pulses of radiation into flashes of light, called scintillations. The machines used to detect the radiation are called scintillation detectors. Some are stationary, some move, and some make use of cameras. The most widely publicized form of scanner is the CAT Scanner (Computerized Axial Tomography); it is also called the EMI scan, ACTA scan, Computerized Transverse Axial Tomography (CTT), Computerized Tomography (CT), and Computer-Assisted Transaxial Tomography.

People are often afraid that a scan will expose them to high levels of radiation. In fact, because the radioactive material is inside the body and the machines are used only to detect this radiation, the average dose does not exceed what you would be exposed to in a regular chest X ray.

Besides CAT scans, there are thyroid scans, brain scans, liver scans, bone scans, and gallium (or total body) scans.

Diagnostic Ultrasound (sonogram, echo): These are tests that examine many parts of the body, using a machine that works on the same principal as sonar and radar: A picture is made using the echoes of pulsating high-frequency sound. Ultrasound is used to get a picture of soft tissues, such as the kidneys, liver, spleen, pancreas, gallbladder, thyroid, heart, eye, female reproductive organs, lymph nodes, and aorta. Several types of "pictures" can be presented on the oscilloscope, and, with the addition of a scanning device, what looks like a cross section of the organ being studied appears on the screen. Ultrasound has the advantage of being noninvasive, painless, and, it is believed, completely harmless.

Laboratory tests: These tests require only minimum participation by the patient: the donation of a few cubic centimeters of blood and urine; a stool sample; a few cells that the doctor has wiped, brushed, or scraped from an accessible part of your body. Included in this group are the CBC, other specialized analyses, cytological tests (the examination of cells), and cultures.

Where the Tests Are Done

Finding your way around the hospital to get tests done can be more bewildering than the tests themselves. Some tests can be performed in the patient's room, in a regular examining room, or in the doctor's office. Most are done in special areas within the hospital.

X-rays, fluoroscopies, and tomograms are done in the Radiology or Diagnostic Radiology Department. Scans are done in the Nuclear Medicine Department. Surgical procedures and others that require a sterile environment may be done in the operating room. Blood tests are handled by the Phlebotomy Department—although the testers often come to you, rather than you going to them.

Many specialized tests have become such a frequent part of the diagnostic procedure that they now have their own headquarters: the Endoscopy Suite, the Ultrasonography Suite, the Electroencephalography Suite, the Cystoscopy Suite, and the Cardiac Catheterization Lab.

As you prepare to go through the diagnostic process, you should discuss every procedure very thoroughly with your doctor so you will know what is being done to you and what will be expected of you. In the next chapter each procedure will be discussed in detail, but there are a few considerations that apply to most of the procedures.

Jewelry. It is generally advisable not to wear any jewelry while you are going through the diagnostic process. This is particularly true when procedures involve the taking of pictures (X-rays and scans).

Dentures. These can cause problems if general anesthesia is being used or in diagnostic procedures involving the mouth and throat. You will be asked to remove them when such procedures are being done.

Anxiety and Anesthesia. Certain types of tests—particularly those

35

involving the reproductive system and the excretory system—can cause much anxiety. Since most tests require that you be relaxed, you should discuss any anxiety with your doctor. Many procedures can be performed either with an anesthetic that puts you completely to sleep or with one that numbs a part of the body while you remain awake. It may seem to you that a general anesthetic would solve your anxiety problem, and in some cases it will, but most of the time the doctor will try to convince you that this is not the best course of action: first, because your cooperation may be needed in order to perform the test properly; second, because anesthesia itself carries certain risks, which the doctor would like to avoid whenever possible. (See chapter 8 on surgery for a full discussion of anesthesia.)

Discomfort vs. *Pain.*   Medical personnel rarely use the word "pain"; they use the word "discomfort." This may pose a communication problem between patient and staff because patients make a definite distinction between discomfort and pain. In this book, the two words are used in the usual sense: Discomfort is a mild sensation, mostly an annoyance, while pain is a more severe physical distress. If doctors and nurses start talking to you about "discomfort," ask them to be specific so that you have realistic expectations.

Basic Vocabulary

Some instruments, materials, procedures, and body parts are involved in a great many tests, and are a part of the medical vocabulary with which you should become familiar.

anesthetic—a gas or drug that produces the loss of sensation. Most of the invasive tests require the use of some kind of anesthetic. There are four types:
  General—an anesthetic which puts the patient to sleep. It is given intravenously or inhaled.
  Local—an anesthetic that deadens sensation in a small area by acting on the nerves in that area. There are three types: (1) *topical,* applied directly on the skin; (2) *block,* which is injected near a nerve trunk and blocks the sensation passing through the nerve; and (3) *infiltrative,* which is injected into the tissues (like the novocaine that you get at the dentist).
  Regional—an anesthetic that is injected into the nerve and anesthetizes a larger area than the local, but does not put the patient to sleep.
  Spinal—an anesthetic that is injected into the spinal cord. There are two types: the *saddle block,* which anesthetizes everything below the waist; and the *caudal,* which anesthetizes the base of the spine. With both types the patient is awake.

arteries—the channels in the circulatory system that take blood, which has been filled with oxygen, away from the heart.

aspiration—the removal of fluid to see if cancer cells are present. Usually a needle is inserted into a cavity (the abdomen, the pleural cavity around the lungs, the cavity around the spine) and a sample of fluid is drawn out for analysis in the laboratory.

catheter—a small tube inserted into a structure (vein, artery, bladder, etc.) for removing or inserting liquid.

contrast material—liquid, gas, or air that blocks X-rays, creating a white image on the film. Usually in liquid form, it may be swallowed or injected, depending on the test.

cutdown—a slit made in the skin in order to reach a vein so that a needle or catheter may be inserted.

dilation—expansion.

drape—sheeting or towels used to cover the part of a patient that is not being examined.

filament optics/fiber optics—a type of technology that relies on the physical properties of light waves transmitted through thin glass fibers. Because the beam of light will pass through the fibers from one end to the other, no matter how that fiber is bent or twisted, it allows the doctor to both send light into the dark recesses of the body and, by using a tiny lens attached to one end of the fibers, actually see what is there when the light travels back.

IV—intravenous. Fluid (saline solution, medication, or blood) administered directly into a vein. The term as used in this section refers to an IV drip: a needle inserted in a vein is connected by a tube to a bottle of fluid hung on a pole. The fluid drips into the vein over a period of time.

NPO—(*non per os*) nothing by mouth; one cannot eat or drink for a specified amount of time.

organ—any part of the body that has a specific function to perform: for example, the lungs, liver, heart, stomach.

organ system—a group of organs and tissues that work together to accomplish a specific body function. Basically, there are eight of these "systems":

1. the musculoskeletal system, including the bones, cartilage, muscle, skin, and fatty tissue
2. the nervous system, which encompasses the brain, spinal cord, and nerves
3. the circulatory (vascular) system, which is made up of the blood, veins, arteries, and the heart
4. the lymphatic system, which includes the lymph channels and lymph nodes (and joins the circulatory system)
5. the digestive system or gastrointestinal tract, which includes the esophagus, stomach, small intestine, liver, pancreas, spleen, gallbladder, and large intestine (colon, rectum, and anus)
6. the respiratory system, which includes the larynx, trachea, lungs, pleura (tissue surrounding the lungs), and mediastina (the space between the lungs)
7. the urinary system, which encompasses the kidneys, ureters, bladder, and urethra
8. the female reproductive system, including the vulva, cervix, vagina, uterus, fallopian tubes, ovaries, and breasts (mammary glands); or

the male reproductive system, which involves the prostate and Cowper's gland, the penis, and testes.

Doctors often regroup these systems into new systems, minisystems, or composite systems for the purposes of diagnosis and treatment. Cancer specialists group the organs and structures of the head and neck (excluding the brain) although the specific sites may be part of other systems. The genital and urinary systems in men are close to one another, and are combined and called the genitourinary system. There are also composite systems, like the endocrine (hormone) system, which includes the adrenal glands, pituitary gland, thyroid gland, parathyroid glands, thymus gland, ovaries, pancreas, and testes; and the immune system, which involves the endocrine system plus the bone marrow, lymphatic system, and spleen.

Some knowledge of organ systems is important for anyone interested in cancer. First, certain cancers—particularly lymphoma and leukemia—are true systemic cancers: Their "site" is the whole system in the body. Second, diagnostic and treatment procedures are often similar for cancers appearing in different locations within one system. Third, all the organs in a system are connected to each other, producing an easy pathway for metastases, which is why doctors finding a primary cancer at one location will examine the whole system for signs of spread. Fourth, the lymphatic system and the circulatory system are interwoven throughout all the other systems: That is why cancers are particularly dangerous when they originate in, or spread to, these systems. Last, by looking at the diagrams in Appendix A, you will notice that many of these systems are packed tightly together in the body: for example, the reproductive system, the urinary system, and the lower half of the digestive system. Cancers that spread by local invasion spread not only to adjoining parts of their own systems but to nearby organs of other systems. Again, doctors will want to examine these adjacent organs and systems for signs of metastases.

puncture site—the location where a needle has entered the body.
radioactive—describes substances that emit radiant energy, such as radium. These show up brightly on X-ray pictures when used as contrast materials.
radioisotope—radioactive forms of an element; used as contrast materials in diagnostic scans.
radionuclides—see radioisotopes.
radiopaque—describes a contrast material that blocks X rays. Areas that have been injected with radiopaque material show up clearly on X-rays as highly defined white areas.
saline solution—a salt solution, given by IV, used to maintain normal fluid levels in the body or to increase fluid levels so that diagnostic or therapeutic chemicals that have been put into the body can be expelled more quickly during urination.
sedative—a drug given to calm the patient, relax muscles, cause sleepiness.
stool—feces, the product of a bowel movement.
veins—the channels in the circulatory system that take blood, whose oxygen has been used by the cells, back to the heart.
void—urinate.
vital signs—temperature, pulse, respiratory rate, and blood pressure.

Chapter Five

DIAGNOSTIC PROCEDURES AND TESTS—WHAT, WHY, AND HOW

In this chapter we will describe the most common diagnostic procedures and tests. Unless otherwise indicated, all procedures can be done on either an outpatient or an inpatient basis.

Acid Phosphatase Test

This laboratory test measures the amount of acid phosphatase in the blood. Acid phosphatase is an enzyme produced in the prostate gland and gradually released into the blood serum. High levels of acid phosphatase often indicate metastatic prostate cancer or multiple myeloma.

ACTA Scan

See "CAT Scan."

AFP Assay

This laboratory test detects the presence of Alpha$_1$-feto-protein in the blood serum. AFP is an antigen—a substance that stimulates the production of antibodies. The AFP Assay is combined with other tests to detect and monitor cancers of the liver, testicles, ovaries, pancreas, stomach, colon, and lungs. High levels of AFP do not necessarily indicate cancer; AFP levels may be raised due to conditions other than cancer.

Alkaline Phosphatase Test

This laboratory test determines the level of alkaline phosphatase in the blood serum and bone. The normal amount of this enzyme varies with age, but it is known to be elevated in cancers of the liver and pancreas, some nonmetastatic cancers, and in the presence of other diseases of the liver, pancreas, lung, and bone. It is normally elevated in pregnancy.

Aortography

See "Angiogram."

Angiogram (Arteriography)

In this contrast-film procedure, the arteries can be seen after a radiopaque material has been injected into the bloodstream. It is generally used to diagnose problems of the legs, kidneys, pancreas, spleen, liver, gastrointestinal tract, brain, and heart.

Three kinds of angiograms are used in cancer diagnosis: *cardiac catheterization*, which visualizes the arteries going into the heart and is particularly useful for diagnosis of Wilms's tumor; *cerebral angiography*, for diagnosing brain tumors; and *renal arteriography*, used to visualize the kidneys. Renal arteriography is conclusively diagnostic in nearly all cases of cancer of the kidney, and also pinpoints the extent of the cancer.

You may be asked not to eat anything after midnight the day before the test. Blood tests may be done to check your clotting time, and you may get a laxative or enema. A saline IV may be started. The area to be injected with the contrast material will be sterilized and, if necessary, shaved. You may be given a sedative and asked to urinate just before the procedure starts.

You will lie on your back on the examining table, a local anesthetic will be administered, and the contrast material will be put directly into an artery (usually the femoral artery in your groin), either through a needle or a catheter. If a catheter is used, it is threaded through the system of arteries until it reaches the area to be examined. The radiologist will watch and guide the catheter's progress by using a fluoroscope. When it has reached its destination, the contrast material will be injected (which may feel warm) and a quick series of X-rays taken. You will hear a loud click as the film goes into the camera. If you are having a cerebral angiogram, you may see bright lights flash.

After the test, pressure will be applied to the artery to prevent bleeding. When the local anesthetic wears off, you may experience some pain. Ice packs may be used to limit swelling, and you may have a temporary black-and-blue mark. You will stay in bed for at least eight hours while nurses monitor your blood pressure and pulse to check for bleeding.

These procedures must be done on an inpatient basis and take from one-to-four hours. Given preparation and recovery time, it is best to think of them as full-day tests.

Arteriography

See "Angiogram."

Barium Enema

See "Lower GI."

41

Barium Swallow

See "Upper GI."

Biopsy

A biopsy is the removal of a sample of tissue or fluid for examination by a pathologist. It provides the definitive diagnosis for cancer.

To examine a tissue sample, extremely thin slices of the tissue are mounted on slides and dyed to highlight certain areas. The sections are then preserved and examined by the pathologist. There are two methods of slide preparation: permanent section and frozen section.

Permanent Section

This method of slide preparation takes several days. The tissue is preserved in formaldehyde, then very thinly sliced and very precisely stained to produce a highly accurate picture of the cells. Such slides enable the pathologist to give accurate and detailed information about the cancer. These slides can also be sent to another pathologist for confirmation of the diagnosis.

Frozen Section

This can be prepared in a matter of minutes, and is particularly useful during a cancer operation; the surgeon can be notified if the suspected tissue is malignant or benign, enabling him to determine the extent of the operation. It may also eliminate the need for a second operation.

Although extremely useful in this situation, frozen sections have several disadvantages compared to permanent sections. The tissue section is quick-frozen before slicing, with the result that the slices are thicker than those of the permanent section, contain more layers of cells, and are thus more difficult to read. Each slice is then dipped in alcohol and quickly stained, which may damage the cells. The pathologist must therefore decide which abnormalities are part of the cell structure and which are the result of the processing. Usually he can tell whether or not the tissue is cancerous, but cannot analyze the type of cancer. Also, these slides cannot be passed on to a second pathologist.

Biopsies are generally classified by the procedures used to get the tissue samples. Unless otherwise noted, biopsies can be done with either a local or general anesthetic and may be done either in the doctor's office or the hospital.

Aspiration or Needle Biopsy

A hollow needle extracts a sample from the tissue or fluid. Suction (aspiration), is the usual method, but sometimes the needle is twisted to cut away a core of tissue. These generally require a local anesthetic and, depending on the site of the tumor and the other tests scheduled, may be done either in the doctor's office or in the hospital. The site discussions in part II contain more detailed information on needle biopsies.

Endoscopic Biopsy

Small tissue samples are taken during an endoscopy. See "Endoscopy" on page 56 and the different types of endoscopies for more information.

Excisional Biopsy (also called "Total Biopsy")

If a tumor is very small, all of it may be surgically removed for examination. Depending on the tumor's location, a local or general anesthetic may be administered and the biopsy performed in either the doctor's office or the hospital.

Incisional Biopsy (also called "Wedge Biopsy")

Part of the tumor is surgically removed along with adjacent normal tissue for comparison.

Open Biopsy

An open biopsy is a major surgical procedure during which the patient is "opened up," a tissue sample taken, and the tumor and adjacent area visually inspected and palpated.

Punch Biopsy (also called "Trephine Biopsy")

A special instrument called a punch is used to pierce an organ either directly or through the skin, or through a small slit made first in the skin. A cylindrical tissue sample is obtained.

Trephine Biopsy

See "Punch Biopsy."

Wedge Biopsy

See "Incisional Biopsy."

Biopsies may also be classified according to the organ or tissue being examined:

Bone-Marrow Biopsy

Bone marrow—the soft material at the center of the bone—produces many of the necessary components of the blood. A sample is obtained usually from the sternum (chest bone) or the ilium (hip bone) using special needles. The test is done by a doctor (usually a hematologist) and an assistant, using a local anesthetic, and takes about forty-five minutes.

The patient may undergo this test as either an inpatient or outpatient, in a clinic, doctor's office, treatment room, or patient's bed. If bone marrow is being taken from the chest, the patient lies flat on his back. If it is being taken from the hip, he may lie in the fetal position on his side. The patient will feel a burning sensation when the anesthetic is injected. As the needle enters the bone, he will feel a sharp pain. For a few seconds he will feel intense pain while the bone marrow is removed. When samples have been taken, the doctor removes the needle and applies pressure over the puncture site. If the procedure is done on an outpatient basis, the patient will remain for about half an hour to make sure there is no bleeding. The area will feel sore and bruised for several days.

This is a routine test for suspected leukemia, Hodgkin's disease, and to determine if cancer has metastasized.

Cone Biopsy

This name describes the shape of tissue samples removed surgically in the cervix. It is done with a local anesthetic. See "Pelvic Examination" for an explanation of the procedure.

Liver Biopsy

Before this needle biopsy is done, the doctor will make sure the patient can hold her breath for the few seconds needed to take the biopsy. Because there is a danger of bleeding, blood tests will be run; the patient's blood will be analyzed to make sure it can clot properly, and will be typed so that reserves will be available in an emergency. The patient may be NPO beginning the night before the test.

During the procedure, the patient will usually lie on her back at the right edge of the bed, with the right arm tucked behind her head, which is turned toward the left. The doctor will thump the liver area to find the dullest-sounding place. The skin over this area will be scrubbed with an antiseptic solution and draped with sterile towels.

Two anesthetics are given: one to the surface area and one in the liver. The first anesthetic will sting a bit, and the second will cause momentary pain. Before the biopsy needle enters, the patient will be asked to breathe out and hold it. She can breathe normally as soon as the tissue sample is taken.

After the procedure, the patient may have pain at the puncture site and also in the right shoulder. This rarely lasts more than twelve hours and can be controlled with mild medication. To avoid bleeding, the patient will be asked to stay on her right side for an hour after the procedure and remain in bed for twenty-four hours. She may remain NPO until all danger has passed. This procedure must be done on an inpatient basis.

Scalene Node Biopsy

The scalene fat pads that drain the lungs are inspected by a broncho-scope (see "Bronchoscopy" for procedure). This biopsy is used to detect lung cancer, to decide if lung cancer is operable, and to determine whether other cancers have spread to the lungs.

Renal Biopsy

This is a needle biopsy of kidney tissue. The actual test takes about fifteen minutes, but if one includes preparation and recovery/monitoring time, the process takes more than twenty-four hours. It is performed by a doctor (usually a kidney specialist: nephrologist) and an assistant.

Blood tests are done to make sure there is no danger of bleeding and that a supply of the right type of blood is on hand in case it is needed. A plain-film X ray or contrast-film tomogram is taken to find out exactly where the kidney is. About an hour before the test is to start, the patient is sedated so he will be comfortable and calm during the procedure.

The patient lies on his stomach and pillows are placed under his abdomen to bring the kidneys closer to the surface. The area will be sterilized, draped with sterile towels, and a local anesthetic given, which will sting for a moment before the area becomes numb. The patient will be told to take a deep breath and hold it as the biopsy needle is inserted. He may feel pressure from the needle, but not pain. After the tissue has been removed, firm pressure is applied to the puncture site.

The patient is required to stay in bed and take plenty of fluids for twenty-four hours while he is monitored for signs of bleeding. Most patients will have a very small amount of blood in their urine. If a clot has formed, the patient may feel extreme pain until the clot is passed in his urine.

Body Scan

See "Gallium Scan."

Body-Section Roentgenogram

See "Tomogram."

Bone Scan

Radioisotopes are injected which are picked up in the bone marrow. Doctors can see abnormal expansion of the bone marrow as well as areas of bone-marrow destruction. This procedure is used to discover multiple myeloma and osteosarcomas, and also evidence of metastasis to the bone by other types of cancer.

The isotopes are introduced through an IV in the arm, three to four hours before the scan. The patient will lie on his back for an hour as the scanning machine passes over him. During this time the patient may be asked to change position. Reference points may be marked on the patient's body with a skin pencil in order to compare the scan with X-ray film.

Brain Scan

After injecting a small number of radioisotopes, the scanner can pinpoint the location of a brain tumor without harming normal tissue. Brain-scanning techniques have revolutionized the process of diagnosing problems in the brain. They are generally 90 percent accurate and, unlike tests such as angiograms, pose no danger to the patient.

The patient is given the radioisotopes either by mouth or through an IV. Depending on the method used, the scan will start either immediately or after a short waiting period, and will take from ten minutes to an hour. The patient will be asked to change positions several times for front, back, and side views. The procedure itself is painless.

The first scan determines whether there is an abnormality in the brain. If an abnormality is found, a second scan may be done immediately, another after twenty-four hours and a third after forty-eight hours, using a different isotope given by IV. Different types of abnormalities become visible at different times: Problems with the brain's circulatory system can be seen immediately; abnormalities caused by cancer show up twenty-four hours later.

Bronchoscopy

In this procedure, a rigid or flexible tube, called a bronchoscope, is passed through the mouth and down the throat to look at the bronchial tubes leading to the lungs. It enables the doctor to visually examine the breathing passages and take tissue samples for biopsies.

The patient will be NPO after midnight before the procedure. The personnel involved include the physician (endoscopist), an assistant, a scrub nurse, a circulating nurse, and an anesthesiologist, if a general anesthesia is given. A local anesthetic is preferred so the patient can help with the examination—by changing position, coughing on command, etc.

If a local anesthetic is used, the patient will first receive tranquilizers and sedatives to relax and calm him. The most difficult part of the procedure is the application of the local anesthetic, which is sprayed in the throat and bronchial tubes. This stimulates the gag and cough reflexes. As the anesthetic numbs these surfaces, the patient feels as if the tongue and throat are swollen, and concludes that he is not able to breathe and swallow, although he can breathe and swallow normally.

After the anesthetic has taken effect, the patient will be positioned. If a rigid bronchoscope is used, he will lie on his back with his head tilted backward, helped by the assistant. This position straightens out the airway and makes it easier to slide the tube in. If a flexible tube is used, the patient will be in a more comfortable position—either lying on his back or sitting up. The patient will feel the pressure of the bronchoscope being inserted, and may cough or gag.

The procedure takes thirty to forty-five minutes, and the anesthetic wears off sixty to ninety minutes later. The patient will not be allowed to eat or drink until sensation has returned. There will be some soreness in the throat, the larynx, and the side of the mouth once the anesthetic has worn off.

Cardiac Catheterization

See "Angiogram."

CAT Scan

The CAT scan visualizes the brain and the torso. Although your doctor will usually scan only one part of your body, the process is the same for all areas.

The equipment is located in two adjoining rooms. The patient will lie on her back on an examining table that is positioned in the hole of what looks like a giant metal doughnut. The doughnut is the CAT scanner, which passes X-rays in a 180° arc through the part of the body being examined. The X-rays meet tissues of different densities as they pass through the body to the detectors. The detectors relay the information to equipment in the adjoining room. A computer translates the information into an image which appears on a screen and can then be printed on paper or photographed by a Polaroid camera.

A series of pictures is taken at one-inch intervals; your body may be marked with a skin pencil for comparison to later X-rays. The technician will move the examining table for each cross-section picture.

No special preparation is needed, though sometimes the contrast material is injected and a sedative may also be given. The procedure is painless and has no aftereffects. The length of the scan varies. Brain scans usually take about half an hour, while scans of the abdomen require at least an hour.

CBC (Complete Blood Count)

The CBC is a series of laboratory tests that analyze various parts of the blood and other substances found in the blood. It is a critical procedure, but simple from the patient's point of view. The patient gives two samples of blood. The first sample is withdrawn from a vein to fill several small (three-inch) test tubes. The patient feels the slight prick of the needle, and the process is completed in seconds. The second sample is taken from a prick of a finger and immediately placed on a slide; this is called a blood smear.

The various parts of the blood are produced in the bone marrow, lymph nodes, and spleen. These blood-producing tissues make the white blood cells (leukocytes) which fight infection; the red blood cells (erythrocytes) which transport oxygen and dispose of wastes such as carbon dioxide; the platelets (thrombocytes) which are necessary for clotting; and the hemoglobin, an oxygen-carrying protein found in red blood cells. These components are carried in fluid made up of blood plasma and blood serum.

The CBC registers the count of each blood component in a given volume of blood, or presents the result in percents; an absolute numerical count of the white and red blood cells and platelets is given; and the hemoglobin is weighed. The test will also show a differential count—the ratio of mature cells to immature cells—and a hematocrit—the percentage of red blood cells. These counts and tests are done by sophisticated machines and computers. The normal ranges for these tests are given in table 3.

TABLE 3
Complete Blood Count: Normal Range of Results

Test	Normal Range
Blasts (abnormal cells in marrow)	Less than 5%
Differential Count	100
Erythrocytes (red cells)	4.5–5 million
Granulocytes (white cells that fight infection)	2000–4000
Hematocrit	Men: 42–46%
	Women: 38–42%
Hemoglobin	13–16 gm/100 ml
Leukocytes (see WBC)	
Reticulocytes—"retic" (young red cells)	0.5–1.5% of red cells
WBC (white blood count: total)	Average: 5000–10,000

The presence of cancer, or a particular type of treatment, will make your counts different from "normal." However, the patient is not necessarily in immediate danger if he is outside the normal range. For example, while the normal count of the white blood cells that fight infection is 2000–4000, the count may go as low as 500 before the situation becomes life-threatening. In any patient, the doctor will be watching the results of the CBC for different significant signs.

The CBC can indicate anemia (low-volume hematocrit—low red blood count, high white blood count), the presence of infection (high white blood count), and problems with blood-clotting (platelet count). It also helps determine whether there has been bone-marrow failure caused by cancer, chemotherapy, or radiation, and it helps monitor lymphomas and leukemias.

The tests discussed thus far have been those done by computer on the large sample of blood. The blood-smear slides prepared from the smaller sample are reviewed by technicians under a microscope and provide additional information about any anemia, infection, or blood-clotting problem.

CBCs are repeated during the course of diagnosis and treatment.

CEA Assay

This is a laboratory test that looks for the presence of carcinoembryonic antigen in the blood serum. An antigen is usually a foreign substance, such as a poison or virus, that stimulates the production of antibodies. High levels of CEA strongly indicate digestive-system cancer, but it has also been found in the blood serum of patients with lung and other cancers, as well as patients with noncancerous chronic liver disease, kidney disease, and inflammatory diseases of the colon. As a result, the CEA Assay is used in combination with other tests. It is also used to monitor a patient's response to treatment: After the tumor has been destroyed, the CEA level returns to normal. If the cancer should recur, the level will rise again.

Cerebral Angiography

See "Angiogram."

Cholangiogram (IVC)

This is a contrast-film tomogram of the gallbladder and bile ducts.

You may be placed on a high-fat diet several days before the test in order to empty the gallbladder of bile. (Bile is used to digest fats. A high-fat diet causes the gallbladder to release the bile to digest the fat.) The afternoon before the test you may get a strong laxative. You cannot eat after midnight, although you may be allowed to drink clear liquids.

The test is done in the Radiology Department. You will be asked to lie on your stomach with your right side raised. Plain-film X-rays are taken and a small amount of contrast material is injected into a vein.

The radiologist will watch you for a few minutes to see if you have an allergic reaction to the contrast material. If there is no reaction, the rest of the contrast is injected and a series of pictures are taken, beginning twenty minutes after the injection and continuing until the contrast material has gone through the gallbladder. This can take over two hours, but, although lengthy, a cholangiogram is almost painless; the hardest part is staying still.

If a cholangiogram is part of a battery of tests that include barium studies, the cholangiogram will be done first.

Cholecystogram

This is a contrast-film examination of the gallbladder.

The night before the test, you will eat no fats, and after dinner you will be NPO except for clear liquids. You will take six tablets—one every five minutes—which contain both the contrast material and a laxative to ensure clear X-rays.

You will lie on your stomach while the X-rays are taken. You will then eat a fatty meal. Twenty minutes later another set of X-rays will be taken to see how well the gallbladder is working. The procedure takes an hour.

Cisternal Puncture

This is the withdrawal of spinal fluid by insertion of a needle in the space between the base of the skull and the first vertebra. It is usually done when the condition of the patient does not allow a spinal tap, and is also used to give anesthesia, and for other diagnostic procedures.

The patient lies on her side with her chin resting on her chest. The nape of the neck is shaved, the area sterilized, and a local anesthetic administered. There will be a stinging sensation as the anesthetic is injected, and a dull pressure as the needle is inserted. The procedure takes between ten and thirty minutes and is done by a doctor and an assistant.

The patient will be watched during and after the procedure for difficulty in breathing and changes in blood pressure and pulse. Once vital signs are stable, the patient may return to normal activities.

Colonoscopy

A type of endoscopy, this procedure allows the doctor (surgeon, gastroenterologist, endoscopist, etc.) to look at the entire large intestine (five to seven feet) using a flexible fiberoptic tube. Tissue and cell samples may also be taken.

The patient's diet is limited to fluids for twenty-four hours before the test. The evening before, a strong laxative is given, and enemas are given at least two hours before the procedure. The patient is sedated, the tube inserted, and the colon examined as the colonoscope is drawn out. The procedure may take thirty minutes to three hours.

If the test is scheduled on an outpatient basis, someone should accompany the patient to assist in getting home. It is not a painful procedure, but discomfort arises from two sources:

First, after the colonoscope is inserted through the anus, air is put into the tube to slightly "blow up" the colon and allow for a clear view. The patient will experience cramps that will go away quickly as the examiner removes the air or it is expelled naturally.

The second source of discomfort is psychological—it is an "embarrassing" part of the body to have examined, although it is a routine procedure for the doctor and assistant.

Colposcopy

The colposcopy is the only form of endoscopy in which the scope does not enter the body. It is performed during a pelvic examination to examine the vagina, cervix, and vulva, and uses an instrument called a colposcope—a magnifying viewer and light source mounted on a stand.

With a speculum in place (the instrument used to spread the walls of the vagina), the area is swabbed with a dye. When viewed through the colposcope, abnormalities show up as white spots. This staining procedure is called the Schiller test. The doctor will take samples for biopsies.

The area viewed by the doctor is transmitted to a TV screen. Videotapes can be made to use for comparison of the area over time. The procedure takes ten to fifteen minutes and is done without anesthetic. The discomfort produced by taking samples for biopsies is similar to menstrual cramps.

There may be some discharge for a few days after the examination because of the brown-colored solution put on the tissues after biopsies are taken. Several days of sexual abstinence are usually suggested since the brown solution may be irritating to your partner. This test does not impair a woman's ability to have children.

A colposcopy is done if there has been an abnormal Pap smear, and also on girls whose mothers took DES during pregnancy.

Computer-Assisted Transaxial Tomography

See "CAT Scan."

Computerized Tomography (CT)

See "CAT Scan."

Computerized Transverse Axial Tomography (CTT)

See "CAT Scan."

Cultures

These are laboratory tests designed to detect and help identify disease, and to indicate the response of the disease to various kinds of treatment. Microorganisms or cells are grown in a special medium, and are obtained from samples of spinal fluid (taken during a spinal tap or cisternal puncture); from feces taken from a stool sample or acquired during a proctoscopy; and from sputum (mucus) obtained by deep coughing, or via washings of the trachea, bronchial tubes, pharynx, or esophagus.

Cystoscopy

A form of endoscopy used to examine the lining of the bladder, this test is done if the patient has had repeated urinary-tract infections or if blood has been found in the urine. It may also be done in preparation for a contrast-film study of the urinary tract.

This procedure is done on an inpatient basis by a urologist, anesthesiologist, nurse, and assistants. The medical personnel are dressed as they would be for an operation in masks, caps, and gowns. The procedure takes from five to forty-five minutes. It is generally faster for women than for men since the tubes from the bladder to the urethra are shorter in women.

If the procedure is being done under a general or spinal anesthetic, the patient will be NPO for twelve hours before the test. Before receiving the anesthetic, he will be given a sedative. A special table with leg supports helps him stay in the proper position—on his back with his knees flexed. His body will be draped (covered) except for the genital area. This area will be cleansed and, if a general or spinal anesthetic has not been used, a local will be given. The cystoscope, a very thin, lubricated tube, will then be inserted gently into the urethra. Sterile fluid may be introduced through the cystoscope into the bladder to permit a better view. The doctor will make a visual examination and may take a tissue sample. Using the cystoscope, a catheter may also be inserted to inject contrast material for other tests and for drainage.

The thought of this test may produce considerable anxiety. Men often have fears of castration, which, in reality, is impossible. There may be a general feeling of embarrassment because of the part of the body being examined and the position. Your doctors and nurses understand and expect these feelings and will be glad to talk with you.

If a spinal or local anesthetic is used, there may be some discomfort as the cystoscope is inserted, during the dilation of the bladder, and if biopsies are taken. There may also be fatigue and discomfort from maintaining the position. These problems will not affect those who have a general anesthetic.

For twenty-four hours after the test, you will be monitored for signs of edema (swelling caused by excessive fluid in the cells), hematuria (blood or red blood cells in the urine), and urinary sepsis (infection in the urinary system). You will be asked to urinate into a special container and to notify the nurse whenever you urinate so that urinalysis (see below) can be done. This will also let the doctor know that your system is functioning normally. Vital signs will be checked frequently.

Duodenoscopy

A form of endoscopy using flexible tubes passed through the mouth to examine the duodenum. See "Upper GI Endoscopy" for a description of the procedure.

Electroencephalogram

A painless procedure taking one to two hours (three or more hours for a sleep EEG), in which wires are attached to the head and the electrical activity of the brain is recorded. It is used in diagnosing brain tumors, but can only show that the brain is functioning abnormally; it cannot give specific information about the abnormality.

Before the test, you may eat, but you may not take any medications or drink any stimulants (coffee, tea, cola) or depressants (alcohol). Hair should be clean.

The test will take place in the hospital's Electroencephalography Suite. You will go to a small room that has either an examining table or a dentist-type chair. Nineteen to twenty-one electrodes will be attached to your head with paste or needles. As the needles are inserted, the feeling is similar to a quick yank on a single hair. The test is painless.

Each electrode picks up the electrical activity from a specific part of the brain. It passes this electrical activity to a pen, which transcribes a line on a moving piece of graph paper. This device is called an electroencephalograph. The lines produced on the paper are wavy, hence the term "brain waves." When one wave does not have a normal pattern, it indicates which part of the brain is experiencing a problem.

The test can be done while you are awake or asleep. If you are awake, you can function normally as soon as the test is over. If you have a sleep EEG, a sedative will be given and you will probably sleep for several hours and be groggy when you awaken. You should arrange for someone to take you home.

EMI Scan

See "CAT Scan."

Endoscopy

This is the general term for all the tests in which a doctor puts a rigid or flexible tube into the mouth, rectum, vagina, or urethra, in order to look at internal tissues and get cell samples. A light, a viewing lens, or other instruments can be passed through the tube. The picture can be displayed on a TV monitor and videotaped for future reference. The term is often used as a short form of "Upper GI Endoscopy" (see below).

Discussions of specific procedures can be found under the listing for each type of endoscopy:

BRONCHOSCOPY (bronchial tubes/lungs)
COLONOSCOPY (large intestine)
COLPOSCOPY (vagina, cervix, vulva)
CYSTOSCOPY (bladder, urethra)
DUODENOSCOPY (duodenum/pancreas): See "Upper GI Endoscopy."
ESOPHAGOSCOPY (esophagus): See "Upper GI Endoscopy."
GASTROSCOPY (stomach): See "Upper GI Endoscopy."
LAPAROSCOPY: See "Peritonoscopy."
LARYNGOSCOPY (larynx)
PERITONEOSCOPY (abdominal cavity/female reproductive system)
PROCTOSIGMOIDOSCOPY (lower portion of the colon)
UPPER GI ENDOSCOPY (duodenoscopy/esophagoscopy/gastroscopy)

Esophagram

See "Upper GI."

Esophagoscopy

See "Upper GI Endoscopy."

Fluoroscopy

A set of procedures using contrast material, X rays, and a fluoroscope to monitor the progress of the contrast material through a body system. Still pictures may be taken at various times for a permanent record.

56

The patient is placed between a special fluorescent screen and an X-ray tube. The X rays are continuously beamed through the patient until the examination is finished.

The IVP and blood-flow tests are fluoroscopic examinations. In addition, fluoroscopy may be used as a part of all contrast-film procedures.

Gallbladder Series

Refers to those tests that examine the gallbladder. See "Cholangiography" and "Cholecystogram."

Gallium Scan (Total Body Scan)

Gallium-67 is a radioactive contrast material that is picked up by rapidly dividing cells. It helps detect the spread of cancer, particularly in the lymph nodes.

Before the test, you may be given a laxative, enemas, and/or a suppository, and you will be asked to urinate just before the scan. There is no restriction on food or drink.

A small amount of gallium will be injected into your vein. The scan may be done immediately or forty-eight hours later. Sometimes the scan is repeated over a four-day period, but you will not need any more injections of gallium.

There will be a slight stinging sensation as the gallium is injected into your vein. You will have to lie still during the scan (up to an hour). It is a painless procedure with no aftereffects.

Gastrointestinal Series (GI Series)

This is a contrast-film study of the whole gastrointestinal tract: from the mouth, through the esophagus, stomach, duodenum, small and large intestines, to the rectum. The series is divided into two parts: The upper GI looks at the top half of the system, from the mouth through the duodenum; the lower GI looks at the bottom half of the system—intestines, colon, and rectum. See the individual descriptions of these two procedures for detailed information.

Gastroscopy

A type of endoscopy used to examine the stomach. See "Upper GI Endoscopy."

HCG Assay

A laboratory test done on a urine sample. HCG (*h*uman *c*horionic *g*onadotropin) is a sex hormone that is sensitive to radioassay techniques. These techniques measure minute amounts of substances that are not detectable in any other way. The test helps monitor ovarian and testicular cancers and choriocarcinomas. (This test is also used to detect pregnancy.)

Intravenous Cholangiogram (IVC)

See "Cholangiogram."

IVP (Intravenous Pyelogram)

A fluoroscopic X-ray examination of the kidneys, ureters, and bladder.

The day before, you may be given a laxative, enemas, and/or suppositories, and you will be NPO after midnight. Before the test, you will be asked to urinate, then a dye will be injected by IV. The dye collects in the kidneys, bladder, ureters, and urethra. At first only a small amount is injected, and the radiologist will wait several minutes to make sure there is no allergic reaction. While the dye is going into your arm, you will stand behind the fluoroscopy screen. The technician watches the dye move through your system on a TV screen in a control booth and looks for any places where its movement may be obstructed. Spot X-rays are taken at various times.

The IVP takes about forty-five minutes. The only pain will be the prick of the needle being inserted. Sometimes the contrast material feels warm, and you may have a metallic taste in your mouth. The dye leaves your system through the kidneys, so your urine will be a yellowish pink for two days.

The IVP is used both for cancer detection and to make sure your urinary system functions properly; complications associated with some types of chemotherapy may thus be avoided.

Laminogram

See "Tomogram."

Laparoscopy

See "Peritoneoscopy."

Laparotomy

In this diagnostic surgical procedure (major surgery), the abdominal wall is opened so the surgeon can examine and palpate the organs deep inside and take biopsies. Patients refer to the operation as "the big zipper" because the scar runs up the stomach. This procedure is usually done as part of a larger "cancer operation," which has both diagnostic and treatment components. See chapter 8 on surgery for a complete description.

Laryngoscopy

A form of endoscopy used to examine and/or take biopsies from the larynx (voice box). The procedure is done in the hospital, but can be done on an outpatient basis. It takes thirty-five to forty minutes.

You cannot eat just before the test. You may be given sedatives and also drugs that inhibit the secretion of mucus and saliva; this facilitates the insertion of the tube down your throat.

The procedure can be done with either a local or a general anesthetic. Local anesthetic is usually preferred so you can cooperate with the doctor by making certain sounds; this moves your vocal chords and allows the doctor to see clearly. The local anesthetic will be sprayed on your throat and vocal chords, either with a separate syringe or with a sprayer attached to the laryngoscope. You will feel

59

the urge to gag and cough. Your head will be raised and held by an assistant. You will not be allowed to eat or drink until the anesthetic wears off (about two hours).

If a general anesthetic is used, you will not be aware of the procedure and will wake up with a mild sore throat. If a biopsy is taken, you may spit up some blood. You should inform your doctor if this occurs.

Liver Biopsy

See "Biopsy."

Liver Scan

A type of radioisotope scan that maps the liver. This test is used to detect cancer in the liver, both as a primary site and as a metastatic site. The spleen is also evaluated during this procedure.

The scan evaluates the liver structure and the liver function. The liver-structure scan will take about thirty to forty-five minutes. A spleen scan usually follows immediately, adding another twenty minutes. The contrast medium is injected by IV, and several scans are taken with the patient in different positions: standing, sitting, lying down on the stomach, back, and left side. The liver-function scan usually requires three scans: one immediately after the injection of contrast material; one later to see if the gallbladder has filled; and a final scan twenty-four hours after the injection of the contrast material.

The only sensation you will feel is the prick of the needle and a possible warm sensation in your veins from the contrast material.

Liver-Spleen Scan

See "Liver Scan."

Lower GI (Barium Enema)

A contrast-film study of the lower GI tract (intestines, colon, rectum) using a radiopaque material called barium sulfate introduced by enema into the rectum. Its progress may be followed with a fluoro-scope. X-rays are taken when the barium has worked its way through the intestines.

Before the test, you will be given laxatives, enemas, and/or supposi-tories. Sometimes several are used because feces or gas will produce inaccurate pictures. You cannot eat or drink anything for twelve hours before the test.

To start the test, the nurse will give you a barium enema (about twelve ounces). This will give you a full feeling and you will have the urge to defecate. You may be asked to move around, and slight pres-sure may be applied to your stomach to help the barium move into position. If you are only having still pictures taken, front and back views will be taken as soon as that happens. If fluoroscopy is being done, still pictures will be taken periodically during the procedure. You may then be asked to go to the bathroom and expel as much of the barium as possible. A second set of pictures will be taken, and an air-contrast study may be done: A small amount of air is forced into the rectum and more pictures are taken. This may cause some tem-porary cramping, but the procedure is more tiring than painful.

You will expel the barium for three to five days after the test. Dur-ing that time feces will look chalky and might be hard, so a laxative may be prescribed.

Lymphangiogram

Using a dye injected into the lymph channels in the feet, the lymph system is clearly outlined for examination by X-ray pictures. Because the dye stays in your system for months, one injection allows doctors to monitor the effects of treatment and the progress of disease during and after treatment. This test is used in the primary diagnosis of lymphomas and leukemias, and also to determine the spread of other cancers to the lymph system.

The procedure takes place in the Radiology Department. The injec-tion process takes about two hours, and the pictures about thirty minutes. You will have to come back the next day for another set of X-rays, which also take thirty minutes.

At the start of the test, your feet will be shaved and cleaned with an antiseptic. A local anesthetic will be injected, which may sting. Then the doctor will make a small slit, or cutdown, in the skin on the top of each foot near the toes or between the toes. A needle will be placed in each lymph channel, the contrast material slowly injected, and X-rays taken as the contrast material moves through the lymph system. Some

61

patients may feel some discomfort at the back of the knees or in the groin at the start of the injection. When the test is done, a stitch or two closes each slit.

The blue dye may cause your urine and bowel movements to be blue for several days, and your feet and legs may be blue for several weeks. There may be some soreness around the slits. You must keep the area around the incisions clean and dry until the stitches are removed, about a week after the procedure.

Mammogram

A type of plain-film, soft-tissue X-ray used to detect cancer in the breast: It can detect 90% of breast cancers. It takes about twenty minutes and is painless.

In the X-ray room, you strip to the waist and one breast at a time is put on a "tray." Several pictures are taken at different angles to make sure the X rays pass through all the tissues. It may be done on one or both breasts.

Needle Biopsy

See "Biopsy."

Open Biopsy

See "Biopsy."

Oral Gallbladder Test

See "Cholecystogram."

Paracentesis

This is an aspiration procedure in which fluid is removed from the abdomen—both for diagnostic purposes and as a treatment when excess fluid builds up in the abdomen causing pressure and pain.

The patient lies flat on her back in bed or on the examining table. The abdomen will be cleaned with an antiseptic and a local anesthetic will be injected. This will sting. When the area is numb, a needle is inserted and fluid withdrawn. Afterward, a pressure bandage is applied. The procedure takes fifteen to thirty minutes. You may feel a little dizzy, depending on the amount of fluid that was taken out.

Pelvic Examination

A pelvic examination is a specialized physical examination of the female reproductive system: ovaries, fallopian tubes, uterus, cervix, vagina, and vulva. It is usually done by a gynecologist as an office procedure taking about twenty minutes. Organs and structures are examined visually and manually, and tissue and cell samples are usually taken. When done in the doctor's office, no anesthesia is used. It may be done in the hospital, under general anesthesia, as part of the normal staging procedure for cancers of the female reproductive system; in this case the patient will be hospitalized for twenty-four hours. Nearly half of all cancers in women are cancers of the reproductive system; many other cancers, particularly cancers in the abdominal cavity, routinely spread to these organs. For all these cancers, pelvic examinations are routine diagnostic procedures.

The doctor will ask you to lie on your back on the examining table with your buttocks at the edge closest to him. A hospital gown or a sheet will have been draped over you, and a nurse will be in the examining room with you. (If your doctor normally does not have a nurse in the room and you feel uncomfortable, request one.) You will spread your legs and put your feet in stirrups so that your knees are in the air. The doctor will then insert a spreader (speculum) to keep the vagina open. (Speculums are now made of plastic and are fairly comfortable after being inserted; older models are made of metal and can be very cold when inserted unless warmed first with water.) After examining the vagina, he will remove the speculum and palpate the ovaries, fallopian tubes, and uterus. He will then gently scrape part of the cervix with a curette to get cell samples for a Pap smear.

Peritoneoscopy

A type of endoscopy used to look at the abdominal cavity. Tubes are inserted through half-inch slits made in the abdominal wall. Usually two slits are made: one for insertion of the tube containing the light source and viewing lens; the other for the tube containing cell- and tissue-sampling instruments.

This is an inpatient procedure that takes a full day from preparation to complete recovery. The patient will be NPO after midnight, and blood tests will be done to make sure the patient's blood is clotting properly and that a supply of blood of the same type is on hand if any emergency arises. Chest X-rays will be taken the day before the procedure as well as the day after.

The procedure is done in an operating room. The patient is given a sedative and a local anesthetic, then a slit is made and air is injected into the abdominal cavity so the doctor can see vital organs more clearly. This can cause pain in the right shoulder. After examination, fluid may be injected to get cell samples, and biopsies may be taken.

The peritoneoscopy takes from two to four hours. The patient may feel discomfort from gas and mild abdominal cramping, a temporary feeling of pain in the right shoulder, and mild discomfort from the stitches used to close the slit(s). For six hours after the peritoneoscopy, the patient's vital signs will be monitored and she will have a saline IV in her arm.

The peritoneoscopy allows doctors to examine the female reproductive system and certain organs in the abdomen, particularly the liver, without subjecting the patient to major surgery.

Pneumoencephalogram

A form of contrast-film X-ray used to diagnose tumors in the brain. After a local anesthetic has been administered, a needle is inserted into the spinal cord and a small amount of fluid is removed. This is replaced with gas or air, and then pictures are taken. The process takes one to three hours, but the patient may have side effects (headaches, nausea, vomiting, fever) which can last several days. This is a high-risk, inpatient procedure that is done only when absolutely necessary. When equipment is available, the CAT scan replaces this test.

For several hours before the test, the patient will not eat or drink. A sedative may be given and an IV started in the neck. If the anesthetic is to be given in the neck, the back of the neck will be shaved. The patient will sit in a somersault chair, securely fastened in so he cannot fall out. After the contrast material (air or gas) is injected, he will be tilted upside down so the ventricular system is filled with the contrast material. More contrast material may be injected and pictures are taken.

This is a painful procedure; administration of the anesthetic causes pain, and the contrast gas or air causes severe headaches and nausea. Some people are frightened by the movement of the chair, although there is no danger of falling out.

The headache may last a day or two, but can be eased by staying flat on one's back in bed, drinking fluids, and taking medication.

Proctosigmoidoscopy

A type of endoscopy that examines the final ten to twelve inches of the colon. Inserting the rigid viewing tube through the rectum, the doctor can see the final, straight ten inches of the rectum and around the bottom curve of the sigmoid colon. This is the area where most cancers and polyps of the colon are found.

This is a quick procedure, about ten minutes, performed by a doctor and an assistant without anesthetic. Before the procedure, the patient is given an enema or a suppository. When the procedure begins, the patient will be positioned either on hands and knees with his head down on the examining table and buttocks raised in the air, or on his side in the fetal position. The patient will be draped to minimize embarrassment.

The doctor, who wears rubber gloves, will manually examine the patient's rectum. This is done to expand the sphincter muscle, which normally keeps the rectum closed, and also to check for any obstruction. The endoscope is then inserted to its full length and the examination of the colon takes place as it is withdrawn. Air is introduced to straighten out the natural folds in the colon and give the doctor a full view. Biopsy samples will be taken of suspicious tissue, and some polyps may also be removed.

During the manual examination and the insertion of the endoscope, the patient will feel an urge to defecate. This feeling can be counteracted by breathing slowly and deeply with the mouth open. Because of the head-down position and deep breathing, the patient often experiences dizziness. He will be asked to lie down and rest for a few minutes after the examination. Once his head clears, he can leave. In the un-

65

likely event that he experiences rectal bleeding or severe abdominal pains, he should contact his doctor at once.

Pyelogram

See "IVP."

Renal Arteriogram

See "Angiogram" (also "Renal Blood Flow Study").

Renal Blood Flow Study

A fluoroscopic examination to check the flow of blood through the kidneys after contrast material has been injected into the veins. Because a large volume of blood flows through the tissues of the kidney, the organ is easily seen using this type of procedure. The differences observed by the radiologist indicate normal and abnormal tissue, and also tell him the type of abnormality (a cyst looks very different from a tumor). See "Angiogram" for the actual procedures involved.

Retrograde Urethrography (Pyelogram)

A fluoroscopic X-ray examination of the urethra (the tube that carries urine from the bladder to the outside of the body). The procedure takes about twenty minutes and is done by a radiologist and a technician with the patient lying on his/her back. Because the anatomy of males and females is different and the procedure has very different psychological effects on women and men, we will discuss the process separately for each sex.

Women

An instrument called a double-ballooned catheter is inserted into the urethra. This is a thin tube that can be blown up at both ends: one end in the bladder, the other right inside the outer opening of the urinary tract. Once the contrast material is injected directly into the urethra, pictures are taken. The patient should immediately tell the doctor of any discomfort. A local or spinal anesthetic may be used, although in women this is usually not necessary.

Men

The urethra (which comes out through the penis) is kept in position by a Brodney clamp. The Brodney clamp is attached to the base of the penis while the other end allows the injection of the contrast material at the head of the penis. After the contrast medium is injected into the urethra, pictures are taken. Although not painful, the idea of the placement of the instrument on the penis may cause fears of castration (which cannot happen). A local, spinal, or general anesthetic may be used. Any discomfort should be reported immediately.

Scalene Node Biopsy

See "Biopsy."

Schiller Test

See "Colposcopy."

Serum Calcium Test

A laboratory test on the blood serum to determine the amount of calcium in the blood. Calcium is vital for the growth and normal repair processes of the bones. Calcium levels are elevated in patients with leukemia and with metastases in the bones.

Sigmoidoscopy

See "Proctosigmoidoscopy."

SMA-12

In this laboratory test, smooth-muscle tissue obtained during a biopsy is stained with a fluorescent dye to detect the presence of certain antibodies. These antibodies are usually found in patients with hepatitis, but may also be found in patients with infectious mononucleosis and such cancers as soft-tissue sarcomas and cancer of the esophagus.

Sonogram

See "Ultrasound."

Spinal Tap (Lumbar Puncture)

The insertion of a needle into the cavity surrounding the lower part of the spine. It may be done for the purpose of obtaining fluid samples for diagnosis (this is a type of aspiration) or for administering medication or an anesthetic.

You will lie on your side with knees tucked up and your chin touching your chest. The lower part of your back will be cleansed and a local anesthetic will be injected. The injection will sting before the area becomes numb, but there will be no pain after this point. A needle is then inserted into the spinal cavity and you may feel a slight pressure. If the purpose is to obtain a fluid sample, a small amount of spinal fluid—usually no more than two teaspoons—is removed. After the procedure, you may be asked to lie on your back to avoid developing a headache (this is caused by the slight decrease in fluid in the spinal canal).

Sputum Test

A laboratory test done on the mucous lining of the bronchial tubes. The sample is usually taken by asking the patient to cough deeply. These cells can be observed under a microscope and used to grow cultures. (See "Cultures.")

Thermogram

A test that pictures the normal and abnormal tissues in the breast. A camera with heat-sensitive film detects the temperature differences in various types of tissues. It is used to find primary breast cancers and cancers that may have spread to the breast.

You are asked to strip to the waist and put your hands on top of your head in a cool (65°) room. You must stay in that position for about twenty minutes to let your body cool before the pictures are taken. The test is painless and uses no radiation.

Thoracentesis

An aspiration procedure using a hollow needle to remove fluid from your chest. The fluid may be taken to provide samples for diagnostic laboratory tests, or as a treatment procedure to ease breathing when there is excessive fluid accumulation.

You will be asked to sit on the side of your bed and lean over the bedside table for support. For comfort, a pillow will be placed under your arms and chest. You must stay still. Your back will be cleaned with an antiseptic, and a local anesthetic will be given; the latter stings. Once the area is numb, the needle will be inserted and fluid taken out. The procedure will take from fifteen to thirty minutes.

After the needle is removed, a small pressure bandage will be put on. A chest X-ray will be taken and your vital signs monitored. Once the anesthetic wears off, your back may feel sore where the needle was inserted.

Thyroid Scan

A scan of the thyroid gland using radioactive iodine or other radio-contrast material. The scan may reveal "hot" or "cold" spots (nodules). Cold nodules will be carefully examined by other tests to check for possible cancer.

The patient will lie on his back with his neck hyperextended backward. (This may cause you to feel you are choking. If this happens, tell the technician so you can be positioned more comfortably.) The scanner is positioned over the thyroid and passes back and forth across the neck. The patient should not swallow or cough when the scanner is directly over the thyroid.

The procedure takes about fifteen minutes. Afterward, the doctor may feel the patient's neck in order to compare any lumps with the information provided by the scan.

Tomogram

A special type of X-ray that provides a clear view of one section of an organ while blurring everything else. These pictures are also called tomographic cuts.

Although painless, the movement of the equipment can be startling. Two X-ray tubes move above the patient in a single plane. While the cuts are made, these tubes swoop abruptly above the patient, coming together and flying apart.

Tomograms, like regular X-rays, can be done on many parts of the body and are usually a contrast-film procedure. The contrast material is administered in various ways, and the procedure can be done on an outpatient basis.

Ultrasound

The use of high-frequency sound echoes to get a visual picture of soft tissues.

Preparation for the procedure is minimal and depends on the organ being examined. For examination of the female reproductive system, a woman will be asked to drink three or four glasses of water before the test; a full bladder helps the transmission of sound and gives clearer pictures. Fasting is sometimes necessary if the gallbladder is being examined. All patients must be able to lie still during the procedure; if this is difficult, a sedative may be given beforehand. Ultrasound will precede any tests involving barium, since barium affects sound waves.

Depending on the organ being examined, the patient will lie down either on his back or stomach. A gel, like Vaseline, is put on the skin to ensure airtight contact with the small round "microphone," called a transducer, which transmits the sound waves and picks up their echoes. The transducer is moved back and forth over the area while the doctor watches the pictures made by the echoes on an oscilloscope screen. When a significant picture emerges, he (or an assistant) will take a Polaroid picture of the oscilloscope display for a permanent record.

The test takes fifteen minutes. The patient feels only the slight pressure that must be applied to keep the transducer in airtight contact with the skin.

Upper GI

Part of the gastrointestinal (GI) series, this test uses a contrast-film X-ray and/or fluoroscopy to get an accurate picture of the esophagus, stomach, and small intestine.

You will not eat or drink for twelve hours before the test. Shortly before the procedure, you may be given a sedative. You will then be given eight ounces of a liquid that tastes like strawberry or chocolate chalk; this is the barium contrast material. In about two hours, the barium will work its way down through the small intestine. If you are only having X-rays, you will lie down and wait during this period, and then front and back pictures will be taken. If fluoroscopy is being done, doctors will watch the progress of the barium and take spot films during the whole two hours.

Although it is a painless procedure that is technically over after the pictures are taken, the process is not actually complete until the barium leaves your system. Barium tends to make you constipated, so the doctor will give you a laxative. For three to five days your bowel movements will be hard and grayish in color.

Upper GI (UGI) Endoscopy

This procedure allows the doctor to take small tissue samples from the esophagus, stomach, and duodenum. It is usually performed by a gastroenterologist and a nurse in the Endoscopy Suite of the hospital, although it can be performed at beside.

The patient will not be allowed to eat or drink after dinner the night before the examination. This is to permit clear viewing of the tissues. Dentures must be removed before the procedure. A local anesthetic will be applied to the throat, either by gargling or by swabbing it on. As it takes effect, the patient's tongue and throat will feel swollen. A sedative will also be given by IV, and will take effect in five to ten minutes. A bite block (mouthpiece) will be placed in the patient's mouth to prevent him from biting the tube of the endoscope, and he will lie on his left side. The doctor will guide the tube down the patient's throat and will ask him to swallow it, allowing it to pass into the esophagus. The patient will want to gag while this is happening, but vomiting is unusual. The doctor gently feeds the tube down to the lowest part of the system to be examined.

During the examination, the patient may feel unable to swallow, although he actually can. He will be given a small bowl or tissues to catch his saliva, or a small suction device will be put in the corner of his mouth. The patient will feel a cramplike pain if the endoscope must be passed through the lowest part of the stomach in order to view the duodenum.

The time involved will vary depending on the part of the upper GI tract examined. An esophagoscopy takes about fifteen minutes, a gastroscopy takes fifteen to thirty minutes, and a duodenoscopy takes fifteen to forty-five minutes.

After the endoscopy, the patient may have a sore throat, which can be helped by lozenges. The patient's vital signs will be monitored for three to four hours, until the anesthesia wears off completely and the gag reflex returns to normal. No food or fluid will be allowed during that time. If this procedure is to be done on an outpatient basis, arrangements should be made to have someone take the patient home.

Urinalysis

A laboratory examination of a urine sample. This includes a description of the urine's physical qualities—color, odor, quantity, specific gravity—and a microscopic and chemical analysis of the urine. These tests are a routine part of a physical examination and provide information for the diagnosis of many diseases. They are particularly helpful in the diagnosis of kidney cancer, which produces an abnormal number of red blood cells in the urine.

Venacavogram

See "Angiogram."

Ventriculogram

An X-ray of the small cavities of the brain. Contrast pictures are taken after the doctor drills a small hole in the skull, removing a small amount of fluid with a needle and replacing the fluid with air or gas. This is a high-risk procedure done only when absolutely necessary. Where equipment is available, the CAT scan replaces this test.

Xerography

A type of mammogram developed by the Xerox Corporation. Also called Xeroradiograms or Xerograms. See "Mammogram" for the procedure.

X-rays

X-rays are a type of electromagnetic radiation which can go through soft tissues but are blocked by dense materials like bone. Tissues with different densities show up as different shades of gray. The X-rays are generated by a machine on one side of the patient and pass through a designated part of the body, making an impression on a film on the other side.

Further Reading

Judith Nierenberg and Florence Janovic, *The Hospital Experience: A Complete Guide to Understanding and Participating in Your Own Care* (New York: Bobbs-Merrill, 1978).

Written specifically for patients, this book is easy to read and provides a wealth of information. Of particular interest are chapter 5 ("A guide to the language, or, Why your CC is important to your Px") and chapter 7 ("Pinpointing the Problem. The thirty-eight most frequently performed diagnostic tests: when a negative result is a good thing").

Barbara Skydell and Anne S. Crowder, *Diagnostic Procedures: A Reference for Health Practitioners and a Guide for Patient Counseling* (Boston: Little, Brown, 1975).

This is a professional book, written in technical language; the layman should not attempt to read it without a medical dictionary. Nevertheless, if you are interested in understanding the complete, technical aspects—including descriptions of the equipment—of nearly seventy diagnostic procedures, this is the easiest book to use. Besides general discussions of major issues, each procedure is described in terms of purpose, time, location in the hospital, personnel involved, equipment, technique, patient sensations, preparation, and aftercare.

Chapter Six

HOW TO FIND HELP

Once the initial diagnosis has been made, the patient enters the most crucial and psychologically difficult period of the cancer experience. Decisions must be made quickly about what kind of treatment to get and where to get it. These decisions can make the difference between living and dying.

If your type of cancer is rare, fast-growing, difficult to diagnose, difficult to treat, or Stage III or IV, gather information as quickly as possible and go to the best treatment team at a major cancer center experienced in dealing with your type of cancer. This must be done within a week.

If your type of cancer is Stage I or II, slow-growing, easy to diagnose, and responsive to standard treatments, you should still move quickly, since delay can allow the cancer to spread, which lessens your chances for cure. However, you will have a broader choice of places to go for treatment. Your case can probably be handled by any qualified cancer specialist, or possibly by your own physician if the treatment is supervised by a cancer specialist.

The first question to ask the doctor who made the initial diagnosis is: How much time do I have to decide? If you have a slow-growing thyroid cancer, you may have years before the situation becomes life-threatening. If you have a fast-growing, Stage IV lymphoma, a few days can make the difference between life and death.

What You Need to Know

Before you make any decisions, you must have the following information: a correct and complete diagnosis; the treatment alternatives for your type of cancer; the best doctors and hospitals for each type of treatment alternative. In addition, you must weigh any personal considerations that may limit your choices.

Since you must collect a mass of information in a short amount of time, it is best not to attempt it alone. In this chapter we will show you how to form your own information-gathering, decision-making network, and how to acquire your information.

Building Your Own Network

Your network should be composed of two types of people. First, two or three medical people—not necessarily cancer specialists—whose judgment you trust. These can be doctors (your family physician, a friend of the family, a member of the family), nurses, or hospital social workers. These people have access to specialized networks. Though they themselves may not be professionally involved with cancer, they know people who are; they went to school with them, and they work with them. They can gather basic information, or can use their sources to check information, particularly conflicting information, that has been gathered by others. The doctors in this group can also use their professional judgment to evaluate or "translate" technical information.

The rest of your team should be composed of two or three close friends and family members who do the legwork and help in the decision-making. These decisions are not technical decisions but ones of judgment. Technical problems have one correct answer; problems of judgment have many possible answers, some better than others. Experts have found that groups of people make better judgments than individuals. Of course, the final decisions must be made by the patient, but a small group of trusted family and/or friends can help with the process.

How to Use Your Team

Step 1:   Confirming the Diagnosis

You should have the initial diagnosis confirmed. This can be done at a comprehensive cancer center, a major medical center, or a uni-

75

versity medical center. See "Treatment Information and Resources" in part III for a listing of these hospitals by state.

If yours is a rare cancer (one that most pathologists do not encounter), if it is difficult to identify under a microscope, and/or if the way the cancer appeared in your body is "unusual," your effort must be greater to find people who have experience in dealing with it. This will be discussed fully in "Locating the Best Doctors and Hospitals," later in this chapter.

To confirm a diagnosis, the results of your tests, including the pictures and the slides made of the tissue samples taken during the biopsy, must be observed by a second pathologist. At this stage, particularly if you have a cancer that is in any way unusual, a comprehensive cancer center may want you to have additional tests before confirming the diagnosis. They may make this request because some of the test results are ambiguous, or because they feel that more tests are necessary to confirm how far the cancer has spread.

In order to proceed with steps two and three, you and your assistants must have the following information:

- the primary site of the cancer
- the specific cell type of cancer
- the extent of metastasis (where it has spread to and the stage of the cancer)
- how fast it is growing, and when the first symptoms appeared
- general state of the patient's health, including special problems that may affect treatment options
- the patient's age
- any previous treatments (if this is a recurrence, or if the patient has had another type of cancer in the past)
- a list of all diagnostic tests done

Step 2: Discovering Your Treatment Alternatives

Begin with the information your doctors give you, the information in the site discussions in part II of this book, and the relevant chapters on treatments. We have tried to discuss all treatment options, including experimental programs (discussed later in this chapter and also in chapter 11). Your team can save you time by researching information using the following resources:

- Your own physician and the specialists she recommends

- Cancer Information Service
- American Cancer Society
- Comprehensive Cancer Centers

Phone numbers are listed by state in part III under "Treatment Information and Resources"

- Your local medical association   Listed in the white pages of
  your phone book under
  "American Medical Association"

- Your local public library

- Medical libraries   Ask the librarian at your local
  library for the nearest medical
  library

The Cancer Information Service is a toll-free hot line that is part of the National Cancer Institute (NCI). NCI is one part of the National Institutes of Health. NCI coordinates, conducts, and funds many of the treatment, research, and communications programs in the United States. (We will be referring to the different activities of NCI throughout the book.) The Information Service has information on a wide range of topics, including diagnosis, treatment, rehabilitation, home care, counseling services, financial aid, patient referrals (for experimental programs), causes and prevention of cancer. Most important, they have lists of all the types of cancers currently being studied, and the hospitals and doctors involved. They will also do research for you. To make the best use of this resource, make your questions as specific as possible. They have printed information that they will send you, and will also answer questions over the phone.

The American Cancer Society provides similar information services, as well as a wide range of basic assistance programs. These will be described in chapter 15, "Living with Cancer."

The Comprehensive Cancer Centers are twenty-one hospitals designated by the National Cancer Institute as regional centers for cancer research and treatment. These are the best sources for confirmation of your diagnosis. Ask if they have ongoing treatment programs (not just experimental) for your kind of cancer.

As of this date, there is no central list of qualified cancer specialists and there is no easy way to find them in the physician directories. Therefore, your medical association can be of great help in finding qualified people in your area.

There are two national physician directories in your local public library: The *American Medical Directory* and the *Directory of Medical Specialists*. Although similar, the latter is the most useful. It lists, by specialty and by state, each doctor's name and certification, birthdate and birthplace, education, career summary, teaching positions held (doctors who teach must keep up-to-date), military record, professional memberships, office address, and office phone. Do not attempt to use these directories to create a "master list" of cancer specialists— their organization makes this impossible. Use them to look up the credentials and experience of doctors whose names have come from other sources.

Medical libraries are a good source of professional, technical articles about your type of cancer. You probably will not be able to understand the articles, but your goal is to get a list of the articles about your type of cancer published in the *last three years*, the names of the authors, and the names of the institutions with which the authors are affiliated. These people have the most experience with your type of cancer and have the most up-to-date information. You may want to use them as:

1. second-opinion consultants for treatment options;
2. the team who should possibly treat you;
3. a resource to find out the names of pathologists who are experts on your type of cancer, and where the nearest excellent treatment center is.

The National Library of Medicine has a computerized system that can locate things quickly. Part of the International Cancer Research Data Bank Program of the National Cancer Institute, it includes the MEDLARS program (a general medical program that can provide lists of articles), CANCERLIT (170,000 citations and abstracts from professional articles on cancer since 1963), CANCERPROJ (summaries of 18,000 ongoing cancer-research projects), CLINPROT (a specialized list for clinical oncologists of new treatment protocols), and MEDLINE (lists of medical articles since 1969). If you use the computer search programs, there may be a fee.

Step 3: Locating the Best Doctors and Hospitals

The medical name for the study of cancer is "oncology"; cancer specialists are called "oncologists."

Oncology, as a specialized field, is only eight years old. Until recently, cancer was not treated by cancer specialists but by the doctors who specialized in the parts of the body where it appeared. For example, cancer of the stomach was treated by a gastroenterologist (stomach specialist), and cancers of the head and neck by an otorhinolaryngologist (ear, nose, and throat specialist). These specialists are still a vital part of the diagnostic process, and often the treatment process as well.

Although the American Medical Association recognizes over sixty areas of specialization, the American College of Physicians and Surgeons has set professional standards—with accompanying training programs and examinations—in twenty-two specialty areas. An additional eighteen areas have been designated as more advanced sub-specialties. When a doctor has successfully completed these require-ments, he is called "board-certified" in a given field. Many doctors are certified in more than one area. (See "American Specialty Boards" in part III for a complete list.)

You might assume that all doctors who call themselves specialists in any of the forty board-certified areas are, in fact, board-certified. They are not. Any M.D. can legally call himself a specialist in any-thing. That is why it is important to check the credentials of the doctors who might be treating you. Board certification is not a guarantee of receiving the best possible care, but it at least shows that the doctor has been through a rigorous training and examination process in the field in which he calls himself a specialist.

There are three standard treatments for cancer (all forms of treat-ment will be explained in the next seven chapters): surgery, radiation, and chemotherapy. Oncologists subspecialize in these areas, but the names of subspecialties can be confusing. Let us look at the credentials that would be found for qualified oncologists in each of the standard treatment areas.

Chemotherapy. Two subspecialties treat cancer with drugs: medi-cal oncology (a subspecialty of internal medicine) and hematology-oncology (a subspecialty of pediatrics; these doctors may also call themselves pediatric oncologists). Qualified doctors in this area have their M.D., have received advanced training in either internal medicine or pediatrics, and have had further training in medical oncology or hematology-oncology. Hematologists-oncologists do not restrict their practice to children. This specialty grew out of hematology, so these doctors are particularly qualified to treat leukemias and lymphomas, no matter what the age of the patient, and may be called to supervise chemotherapy in other forms of cancer.

Radiation. Although you can find textbooks entitled *Radiation Oncology*, and medical-school training programs in "radiation on-cology," and hospital departments of "radiation oncology," there is no official specialty that is actually called radiation oncology. There is only one general board-certified field of radiology, so you must check the radiologist's further training and experience. Diagnostic radiologists only use radiological techniques to make diagnoses. Therapeutic radi-ologists specialize in using radiation as a cancer treatment. Pediatric radiologists specialize in giving radiological treatment to children. Another certified field used to diagnose and treat cancer, nuclear medicine, is explained in chapter 4.

Surgery. Since surgery is the primary form of treatment for most cancers, it is astonishing that there is no subspecialty of surgical oncology. The patient must find a surgeon who not only has good credentials and a good professional reputation in his surgical subspecialty but also has extensive cancer experience.

Gynecologists are particularly involved with cancer; cancers of the reproductive system account for the majority of cancers in women. A board-certified gynecologist has had training in treating cancer, and is qualified as a surgeon for his area of the body. A handful of gynecologists have taken advanced training and have become certified in medical oncology as well as obstetrics and gynecology. Most gynecologists who specialize in cancers of the reproductive system have not had such training. There is no special certification in "gynecological oncology," although some doctors call themselves gynecological oncologists. Just as with surgeons, you must check their training and experience to see whether they are qualified to treat you.

Many types of cancers respond to only one type of treatment. In this case, you will look for the best doctor to give you that treatment. For some types and stages of cancer, however, a variety of treatments may be given by equally qualified doctors. Your first oncologist may recommend surgery, chemotherapy, and/or radiation, either alone or in combination. When you get a second opinion, especially if there is more than one primary treatment for your cancer, it is wisest to consult an oncologist whose specialty is different from that of the first. For example, if your first oncologist is a medical oncologist (chemotherapist), you might want a second opinion from a radiation oncologist. If you have a type of cancer that is being investigated in clinical research programs, you may want a consultation from that kind of team.

Even if everyone agrees that surgery is the first step in treatment, it is wise to get a second opinion from another surgeon. A situation that has received a great deal of publicity lately is the difference of opinion among doctors regarding breast-cancer surgery. (It is discussed fully in that site discussion.) The range of opinion among equally qualified surgeons goes from simple removal of the lump to removal of the breast, lymph nodes, and muscles.

Experimental Programs

Before making your final decision, one last area should be explored: experimental treatments. For many cancers, these treatment programs offer the "latest" and may give the patient the best odds. The details of the various types and phases of experiments are explained in chapter 10. Here we will discuss the rights, responsibilities, options, and advantages of an experimental patient and how one becomes involved in such a program.

In the United States, most experimental and investigational programs are supervised and/or coordinated by the National Cancer Institute and must meet very strict criteria. (Other, privately supported programs are being conducted, but there is no central clearinghouse for information or patient referral for these programs.) Experimental programs (the specific treatment plans are called protocols, or regimes) are being conducted in chemotherapy, radiation therapy, nuclear medicine, and surgery. All treatments involving immunotherapy, hormone therapy, hyperthermia, bone-marrow transplants, and nutrition are considered experimental. In order to participate in these programs, you must be fully informed about the nature of the experiment, possible risks, side effects, and gains. The risk/benefit ratio varies enormously.

Rights, Responsibilities, and Options of Patients in Experimental Programs

Any patient involved in an experimental or investigational program must be told, both verbally and in writing, the purpose of the treatment; the details of treatment; the tests done before and after treatment (experimental programs require more thorough testing than normal treatments); the risks and side effects of the treatment, the testing, and the monitoring procedures used; the level of the experiment; and the projected chances of the individual patient's being helped by the treatment. The patient will then sign a consent form, which means he understands all that is involved.

If there is anything you do not understand, ask questions. There is no such thing as a "trivial" question. The doctors know that this is completely new to you and that there are many things you will not understand.

As part of a tightly controlled scientific experiment, the patient also has responsibilities. You must come for treatments and tests when they have been scheduled. If any part of treatment is to be carried on at home (for example, taking pills on schedule), you must carry out that part of your treatment exactly as the doctor tells you. You must also call your doctor immediately if you have forgotten to do part of the treatment program on schedule, and to report any strange, unexpected physical changes (fever, local reaction where drugs were given, rashes, fatigue, etc.). Exposure to illness must also be reported, as well as anything you are doing outside the treatment program to improve your health or general well-being: any outside medication or vitamins, special diets, counseling, therapy, biofeedback, etc.

You should never become involved with an experimental program until you have explored all the standard treatments available. But even after you have decided to enter an experimental program, you are not locked in forever; you can withdraw at any point in the program.

Should you decide to withdraw, your doctors from the experimental program will oversee your transfer to another qualified doctor of your choice.

You can also decide to discontinue all forms of treatment. The only option you do not have is to modify the experimental treatment. Although the doctors make some adjustments based on your individual reactions (this type of flexibility is built into the protocols), there is a point beyond which they cannot go and still consider you a part of the program.

Advantages of Being a Guinea Pig

If you have a type of cancer that has not had a high response and/or cure rate from standard treatments, experimental treatment can offer you a greater chance. Also, as part of an experiment, your treatment is conducted under the best of circumstances: You are watched very closely, and everything possible is done to make sure you respond well. There is the additional advantage of being treated by a team of experts should any unusual or dangerous physical problems arise.

Any program conducted directly by the National Cancer Institute in Bethesda, Maryland, is completely free. This includes treatment, all transportation, lodging (most patients are treated on an outpatient basis), and any testing that may be done at your local hospital between treatments. They will also treat any other medical or dental problems you may have free of charge while you are involved with the experiment. Many of the other comprehensive cancer centers also offer free treatment.

How to Become a Part of an Experimental Program

The information in this book and a call to the Cancer Information Service hot line will tell you whether there are experimental programs for your type of cancer, and whom to contact.

Treatment programs (clinical trials) are either carried out directly by the National Cancer Institute (in Bethesda, or at the Baltimore Cancer Research Center and the Veterans Administration Hospital in Washington, D.C.); or supervised by the NCI and carried out by groups of doctors investigating certain types of cancer; clinical cooperative groups; and organ-site programs (interdisciplinary programs that focus on the cancers of the large bowel, bladder, prostate, and pancreas). All of these programs and groups of people are described in part III under "National Cancer Institute Programs/Clinical Cooperative Groups."

You or your doctor may contact the appropriate people to see if you are a candidate for one of the programs. If you are, have your doctor contact the Office of the Director, The Clinical Center, National Institutes of Health, Bethesda, Maryland 20205. Phone: (301) 496-4114. Your medical report should be sent, as they will only admit on the basis of a confirmed diagnosis. They will decide within days if you are an appropriate patient.

Step 4: Personal Considerations

If your research team keeps producing redundant information—if certain oncologists, treatment centers, and treatment plans recur as the best in the field—the choice is clear. However, you often find yourself faced with a less obvious choice.

One of the most exasperating situations is trying to sort out conflicting medical opinions of equally qualified people. But by the time you reach this point, and have taken this conflicting information to your own network, you will probably find that some of these doctors are "more equal" than others. This is also the time when personal considerations come into play.

Most people feel more comfortable being treated as close to home as possible; indeed, economic and family considerations may make treatment impossible far from home. You may also feel more comfortable with a particular doctor—although, given the seriousness of the disease, it is usually advisable to go with the doctor and facility that give the best medical treatment. Financial considerations will play an important role, too—although, as you saw in the last section, some of the best treatment available is free. (Also see chapter 15 for discussions of financial help available.)

The growth of the consumer health movement, the increasing level of technical knowledge that patients have, and the growing awareness that there *are* choices open to the patient have made many patients insist on their full right to make the final decisions. This becomes an increasingly important issue when one is contemplating treatments that will effect the reproductive or excretory system, or treatments that may be disfiguring or seriously debilitating. As one person asked, "How much can be negotiated?"

The answer depends on the specifics of each case: the nature of the cancer itself, the treatment options available, and the doctors involved. We have already mentioned that experimental treatment protocols are not negotiable. We have also mentioned that there may be some choice of surgical procedures. How much freedom you actually have depends on the medical imperatives of the treatment design (all of the treatment plans have been carefully designed with a set of goals; modifying one part may ruin the effectiveness of the whole treatment), the flexibility of your doctors, and their willingness to cooperate with your wishes.

Some general questions can serve as a framework for discussions with your physicians:

Are the options I am considering equal? What are the possible risks and gains associated with each treatment? Can the same treatment be given in different places? Do each of these places have the backup systems necessary to handle crises?

Do I understand each part of the proposed treatment? When patients negotiate treatment plans, they usually try to scale them down. You need to understand how the plan has been designed, what part each treatment plays, and what the immediate and long-range impact will be. A question that often comes up is why a patient who has had successful cancer surgery should submit to follow-up chemotherapy or radiation. Such adjuvant therapy is recommended because doctors cannot be absolutely sure they have removed the last cancer cell, and the chances for long-term remission or cure are significantly increased with backup treatment. A few months of discomfort and inconvenience now can prevent a much more serious situation in the future.

These kinds of questions also arise when dealing with combination chemotherapy. As you will see in chapter 10 on chemotherapy, the combinations have been chosen very carefully; you are not free to pick and choose which drugs you want to take. For some cancers, however, there may be a choice of combinations, and these you will want to discuss fully with your doctors.

Are my options created by differences of opinion among qualified physicians? In this case you can select the doctor whose opinion most closely coincides with your own.

Do I understand that there are situations in which I cannot be consulted? Have I made my position known to the doctor beforehand? Certain decisions must be made during surgery when the patient is asleep. You and the surgeon should have discussions beforehand, at which time you should express your opinions and wishes.

In this chapter we have tried to give you guidelines for making crucial decisions about where to be treated: the kinds of information you need to gather; the criteria for deciding whether you need the services of the most qualified cancer treatment facilities, and whether you should consider an experimental treatment program; how to build and use your own information-gathering/decision-making network; where to go for the information you need; and the questions you should ask before making a final decision.

Look in the appropriate site discussion in part II to see what kinds of treatments are given for your cancer. Read the relevant chapters of the next eight. Chapter 7 should be read by everyone—it provides an overview of all treatment options; chapters 8–12 discuss standard, experimental, and supportive treatments available at the leading cancer centers; chapter 13 discusses the special considerations for children with cancer; and chapter 14 briefly outlines unorthodox therapies, which are not available at the major cancer centers. (Note: The site discussions do not include any references to unorthodox therapies; the reasons for this are discussed in chapter 14.)

Further Reading

Norman Cousins, *Anatomy of an Illness* (New York: Norton, 1979).
How a patient can help design and implement his own treatment plan in collaboration with a cooperative physician.
Harold Glucksberg and Jack W. Singer, *Cancer Care: A Personal Guide* (Baltimore: The Johns Hopkins University Press, 1980).
See especially chapter 4, "Who Should Treat You? Where Should You Be Treated?"
Marion Morra and Eve Potts, *Choices* (New York: Avon, 1980).
See especially chapter 1, "Facing the Diagnosis"; chapter 2, "Deciding on Your Doctor and Hospital"; chapter 5, "Treatment"; and chapter 23, "Where to Get Help." Good checklists for evaluating doctors and hospitals, good lists of specific questions to ask.
Lawrence Galton, *The Patient's Guide to Surgery* (New York: Avon, 1976).
See chapters entitled: "Some Important Facts about Surgery"; "Is Your Operation Really Necessary"; "Choosing a Surgeon"; and "The Hospital."

Chapter Seven

TREATMENTS—
AN OVERVIEW

Introduction

Almost all cancers are treatable, and 33% are cured. For those it cannot cure, treatment has significantly lengthened and improved the quality of the patient's life. This is important, since improvements in cancer treatments are being made at a rapid rate; you may live to see a cure developed for your cancer.

You and your doctor should discuss the goal of his recommended treatment. A patient generally assumes that the goal is a cure or long-term remission. Doctors, however, have several goals, depending upon the patient, the kind of cancer, how advanced it is, and the treatment options available.

Cure/remission. The goal here is to rid the patient of the disease entirely, or at least to significantly control the growth of the cancer so the person can live a normal life.

Palliative Treatment. The goal is to improve the quality of life even though cure is presently impossible. This means treating the symptoms that cause distress in the patient.

Preventive Treatment. In this case treatment is given to parts of the body that show no signs of cancer but in which cancer is likely to occur.

Types of Treatments Available

The wide range of treatments currently available can be divided into four groups:

1. *Standard treatments.* Surgery, radiation, and chemotherapy are the treatments given at the major cancer centers and supported by the National Cancer Institute and American Cancer Society. These will be discussed in the next three chapters.

2. *Experimental treatments.* These include new developments in the three standard treatments, various combinations of the three, and treatments that use immunotherapy, hormone therapy, hyperthermia, and bone-marrow transplants. The latter areas are considered experimental, although various components have been incorporated into the standard treatments. Immunotherapy, hormone therapy, hyperthermia, and bone-marrow transplants will be discussed in chapter 11. These experimental treatments are supported by the same groups that give standard treatments.

3. *Supportive treatments.* These components of treatment plans make standard and experimental treatments more effective and/or promote a higher quality of life. They include therapies for pain, nutrition, and rehabilitation, and will be discussed in chapter 12. Additional information, particularly about psychological-adjustment support systems, can be found in chapter 13, "Childhood Cancers," and chapter 15, "Living with Cancer."

4. *Unorthodox treatments.* These treatments—also called "nonstandard" or nontoxic therapies—are usually not given by board-certified oncologists. They include therapies based on nutrition, various types of mind control, biofeedback, "natural" drugs (like laetrile), vitamins, and holistic medicine. Many of these techniques will be discussed in chapter 12, "Supportive Therapies," because there is a gray area where some orthodox and unorthodox treatments overlap. The important point is that, when used by unorthodox therapists, unorthodox treatments alone are used as direct curative treatments. Orthodox treatment givers, exemplified by major cancer centers, only use these techniques as supportive additions to standard treatments. These unorthodox cancer treatments are discussed in chapter 14.

Statistics and Other Benchmarks— What Do They Really Mean?

Of most interest to patients are survival rates and response rates expressed in the prognosis. Survival rates indicate the mathematical chances of staying alive from the time of diagnosis to "cure"—usually five years for most types of cancer. But these percentages include everyone with your type of cancer; they tell you nothing about yourself. Let us say that a person has a Stage IV stomach cancer that has an 11% survival rate. The "11%" means that out of every 100 victims, 11 made it to the five-year mark and 89 did not. It does not tell you if you will be one of the 11 or one of the 89.

Statistics are also based on old information. Obviously, if the survival rate is based on a five-year period, the people in the statistical group received their treatment more than five years ago. Since new and more effective treatments are constantly developed, these numbers are not necessarily applicable to you. This will be discussed in more detail in the treatment chapters and in part II.

The same considerations come into play with response rates, which indicate the percentage of people who respond to various types of treatment and how well they respond.

You should also understand the vocabulary used to indicate possible responses to treatment: cure, remission, partial remission, complete remission, clinical remission, histological remission, and NED.

"Cure" does not mean for cancer what it means for chicken pox. When you are cured of chicken pox, the disease has gone away and you will never have it again. If you are cured of cancer, it means (1) the doctors can find no sign of disease in your body, although there is no way to say with absolute certainty that every last cancer cell is gone; and (2) you have been in that condition so long that statistically you are back to square one: for your age, sex, etc., you are no more likely to get cancer or die from it than anyone else.

Doctors use the term "remission" more often than "cure" when describing successful cancer treatment: It refers to the period when the signs of cancer have abated. There are several different kinds of remission. In complete remission, doctors can find no cancer in the body. Complete remission can be either clinical—which means that no signs of cancer show up in any of the clinical tests—or histological—which goes a step further by examining tissue under a microscope and finding no cells in the places cancer is most likely to occur. Some hospitals use the term "NED" (*no evidence of disease*) instead of "complete remission."

"Partial remission" means that some cancer is left after treatment, but its growth has been checked. Since some cancer is left, it is likely that it will eventually start to grow again. "Spontaneous remission" refers to the disappearance of symptoms without formal treatment; the reasons for their disappearance are not known.

Remission can also be described as "short-term" or "long-term"; the latter, for all practical purposes, means about the same as "cured."

Monitoring

In each chapter on treatment, there is a section describing the procedures used in monitoring the course of the disease and the effects of treatment. For many types of cancer, the key to long-term survival is not the initial successful treatment but catching the likely recurrences in time. A dramatic example is provided by testicular cancer, which has a high recurrence rate in the first two years after "successful" treatment. If the recurrence is detected immediately—before any symptoms are detectable by the patient himself—and treated within a month, the long-term cure rate is about 90%. If there is delay in this detection/treatment process, the cure rate falls dramatically to about 30%.

In part II we have indicated which cancers are likely to recur. Always check with your oncologist about your optimal checkup schedule, and adhere to it religiously. For some cancers, the patient may have to spend a year or two having monthly checkups.

You will also have blood tests on a regular basis. Laboratory analysis will determine, for example, the effects of radiation on your bone marrow and other parts of your immune system, and treatments will be stopped or rescheduled if your "counts" become too low. Depending on the type of tumor, doctors may also look for tumor markers.

Tumor markers are chemicals that signal the presence of certain types of tumors. In some cases they are chemicals not normally produced by healthy cells; in others there is a change in the level of regularly occurring chemicals.

The most common tests for tumor markers are the CEA and AFP assays described in chapter 5. Others currently being tested include the TPA (tissue polypeptide antigen). Some scientists feel the TPA, used along with the CEA, is the most effective tool for monitoring cancer therapy. Another tumor marker, the Tennessee antigen, has enabled doctors to detect 75% of lung cancers, 79% of stomach cancers, and 82% of colorectal and pancreatic cancers in preliminary clinical trials. The most exciting tumor marker is the B-protein; it is not linked to any specific type of cancer, but may possibly signal the presence of any tumor. Preliminary results have shown an 87% detection rate for all common types of cancer, with a false/positive rate of only 8% (indicating the presence of cancer when in fact there is none), and nearly 100% accuracy in predicting recurrences.

Other tumor markers are in the early testing stage: beta-glucuronidase (for leptomeningeal carcinomatosis); BCFP (breast-cyst fluid protein, for breast cancer); CMA (colon mucoprotein antigen, for colon cancers); CSAP (colon-specific antigen protein); GT-II (galactosyl transferase isoenzyme-II, for pancreas, stomach, and colon cancers);

POA (pancreatic oncofetal antigen, for pancreatic cancers); PSA (prostate-specific antigen), and ZGM (zinc glycinate marker, for gastrointestinal tumors). In the late 1980s, human testing on these tumor markers will be completed.

Although this line of research may ultimately lead to a quick and simple "cancer test" that can be done on ordinary blood samples and assure early diagnosis, for the foreseeable future the use of tumor markers will be limited to the monitoring of already diagnosed cancers.

Miracles and "The Cure"

The odds are low of finding a single cancer cure in the immediate future. Nevertheless, for many types of cancer, there have been truly miraculous developments in treatment that have turned certain death sentences into 50%, 80%, or even 90% cure rates. These kinds of miracles usually don't make headlines, because they don't happen overnight; they are the products of many years of careful development and testing. You can find out more about these real miracles through the Cancer Information Service, the Clinical Cooperative groups, the major cancer centers, and others who are on the leading edge of the fight against cancer.

There are two groups of more-spectacular potential miracles that do make the headlines, that have become a part of our popular culture, and are of great interest to cancer patients.

The first group is in the realm of unorthodox therapies. We will talk more about the difficulties of evaluating these treatments in chapter 14, but it should be noted here that there is only anecdotal, testimonial-type evidence about the effectiveness of these treatments; there is no scientific proof that they work.

The other group comes out of more orthodox corners of American medicine, but can be even more confusing and disappointing to cancer victims. These are the cancer "breakthroughs" that make headlines. Though the responsible news media do give space to the limitations of the latest developments, they are in fairly small print. Thus it may be helpful, in evaluating such stories, to bear certain things in mind.

· Most of the breakthroughs that become news are the initial results of laboratory experiments. They must still go through the rigorous process of animal and human testing before they become generally available (if, in fact, they actually work). This may take anywhere from two to five years.

· The media often phrase their headlines as if they were reporting *the cure* for all types of cancer. The actual scientific reports (from which the news media get their information) indicate that the scientists and doctors involved see each breakthrough as having a much more limited use.

The questions to ask about any news story are:

1. What specific types of cancer are the targets for this line of research?
2. Who are the researchers, and what institution are they associated with?
3. What scientific or medical journal(s) have the complete story?
4. Is human testing going on? Who is in charge of the testing program? Where will the testing be done? What are the eligibility requirements for becoming a part of this experiment? How does one apply?
5. Does this development offer more hope for effectively treating my cancer than standard or Phase III experimental treatments currently being used?

The answers to these questions may be found by a careful reading of the news story, and from contacting the researchers directly by mail or phone, finding the original scientific reports in a medical library, and calling the Cancer Information Service hot line to find out where experiments are taking place. Most important, you should talk to your oncologist. Promising lines of research are discussed informally among doctors, and items appear regularly in the cancer newsletters and journals. It is very likely that your oncologist has been aware of this "new" research for several years and can help to put things in perspective.

Interferon: A Case Study

LEADING U.S. CANCER DOCTORS AGREE TO ISSUE
WARNINGS ON INTERFERON

The nation's leading cancer doctors have agreed to warn their often frantic patients that the much publicized new drug, Interferon, is far less impressive against cancer so far than they had hoped, and any good results have been very temporary. . . . There is no evidence or even remote suggestion yet to indicate that Interferon may cure advanced cancer, and no acceptable evidence that it can extend patients' lives "regardless of the type or stage" of the cancer they have. . . . Many other new approaches to cancer treatment currently under investigation provide results equally or more favorable.

Washington Post, June 15, 1980

That is the story that should have made the headlines. Instead it was slipped in on page 9, two months after *Time* did a cover story

91

on Interferon and it had made front-page headlines in papers all across the country. Even Madison Avenue had picked up Interferon as the key to a TV ad campaign for a new magazine:

"Do you know what that is?" [Man pointing to a blackboard behind him filled with drawings of test tubes and illegible scrawls] "That's a scientist's way of explaining Interferon—possibly the greatest breakthrough science has ever made in the fight against cancer. . . ."

Interferon *is* a miracle drug, but it has yet to produce miraculous results in the fight against cancer. The case of Interferon is a good example of what happens to a scientific breakthrough that is inaccurately presented to the public.

The discovery of Interferon grew out of the research done in immunology. The original research was completed in 1957 at the National Institute for Medical Research in London, England, by Alick Isaacs and Jean Lindemann, both specialists in the study of viruses. They were exploring a phenomenon called "viral interference," seeking to discover why people seemingly cannot harbor two virus-caused illnesses at the same time. They found that cells attacked by the first virus produced a substance that acted as a messenger to warn the other cells of viral attack; the other cells would then block the attack. They called this chemical messenger "Interferon."

This discovery was exciting because (1) it promised to be the same type of wide-spectrum miracle cure against viruses (colds, flu, chicken pox, etc.) that penicillin was against bacterial diseases; (2) being a substance naturally produced by the body, there would be few, if any, side effects when it was used; (3) it showed some antitumor effects.

Unfortunately, though this was known over twenty years ago, no one could do much with the knowledge because it was impossible to obtain Interferon at a reasonable cost. Until last spring the only way to obtain Interferon was to take it out of human blood, where it was present in only minute amounts. Ninety thousand pints of blood are needed to extract a little more than a tenth of an ounce of Interferon. California Institute of Technology scientists estimated that a pound of Interferon would cost between $10 billion and $20 billion.

The reason for all of the headlines in March of 1980 was not the discovery of Interferon but the announcement by the Massachusetts Institute of Technology of a way to produce it at much lower cost. This went along with the recombinant DNA technique (see the next section for an explanation of this technique) being used by several pharmaceutical companies, which made use of gene splicing: Combining the genes that make Interferon in the human body with the genes in a bacteria causes the bacteria to produce Interferon.

However, it will be years before we know how Interferon can be most effectively used in cancer treatment. First of all, there are several types of human Interferon. We don't know which type is most effective against what type of cancer. We don't know if the Interferon manufactured by the bacteria is really the same as any form of human Interferon. Then there is the fact that while Interferon seems to be good at fighting viruses, very few cancers have definitely been linked to viruses. In the small experiments done so far, there have been results that merit further research: Interferon does slow cell division in both healthy cells and cancer cells; it seems to work best when the cells are in the G_0 phase (a phase in which most anticancer drugs are not effective); it appears able to marshal the natural forces present in the immune system.

From the results so far, it looks as though Interferon may be used primarily to increase the efficacy of other, more standard treatment programs. Right now, it's not known what Interferon will do. Though this area of cancer research is very promising, the results will not be known for several more years.

Developments Reported in 1980

Each year over 10,000 professional articles appear in 900 special publications for doctors and research scientists. Almost all of them deal with the "latest" in their particular areas of cancer research/ treatment. In the site discussions, we have included the most recent significant material as of the date this book went to press. The best way for the layman to keep up-to-date is to contact the teams listed in part III, the National Cancer Institute programs, or those referred to in appropriate chapters.

The news you will want to find is not the theoretical or laboratory-experiment-stage breakthroughs but the much less dramatic gains that are being made in refining treatments. For example, cancer of the rectum has been one of the most stubborn types of cancer to treat, with over 50% of the patients who received the standard surgical treatment showing a recurrence of the disease within two to two and a half years.

In September 1980, the Gastrointestinal Tumor Study Group reviewed a five-year study they have been conducting in which surgery alone was compared with combination chemotherapy alone; radiation alone; and a combination treatment of surgery, followed by four to six weeks of radiation, followed by a year and a half of chemotherapy.

Their findings showed that the recurrence rates were: 52% surgery; 39% chemotherapy; 32% radiation; 21% for combination therapy.

When interviewed by the *Washington Post*, Philip Schein, cochairman of the study group, said: ". . . we stopped doing surgery alone in our study last February. And if one were going to select a therapy today, I think one would go with the triple treatment."

The group will continue the study, comparing this combination with other possible combinations for even better results. They do not yet have figures comparing five-year cure rates among the various treatments. From the point of view of the cancer patient, *this* is news.

In the same way, a combination chemotherapy called MOPP (nitrogen mustard, Oncovin Vincristine, prednisone, and procarbazine) has proven very successful in treating Hodgkin's disease. With both highly successful radiation treatment and chemotherapy treatments for this form of cancer, the cure rate is about 90%.

These two announcements did make it to the press. But most of the real progress, particularly as Phase III testing is under way, is reported only in the special journals or at oncology conventions. Now, at midpoint in the testing of combination chemotherapies for diffuse histiocytic lymphoma, the results of clinical trials are pointing to very optimistic results, with the real possibility of long-term remission rates going from 17% to possibly 60%, even in Stage IV patients.

There is also the field of genetics, and particularly the technology of recombinant DNA, where genes can be transferred from one organism to another. Although a long way from being used in humans, one possible use for this technology is to take genes that are resistant to certain chemotherapy drugs, which have a devastating effect on the bone marrow, and give them to cancer patients; then the patient could receive the anticancer drug in high doses, allowing the cancer to be killed but not affecting the bone marrow.

Another development in immunology is the hybridoma, which combines a cancer cell and an antibody-producing cell. Utilizing the fast reproductive capabilities of the cancer cell, it is now possible to create this special man-made tumor, which has the potential of churning out vast amounts of highly specific antibodies. This may lead to what is called "targeted drug therapy," i.e., it may be possible to create a hybridoma that will only attack a specific cancer, "attach" the chemotherapy (including radioactive) drugs to the hybridomas, and send them on their way to kill the cancer but leave the healthy tissues alone. Hybridomas are also thought to have great potential in cancer diagnosis, in organ and tissue transplantation, in determining a person's disease susceptibility, and other areas.

Further Reading

"Interferon: The IF Drug for Cancer," *Time*, March 31, 1980.

"The Miracle of Spliced Genes," *Newsweek*, March 17, 1980.

Michael Shodell, "Enlisting Cancer: A New Technology Uses Man-Made Tumors Called 'Hybridomas' to Fight Fire with Fire," *Science 80*, September/October, 1980.

Victor Cohn, "Radioactive Treatment Extends Life of Liver Cancer Victims," *The Washington Post* (October 7, 1980), p. A5.

All of the above articles were written for the layman. If you are interested in the more technical side of recombinant DNA, *Science* devoted a whole issue to it (September 19, 1980, Vol. 209, No. 4463).

Chapter Eight

SURGERY

Specific Operations for Specific Cancers

Surgery is the most frequently used form of cancer treatment—either by itself or along with radiation and chemotherapy. Because operations are so specialized, we have discussed them in detail in the site sections. In this chapter we will (1) give you a basic orientation to both cancer surgery and the "rules" that apply to it; (2) discuss anesthesia; and (3) talk about types of cancer surgery that affect the patient long after the stitches are healed—for example, operations that involve the reproductive and excretory systems, or amputations. These operations often have great psychological impact and one should know that support systems are available to help a person adjust.

Considerations and "Rules"

Cancer surgery attempts to remove localized tumors completely or reduce the size of large tumors so that follow-up treatment by radiation or chemotherapy will be more effective. The surgery is often also a diagnostic (staging) process as well as a treatment process, and these two processes may take place simultaneously. For that reason, the surgeon may remove the primary tumor, some normal tissue surrounding the tumor (to make sure that he gets it all, and also to compare the cancer cells with the healthy cells to aid in diagnosis), the lymph nodes near the primary tumor (to detect and guard against the spread of individual cancer cells that may have already lodged in these lymph nodes), and any organs in the body that may already be affected by the cancer. If there is any doubt that all of the primary tumor has been removed, additional biopsies and frozen sections will be done while the surgery is taking place.

Sometimes the surgeon will take out not only the lymph nodes adjacent to the tumor but all the lymph nodes in the region. This may be done to check the spread of cancer or to determine whether the cancer has spread further than the clinical diagnostic tests have shown. There has been some controversy in recent years about the removal of regional lymph nodes, since there is evidence that they may have a function in the body's immune system.

In general, slow-growing cancers have the best chance of being cured by surgery. But it is often impossible to predict before the operation exactly how extensive (radical) the surgery will have to be: The surgeon's experience and knowledge about dealing with cancer, the needs of the particular patient, and the proposed overall treatment plan, as well as what the surgeon actually finds when he goes in, will all be part of the decision-making process.

In addition to curative surgery, surgery may also be performed as a preventive measure (to remove precancerous conditions) and/or a palliative measure (to reduce pain and other symptoms). If curative surgical procedures cause any disfigurement or deformity, reconstructive surgery may be scheduled to repair the damage.

Types of Surgeons

There is no specific surgical specialty that deals only with cancer. You need to find a surgeon who is board-certified, who specializes in the area of the body in which your primary tumor lives, and who is experienced in dealing with cancer. The American Medical Association lists the following surgical subspecialties: Abdominal Surgery, Cardiovascular Surgery, Colon and Rectal Surgery,* General Surgery, Hand Surgery, Head and Neck Surgery, Maxillofacial Surgery, Neurological Surgery,* Orthopedic Surgery,* Pediatric Surgery, Plastic Surgery,* Thoracic Surgery,* Traumatic Surgery, Urological Surgery. Only traumatic surgeons (who specialize in treating the victims of gunshots, knife wounds, and accidents) would not treat cancer patients. In addition, board-certified obstetrician-gynecologists are qualified and trained as surgeons. The specialties marked with (*) have their own separate advanced-certification boards, in addition to the American Board of Surgery.

97

Unusual Surgical Techniques

Most people think of surgery as performed only with some kind of knife. However, technological advances in many areas have made other types of surgery possible.

Cryosurgery is employed to destroy tumors by freezing them with liquid nitrogen. The liquid nitrogen may be sprayed on, or applied with a probe that is either inserted into the tumor or applied to the surface of the tumor. The tumor is killed by several rounds of freezing and thawing, and the body naturally removes the dead cells over a period of time as they are shed. The procedure is done in the operating room. It is a technique used primarily with head and neck tumors, skin tumors, and is also used to stop hemorrhaging. Other uses are being tested.

Chemosurgery kills tumors through the repeated application of a chemical to the tumor's surface, a process that enables the cancer cells to be examined and destroyed one layer at a time. It is used for skin cancers and has as its advantage minimal destruction of normal cells.

Electrocautery or *electrosurgery* kills cancer cells by use of a high-frequency electric current. It is used mainly in cancers of the mouth, rectum, and skin.

Laser surgery destroys tumors through the use of a laser beam. It is used primarily in eye cancers.

Questions to Ask Before the Operation

In some types of cancer, surgery is a regular part of a standard treatment program. In other cases there may be a choice, and it becomes the patient's responsibility (using the advice of competent doctors) to decide between having surgery or opting for treatment with radiation or chemotherapy alone. Even in cases where surgery is agreed upon, there may be a range of choices on the extent of the surgery.

The American Medical Association has been involved in a public-relations campaign that urges people to get a second opinion before undergoing any surgical procedure. Actually, the patient should get two "second opinions": the first to determine whether surgery is indeed necessary (this second opinion should come from a cancer specialist who is not a surgeon); the second to get another surgical opinion on the details of the operation, if one is indicated. All doctors involved in this decision should be asked the following questions:

- Exactly what will the operation involve, and what do they hope to achieve with the operation?
- Is there a less radical procedure that can be done?
- Will the operation deform the patient in any way or cause psychological problems, and if so, how will these problems be dealt with?
- What risks are involved?
- What will happen if surgery is postponed or not done at all?
- Are there any treatment alternatives that don't involve surgery?

Major Surgery: An Overview of the Process

All major surgery involves a hospital stay, the use of anesthesia, and the patient's participation in certain preoperative and postoperative experiences.

Most surgical patients check into the hospital the day before the operation is scheduled. Routine blood and urine tests will be done, and other tests may be scheduled, depending on the type of operation and the general condition of the patient. During this preoperative period, the major focus of tests and conversations with physicians will be on anesthesia. The selection of the proper anesthesia, and the careful monitoring of the patient during the operation and the recovery period, is a complex job requiring a board-certified physician called an anesthesiologist. Anesthesia is given either by an anesthesiologist or by an anesthetist (a specially trained nurse) under the supervision of a doctor. Anesthesiologists are part of a hospital staff and are usually selected by the surgeon (certain surgeons become accustomed to working with certain anesthesiologists).

The four basic types of anesthesia (general, local, regional, and spinal) were explained at the end of chapter 5. All four involve the use of drugs in either liquid, gas, or pill form to achieve a loss of sensation. Although acupuncture is used in China to achieve drugless anesthesia, and has generated interest in this country, it is still not widely used; therefore we will not deal with it in this chapter.

Before surgery takes place, the anesthesiologist will see you for a preoperative evaluation. He will ask you about your medical history, about specific problem areas, treatments you have had, and whether you regularly take any medication that might react badly with the anesthesia. Questions will center on six areas: the cardiovascular system, (heart and/or blood pressure problems, and medication you are taking to control such problems); endocrine system (problems with diabetes, thyroid or adrenal glands); pulmonary system (whether you are a smoker, or currently have any upper-respiratory problems); gastrointestinal system (problems with bowel obstructions, chronic severe diarrhea, liver problems, or malnutrition); neuromuscular system (whether you or any member of your family have had problems with anesthesia; whether you are a nervous or anxious person, and whether you are on antidepressant drugs). He will also examine your mouth, noting dentures (which must be removed before the operation); bridges; caps; crowns; missing, broken, or loose teeth; and the physical contours of the mouth, to be sure there will be no problems if anesthesia is administered through the mouth.

If you have very definite feelings about anesthesia, these will be taken into consideration: Some patients want to be "out" for even the most minor procedure; others don't want to be "out" for even the most major surgery.

Based on your answers to all these questions, he will select the appropriate anesthesia and possibly ask that a few more tests be done. He will explain the possible side effects and will answer any questions.

After the preoperative evaluation is completed, the patient is generally allowed a light supper and then not allowed to eat until after surgery is over and the anesthetic has worn off.

An IV may be started either the night before the operation or the morning of the operation. On the morning of the operation, the patient will be "prepped": Areas of the body that are exposed during surgery will be shaved and cleansed; an enema may be given; a stomach tube may be inserted for patients undergoing abdominal surgery (this is a thin tube which is inserted through the nose, swallowed by the patient and remains in the patient through the operation and often through the recovery period to allow easy removal of unwanted fluids and gas); a urinary catheter may be inserted to allow easy drainage of urine; premedication (a sedative prescribed by the anesthesiologist) may be given (using the IV tube) to relax the patient.

When the operation is completed, the patient will be taken to the recovery room and his vital signs carefully monitored until they return to normal and the anesthesia has worn off. Once back in his room, the specifics of how pain will be managed, how much physical movement will be allowed/required, and when normal eating and elimination will be started will vary from patient to patient. In general, the focus is on having the patient up and around as quickly as possible.

Special Problems: What to Expect and How to Deal with It

Most operations are not pleasant—they involve some pain and discomfort through the recovery period. But they generally do not bother us much after the incisions have healed. That's because our basic identity as human beings is not connected with the functioning—or even the existence—of our internal organs. Most people don't even know where their spleen is, much less have any great attachment to it.

But there are some types of cancer operations that affect parts of the body that have great meaning for the patient. Amputations, and some cancer operations of the head and neck, may leave the patient feeling deformed. The removal of parts of the reproductive system has great impact on a person's sexual—and therefore personal—identity. The operations called "ostomies"—those that divert our waste materials through plastic tubes into disposable plastic bags attached to the outside of the body—can also be very difficult to deal with.

If you are going to have—or already have had—one of these operations, the most important thing to realize is that your anxiety, fear, and depression are perfectly normal, and that the best way of dealing with it is not to try to endure the experience alone. The thousands of people who have already gone through this experience have found that with professional help—and the self-help groups formed by similar patients—people can and do adjust and go on to lead happy, healthy, and productive lives.

The most immediate source of information for any individual patient will be the social workers in the hospital where you are having surgery performed and your local chapter of the American Cancer Society (listed in the white pages of your telephone book). Certain patient groups have grown into nationwide organizations with hundreds of chapters throughout the United States. The support services for people who have undergone specific surgical procedures are listed in part II with the descriptions of each type of surgery. Psychosocial rehabilitation programs are listed in chapter 15, and special support services for children can be found in chapter 13.

Further Reading

Paul J. Melluzzo and Eleanor Nealson, *Living with Surgery* (New York: Lorenz Press, 1979).

An excellent book, written for patients who are contemplating operations difficult to deal with, both physically and psychologically. Of particular interest to cancer patients are the chapters on mastectomies, ostomies, amputations, hysterectomies, and neurosurgery. Each chapter not only gives details on the operations and the technical aspects of rehabilitation, but recounts very personal case histories to illustrate different types of problems that patients face at various points in the process, and what kinds of adjustments families have to make. There is expert commentary by qualified therapists. ($9.95, hardback.)

Lawrence Galton, *The Patient's Guide to Surgery* (New York: Avon, 1976).

A general layman's medical book covering more than 150 operations, including separate chapters on choosing a surgeon, hospitals, fees, costs and insurance, preoperative care, anesthesia, the operating room, postoperative care, and recent advances in surgery. ($2.50, paperback.)

Judith Nierenberg and Florence Janovic, *The Hospital Experience* (Indianapolis: Bobbs-Merrill, 1978).

Part IV explains preparation, procedures, and problems common to all operations as well as providing descriptions of twenty-two operations. Of particular interest are the descriptions of breast surgery, cholecystectomy (gallbladder removal), gastrointestinal surgery, hysterectomy, lung surgery, prostatectomy, and urostomy. ($7.95, paperback.)

Alexander A. Birch and John D. Tolmie, *Anesthesia for the Uninterested* (Baltimore: University Park Press, 1976).

A highly amusing—but technically accurate—introductory textbook for medical students, with hundreds of pictures and diagrams (using pretty models in bikinis whenever possible). Since anesthesia is a subject that puts everyone to sleep—doctors included—the book was written to attract more doctors to the field (which is described as "a discipline based on physiology and pharmacology that encompasses the whole spectrum of medicine" but is generally thought of as "just long boring periods interrupted by crises"). The book covers the history of anesthesia, preanesthetic evaluation, preparation for administration of anesthesia, monitoring, anesthetic administration, extraoperative activities of the anesthesiologist, and anesthesia economics. ($7.50, paperback.)

Chapter Nine

RADIATION

Radiation is the second most common form of cancer treatment, with over half of all cancer patients receiving radiation as part or all of their treatment plan. It was the second type of treatment to be used against cancer: A year after Wilhelm Roentgen discovered X-rays in 1895, a French doctor, Despeignes, used them to treat stomach cancer.

Radiation is used as a primary treatment in certain cancers; in combination with surgery (given before surgery to shrink the size of the tumor, and afterward to clean up cells that might be left, or to sterilize tumors that may have been inoperable); and also in combination with chemotherapy. For some cancers, radiation has been combined with both surgery and chemotherapy to provide optimal treatment.

Just as with other forms of treatment, it can be used to cure cancer or to provide palliation (a reduction of pain and symptoms).

Types of Radiation Therapy

Radiation-therapy techniques can generally be divided into two groups: those utilizing external radiation and those utilizing internal radiation.

External radiation refers to bombarding the cancer cells with some type of ray. There are special machines used to deliver these rays: special X-ray machines (different from those used in diagnostic radiation) called "megavoltage" or "supervoltage" machines deliver high-energy radiation that can penetrate deep into the body without doing great damage to surface tissues. Included in this group are linear accelerators, which produce high-speed gamma rays; *neutron radiation machines* and betatrons, which beam high-speed neutrons or high-speed atomic particles into the tumors; and machines that make use of cobalt. Low-voltage (orthovoltage) machines are now used very infrequently, mainly for treating skin cancers.

Internal radiation is achieved by putting radioactive substances inside the body (in either solid or liquid form). It provides a source of highly localized, constant radiotherapy, causes minimal damage to healthy tissues, and assures the presence of radiation whenever cells are most sensitive. Internal radiation may be given in the form of intracavity or interstitial implants, where the radioactive material, contained within tubes, needles, or "seeds," is placed directly in or on the tumor; or in the form of radioisotopes (see chapter 5 on diagnosis for definitions and explanations), which, when introduced into the bloodstream, seek out and concentrate in the tumor itself. Some of the radioactive substances used in internal radiation treatments are cobalt-60, radium, radioactive iodine, iridium-192, cesium-137, radioactive phosphorus, and radioactive gold.

How Radiation Works Against Cancer

In radiation therapy we do not talk about removing cancer or killing cancer; radiologists use the term "sterilizing the tumor." This is not just a linguistic quirk but reflects how radiation works in stopping the growth and ending the existence of a tumor.

The radioactive particles entering the tumor give off a form of radiation that changes the chemistry of the cell. The changes will either cause the cell to die immediately, or will effectively sterilize it (make it incapable of dividing), or will cause mutations in the genetic material of the cell so that, at some future time, the daughters of that original cell will be unable to divide themselves into exact replicas of the parent cell, i.e., functioning cancer cells.

Limits on the Use of Radiation Therapy

The use of radiation as a treatment for cancer is limited by a number of factors. The first one is that only certain types of tumors are sensitive to radiation. Others are highly radioresistant, and many fall somewhere in between.

For some types of tumors, the location makes a great deal of difference in determining whether or not radiation will be used. Not only must the tumor be located in a place where the radiation can get to it in sufficient quantities, but great care must be taken not to damage healthy tissue. Just as different tumors have different degrees of radiosensitivity, there is variation in the radiosensitivity of healthy tissues: kidneys, liver, lungs, and muscles are particularly sensitive. Also, irradiation of the ovaries and testicles can lead to sterilization, or may effect the still viable sperms and eggs in such a way that genetic mutations will show up in later generations.

Even if a tumor is generally radiosensitive, the cells may only respond to radiation in certain parts of their life cycle. When cells are in their M phase (in the actual process of dividing), they are the most susceptible to radiation. When they are in the S phase, they are the least susceptible. Cells in the G_0, G_1, and G_2 phases are of middling sensitivity. Since all the cells in a tumor are not in the same phase at the same time, any single radiation treatment will cause only partial damage.

Adding to this problem is the natural mechanism in the DNA of the cancer cells which repairs damage. This repair feature causes some strange responses in different types of tumors. Some tumors can be completely sterilized by radiation, but it takes a long time. (The repair mechanisms work well, but the radiation causes damage to the genes so you have to wait until several generations of cancer cells are produced for the tumor itself to become sterilized.) Other tumors, like some sarcomas, have a very dramatic, immediate response—they almost seem to disappear—but grow back again very quickly.

The chemical changes produced by radiation require a fairly good supply of oxygen. Tumors located in places that do not have a good supply of oxygen may not respond well to radiation treatment.

Radiation treatment itself may be carcinogenic: It can cause the development of a totally new type of cancer while successfully treating the original cancer.

Radiation is most effectively used as a localized treatment. It cannot get to metastases, and wide-field irradiation can cause disastrous damage to vital healthy tissues, particularly the bone marrow, which produces the substances necessary to the functioning of the immune system.

Doses and Timing

Radiation must be given in a dose that will damage the cancer cells but will allow the normal cells to recover. Treatments must also be timed to produce the maximum effect while allowing the healthy tissue enough time to repair damage.

The dose of radiation administered is measured in rads (*r*adiation *a*bsorbed *d*oses). A rad measures the actual amount of energy absorbed by the tissues. The higher the voltage of the machine, the greater the penetration of rays, the higher the rads. Dosages vary according to the location of the tumor, its depth, and the type of machine to be used. The radiation oncologist decides on the type of radiation most suitable, the amount or dosage, and the length of the course of treatment. In general, the higher the dosage, the greater the damage to cancer (and normal) cells. The larger the tumor, the more radiation is needed to destroy it. If a malignant tumor is considered "curable," higher doses of radiation will be given to a larger area. Lower doses of radiation may be given to a patient with widespread disease, to try to control pain and symptoms.

Because there are so many variables, ideal schedules for different tumors have not yet been developed. It is imperative that once your dosages and treatment schedules have been worked out, you appear for treatments exactly on time. There may be some adjustments made in your therapy based on your response (that includes how the tumor is responding as well as the type and severity of the side effects that you experience), but these adjustments will be made by your oncologist.

Treatment Procedures: External Radiation

People Involved

Your treatment team will probably include your radiation oncologist (who may also be called a "radiation therapist," "radiotherapist," or "therapeutic radiologist"); a highly-trained technician who actually gives you the treatment and is called a "radiation-therapy technologist"; and radiation-therapy nurses, who are R.N.s with specialized training in caring for patients who receive this type of treatment. The oncologist may also call upon the services of a radiation physicist and/or a dosimetrist to plan treatments and appropriate doses.

None of these people will be in the treatment room with you when you get your therapy, since they need to protect themselves against unnecessary exposure to radiation. However, you will be closely watched via TV cameras, and you will be in voice communication with the technologist in the control booth at all times.

Where Treatments Will Take Place

You will probably receive your treatments as an outpatient in the Radiology Department or Nuclear Medicine Department of the hospital. The treatments take only a minute or two, but you should allow considerably more time for preparations and the normal delays. Until you know how you react to your therapy, you should have someone come with you in case you don't feel well enough to get home by yourself.

Preparation for Treatment

Certain preparations are necessary to make sure that the radiation is always aimed at the proper place on your body, and to make sure that parts of the body that do not have to be exposed to the radiation are shielded. Your skin may be marked with a dye or felt-tip marker to show where the beams should enter the body. These should remain on your skin for as long as you are having treatments. Your radiotherapist will tell you how to bathe in order to leave these markings on. Often they will make a special mold of your body to make an individualized body shield. They cut holes in the shield at the points where the radiation is supposed to enter. Other, localized shields may also be used. All of these shields are put in place just before treatment starts.

Treatment

You will lie down on the treatment couch and it will be rolled into position. The machines that deliver the radiation will be aimed at the appropriate parts of the body. At times only one beam is used. For some treatments, several beams are aimed at the cancer from different directions. When the beams are aimed properly and cover the right amount of area, lights on the machine illuminate an area the same size and position as will be bombarded by the rays. The shields will then be put in place, the technician will tell you to lie still, and he will leave the room and go into his control booth. He will tell you when the actual treatment is about to begin. You may hear some buzzing, whirring, and clicking sounds, but the treatment itself is completely painless.

Treatment Procedures: Internal Radiation

People Involved

Your treatment team may include a radiation oncologist, a surgeon, and specially trained nurses.

Implants

If radioactive material is going to be implanted directly in the tumor (interstitial implants), a surgical procedure will be performed in the operating room. Gold or platinum needles filled with the radioactive material will be placed in rows in the tumor. After about a week they will be removed via another surgical procedure. You must be in the hospital for the entire treatment.

Another type of implant—standard for bladder or cervical cancer—places tiny gold pellets (seeds) filled with radioactive material inside the tumor. They give off radioactivity for about two weeks, after which they are not removed but remain harmlessly in your body. As soon as you recover from the procedure, you can go home.

Intracavity Radiation

This is a set of procedures in which containers are temporarily placed inside the cavity where the cancer is growing. This can be done for cancers of the uterus or the cervix, where the containers are put directly into the vagina. The procedure is done in the operating room while you are asleep. The containers must stay in place for a period of time—usually seventy-two hours—and for the entire time you will remain in bed, moving as little as possible so that the container stays in position. Often a catheter will be inserted to drain your urine so you will not need to move to go to the bathroom. At the end of the treatment the container is painlessly removed, either while you are in your bed, or in the operating room or the Radiology Department (depending on your hospital's usual procedures). No anesthesia is used for removal.

Intracavity radiation also includes the introduction of radioactive isotopes, in liquid form, directly into the bladder. The procedure is similar to that for a cystoscopy, described in chapter 5.

Radiation Given by IV or Pills

Using procedures very similar to those described for the diagnostic tests called bone scans and thyroid scans, radioisotopes can also be introduced into the bloodstream to treat certain cancers, particularly those in the thyroid and in the skeletal system.

108

For some cancers, there has been experimentation with radiation treatments that combine both internal and external radiation. See the site discussions for the type of radiation or combined treatments used in any particular kind of cancer.

Side Effects of Treatment

Side effects will vary according to the type of radiation therapy you receive and the part of the body irradiated. Also, individual reactions vary enormously: Some people have many side effects, some none at all; some people have severe reactions, while others have very mild ones. Your oncologist or oncology nurse will give you a list of the side effects to expect, when to expect them (some occur immediately, some do not appear for days or weeks or even longer), and what you should do about them. If they do not give you a list, ask for one. Below is a list of common early side effects that are only temporary.

GENERAL: skin reactions (dryness, itchiness, change in color); hair loss; fatigue; loss of appetite; constipation

HEAD TO UPPER CHEST: dry mouth; sore throat and mouth; difficulty swallowing; color changes in mouth and tongue (white spots in the mouth, red tongue); thick saliva; sense of taste affected (changed or lost); tooth problems; earaches; change in fatty tissue under the chin (it may sag or get bloated)

BREAST: Skin in armpit or under the breast may become dry or moist, tender, or may itch.

UPPER ABDOMEN: feeling of fullness; nausea; vomiting

LOWER ABDOMEN: cramps; diarrhea; nausea; in rare cases there may be a burning when you defecate or bladder inflammation.

Most of the common side effects are uncomfortable, but patients quickly get used to them. The one really difficult side effect is hair loss, often the most psychologically devastating part of cancer treatment, both for men and women. *It does grow back*, however, and wigs and scarves will help you through the treatment period.

Monitoring the Effects of Treatment

Your oncologist will monitor the rate of tumor shrinkage by periodically taking more diagnostic X-rays and/or scans and actually measuring the size of the tumor on the picture with a metric ruler.

109

In addition to the tests done during the course of treatment, you will be checked periodically after treatment has ended. The schedule of these checkups depends on the type of cancer, how well you responded to treatment, and the kind and severity of side effects you have experienced.

Pushing Back the Limits

Research is constantly being done to make radiation therapy more useful and more effective. New machines have been developed that produce different types of radiation (some cancer cells are sensitive to some forms of radiation but not to others) and deliver a more powerful, concentrated dose of the beams. Such machines have a greater ability to kill cancer while causing less damage to healthy tissue. There are also new machines that can deliver several beams of radiation at the same time from different angles, which means that a greater dose can be administered to cancer cells, while milder doses pass through the healthy tissues.

It is known that certain chemotherapy drugs (antimetabolites and fluoridated pyrimidines) block the cell cycle in phase S. That means that, by using careful calculations, it is theoretically possible to administer these drugs for a certain period of time until all the cells have been synchronized in the S phase. By knowing the timing of the cell cycle for a given type of cancer cell, they can stop administering the drug at the right moment, wait until they all reach the M stage, and then zap them. It is a big job to translate this theory into practice, but researchers are beginning to have some success with it.

Other researchers are working on the "oxygen effect," supplying oxygen to cancer cells that lack enough oxygen to make radiation effective. Tests have been conducted using techniques that both supply massive amounts of oxygen to the patient directly and also (using what is known about the biochemistry of cells) increase the concentrations of already available oxygen. In addition, certain substances that behave like oxygen, such as synthetic Vitamin K, can be introduced into the body, making the cells susceptible to radiation.

Further Reading

Lucien Israel, *Conquering Cancer* (New York: Vintage, 1978).
See chapter 7, "Radiation."

Chapter Ten

CHEMOTHERAPY

Introduction

Chemotherapy is the treatment of cancer using drugs. Usually "chemotherapy" refers to the use of drugs that have direct tumor-killing properties, although professional books often include drugs that are specifically designated as part of hormone therapy and immunotherapy. We have included the drugs used in hormone and immunotherapy in the list at the end of this chapter, since they are often used with chemotherapy drugs; but the general discussions of these two forms of treatment will be found in the next chapter, "Experimental Treatments."

Your oncologist may recommend chemotherapy because he feels it may cure your cancer, or help to maintain long-term remission, or increase the effectiveness of surgery and/or radiation treatments, or help control pain or other symptoms that can debilitate you. Chemotherapy, however, is an area of treatment that is constantly changing and developing. If you have a type of cancer that responds well to drugs, it is well worth your while to find out what the "latest" treatments are. The difference in chances for cure between standard and Phase III experimental treatment is often dramatic.

As of April 1980, there were over 1900 experimental treatment plans (protocols) being tested throughout the world. These tests include new anticancer drugs, new combinations of drugs, and "old" combinations of drugs on untested types of cancer, as well as various combination treatments involving drugs with surgery and/or radiation. The 250 drugs being used in these protocols include the cancer-killing drugs, the drugs used in immunotherapy and hormone treatments, and also

111

vitamins. Some drugs that have been shown to be effective in treating a wide variety of cancers are used in many protocols: Methotrexate is part of 528 separate protocols used in treating cancers of the brain, central nervous system, breast, colon and rectum, esophagus, liver, pancreas, stomach, kidney, prostate, testis, cervix, ovary, uterus, head and neck, lung mycosis fungoides, myeloma, Ewing's sarcoma, neuroblastoma, retinoblastoma, rhabdomyosarcoma, osteogenic sarcoma, soft-tissue sarcoma, melanoma, leukemias, and lymphomas. Other drugs, like OK-432, are only being used in one kind of cancer (in this case, stomach). Most fall somewhere in between.*

The list of most commonly used drugs and their side effects at the end of this chapter has been provided to give you a feeling for what may be involved in your chemotherapy. It is not meant to be exhaustive—an impossible task for a book of this kind. In each site discussion, we have also listed the whole range of drugs being tested for that particular cancer (if there are any), and whom to contact for information about the various programs. Should you decide to become a part of any of these treatment protocols, all the drugs, their effects on the cancer, and their side effects on you and your healthy tissue will be explained fully before treatment starts.

This chapter will offer a general explanation of chemotherapy and what it is like to have chemotherapy as part of your treatment.

How Chemotherapy Works

Drugs that are effective in treating cancer interfere with the natural activity of the cancer cells, either by going in directly to sabotage a specific phase of cell development or by sending confusing messages that cause the cells to do the wrong thing and thereby destroy themselves. Not all drugs are effective against all cancers, and the different groups of drugs act in different ways.

Cancer biologists divide the drugs used in chemotherapy into six groups:

Alkalying agents—which interfere with cell division and affect the cancer cells in all phases of their life cycle (although they may be slightly more effective in some phases). They confuse the DNA by directly reacting with it.

---

* *Compilation of Cancer Therapy Protocol Summaries,* April 1980. Fourth Edition. U.S. Department of Health, Education, and Welfare, Public Health Service, National Institutes of Health. NIH Publication No. 80–1116.

Antimetabolites—which interfere with the cell's ability to make an exact copy of itself; they either give the cells wrong information or block the formation of "building block" chemical reactions which the cell needs to replicate itself. These are phase-specific drugs—they only work in one phase of the cell's life cycle.

Vinca Alkaloids (plant alkaloids—naturally occurring chemicals that stop cell division in a specific phase.

Antibiotics—also made from natural substances that interfere with cell division; they can affect cancer cells in all phases of their life cycle and interfere with DNA synthesis.

Hormones—substances that occur naturally in the human body; they give messages that either encourage or stop growth or activities in certain cells or organs. There are two types of hormones: sex, or steroid, hormones, and glucocorticoid hormones. The sex hormones act on a very specific group of tissues and are useful in treating cancers of the prostate, breast, uterus, and kidney. Glucocorticoid hormones act on a wide variety of tissues and organs and have been used to treat Hodgkin's disease; lymphocytic and histiocytic lymphoma; lymphoblastic, lymphocytic, and acute myelogenous leukemia; and multiple myeloma.

Miscellaneous drugs—those that don't fit into any of the other categories. (See "Major Anticancer Drugs" in part III for a partial list.)

Chemotherapy is most effective against cancers that divide rapidly and have a good blood supply. In twenty types of cancer, chemotherapy (often used in combination with surgery and/or radiation) has contributed to a longer life-span and, in some cases, normal life expectancy. These include gestational choriocarcinoma; Burkitt's lymphoma; Hodgkin's disease; Wilms's tumor; embryonal rhabdomyosarcoma; acute leukemia in children; histiocytic lymphoma; Ewing's sarcoma; retinoblastoma; testicular cancer; lymphocytic lymphomas; osteogenic sarcoma; adult acute leukemias; multiple myeloma; breast carcinoma; neuroblastoma; carcinoma of the prostate; endometrial carcinoma (uterus); carcinoma of the ovary; and small-cell, undifferentiated lung cancer.

Chemotherapy may be given in a single drug or a combination of drugs. Combinations have been developed for several reasons: Different drugs attack the cancer cells in different ways; some drugs may make other drugs more potent; combinations help to avoid the problem of cancer cells becoming immune to a certain drug; using a combination of drugs (rather than a large dose of one drug, or several drugs, that have the same kind of side effects) limits the harmful (toxic) effects on healthy tissues. In other words, for many kinds of cancer, a

113

combination of drugs (each one of which is effective in attacking that kind of cancer) provides more effective cancer-kill with fewer harmful effects on healthy tissues.

Of course, since chemotherapy drugs act on rapidly dividing cells, there is some effect on cells that are normal and healthy. The most rapidly dividing cells in your body are your mucous cells, which line your whole intestinal tract (remember that your intestinal tract is really one long tube that starts at your mouth and ends at your anus); your hair cells, and your bone-marrow cells. The effect on mucous cells is seen in nausea and vomiting, mouth sores, diarrhea, stomach cramps, etc. The effect on your hair roots is hair loss. The effect on your bone marrow is a lowering (or depression) of your ability to produce white cells (which fight infection); platelets (which enable your blood to clot); and red blood cells, which carry oxygen to all parts of your body and carry off certain cell wastes (like carbon monoxide).

Planning Chemotherapy Treatments

Your medical oncologist will recommend chemotherapy for you based on the following considerations:

Responsiveness of the Cancer to Chemotherapy

Only certain types of cancers are responsive to drugs. The cancers most effectively treated this way have large proportions of dividing cells, are usually small tumors (either naturally or because most of the tumor has been removed by surgery or radiation), or are systemic cancers like leukemias and lymphomas.

Location of the Tumor

Even if the tumor can respond to chemotherapy, its actual location will affect the choice of treatment. In some cases, tumor location will make chemotherapy, perhaps combined with radiation, the only treatment option: For example, certain brain tumors cannot be removed surgically, so chemotherapy and/or radiation are the only choices.

General Condition of the Patient

Cancer patients are often shocked when they hear medical personnel refer to them as healthy: How can someone with cancer be healthy?

When they term a cancer patient "healthy," they are referring to how well the body is functioning, except for the site of the cancer. When they speak about a cancer patient being "sick," they are talking about a serious breakdown in the functioning of vital organs and systems: A sick cancer patient is one who is in a life-threatening situation. The evaluation of a patient's condition takes into account the patient's general state of health (cancer aside), as well as specific medical problems he or she may have in addition to the cancer, since such problems may interfere with the specific chemotherapy recommended. In evaluating your condition, your oncologist may use a rating scale similar to the one shown in table 4. In general, if a patient's

TABLE 4
Rating Scale for Evaluating Cancer Patients' General State of Health

Definition	Percent	Criteria
Able to carry on normal activity and to work; no special care needed	100	Normal; no complaints; no evidence of disease
	90	Able to carry on normal activity; minor signs or symptoms of disease
	80	Normal activity with effort; some signs or symptoms of disease
Unable to work; able to live at home and care for most personal needs; a varying amount of assistance needed	70	Cares for self; unable to do normal activity or do active work
	60	Requires occasional assistance; able to care for most needs
	50	Requires considerable assistance and frequent medical care
Unable to care for self; requires equivalent of institutional or hospital care; disease may be progressing rapidly	40	Disabled; requires special care and assistance
	30	Severely disabled; hospitalization indicated although death not imminent
	20	Very sick; hospitalization necessary; active supportive treatment necessary
	10	Moribund; fatal processes progressing rapidly

William B. Pratt and Raymond W. Ruddon, *The Anticancer Drugs* (New York: Oxford University Press, 1979), p. 38.

score is below 40%, it is unlikely that his condition can be improved by chemotherapy.

Once the doctor has made a general evaluation of your condition, and has decided that chemotherapy will be helpful for your type of cancer, he must also look at the specific drugs he wants to use and look at the parts of your body that would be most affected by them. He will determine what organs must metabolize or rid your system of the drugs, and what side effects the drugs might have if you have had problems in any of these organs. The nine systems evaluated are: bone marrow, gastrointestinal tract, oral mucosa (lining your mouth), liver, central nervous system, heart, lung, kidney, and skin. If there are problems, your doctor may reduce the dose of a particular drug or eliminate a drug entirely.

Selecting Specific Drugs

For some cancers, only one drug is needed for effective chemotherapy. For others, a combination of drugs is used. The selection of drug combinations depends on three things: the proven effectiveness of each drug when used alone against that cancer; a difference in each drug's method of attacking the cancer, so that maximum cancer-kill can be achieved in each cycle while minimizing the chance of developing resistance to any one drug; and a difference in the side effects of each drug (minimally overlapping toxicity), so that your healthy tissue will not be badly damaged by the chemotherapy.

Administering Chemotherapy

How a drug will be administered depends on the most effective way to treat your cancer and on the chemical properties of the drug. Some drugs, for example, cannot get into the bloodstream through the stomach—they must be injected directly into the bloodstream; these would have no effect if you took them in pill form.

There are three basic ways to administer drugs:

Injections

Intravenous (IV): Drugs are injected directly into a vein. This is done either in the form of a *fluid drip* (commonly called an "IV" or "drip") or as an *IV push.* If given as a drip, a bottle of the drug is hung on a pole; a tube runs from the bottle to the needle, which is inserted in your vein, and the drug drips in at a specified rate. The IV push is like a regular shot, but directly into a vein. Procedures can take from fifteen minutes to twelve hours.

Intramuscular (IM): A regular shot into the muscle of the arm, thigh, or buttocks.

Subcutaneous (SQ): A shot under the skin.

Intra-arterial (IA): Identical to an IV (drip or push) except that the needle is inserted into an artery instead of a vein.

Intrathecal (IT): Injection of the drug directly into the spinal fluid.

Intracavitary (IC): The drugs are injected directly into a cavity, or "empty space," usually around the lung (pleural space) or into the abdomen.

Regional Perfusion: This technique concentrates certain drugs in one area (usually arms or legs) by creating a closed-circuit system in the bloodstream. A tourniquet is used to stop the blood flow out of the affected area so that no harm comes to other organs. The drug is put into the artery, which carries it to the cancerous area; it is then taken out of a vein and pumped back into the artery for a continuous high concentration of the drug.

Orally

You swallow the drugs either in the form of pills, capsules, or liquid.

Topically

For some skin cancers, drugs are administered in the form of a cream.

How often you get the drugs depends on your treatment program (which may be called a regime, regimen, or protocol), how long your cycle is (from the start of one round of chemotherapy to the start of another), and how many cycles are in your treatment plan. Typical cycles are three weeks, four weeks, or six weeks long, and divided into two parts: the period when you get the chemicals, and the period of recovery from them.

An example is the typical four-week cycle. Each day is assigned a number, from day 1 to day 28. You may get your IV drugs in the hospital (as an outpatient) on day 1 and day 8. You take your pills at home on days 2 to 7 and days 9 to 15. Days 16 to 28 are the recovery period. During this time you return to the hospital several times for blood tests so the doctors can see how you are reacting to the drugs. After day 28, you immediately begin day 1 of the next cycle.

At certain times you might be asked to be an inpatient. If you are being given combinations of drugs, you may be asked to spend part or all of the first cycle in the hospital so your reactions can be watched closely. Specific drugs, like methotrexate, require constant monitoring until they leave your system. In this case, the high doses of methotrexate required for effective cancer-kill cannot be tolerated by the body without some help. After a certain period of time, a drug called leucovorin is given to the patient to counteract (neutralize) the methotrexate. This is called a leucovorin "rescue." If given this particular drug, you would have to check into the hospital for three days of every month.

Side Effects of Chemotherapy

Different drugs cause different side effects. Your oncologist should provide you with a list of side effects of every drug you will be taking. You may also refer to the list at the end of this chapter. This list, however, only tells you what *might* happen, because people react differently to the same drug: Some people have no side effects; some people

117

have all of them; and most people fall somewhere in between. The severity of the side effects also differs from person to person: For example, two people may suffer nausea from the same drug—but one feels slightly queasy for four hours, while the other vomits violently for twelve hours. Even the same individual reacts a bit differently each time he gets the drug—some sessions will be harder than others. There is no way to predict how you will react to the drugs until you take them.

Chemotherapy drug doses and schedules are developed so that the drugs enter the body, kill the rapidly dividing cancer cells, and are expelled before they can damage most healthy cells, which divide more slowly. But the normal cells that make up the mucous lining of the intestinal tract, the hair producing cells, and the bone-marrow cells are also rapidly-dividing cells, hence these, too, are affected by the chemicals, causing the three most common side effects: nausea and vomiting, hair loss, and bone-marrow depression.

Nausea and vomiting can sometimes be controlled by antinausea drugs, or by meditation or biofeedback. Some people just get sick no matter what they do. Again, there is no way to predict. A few things are helpful to remember: You will recover from nausea between four and twenty-four hours after it starts; and severe nausea usually follows a pattern, with the bouts of vomiting coming farther and farther apart. For example, you may vomit every fifteen minutes for two hours, every half an hour for two hours, and every hour for another few hours. You will not go back to the every-fifteen-minutes cycle again. When it finally ends completely, you will be completely exhausted and want to sleep. Do it.

Hair loss (what doctors call alopecia) is mainly a psychological problem; there is no pain and your hair does grow back. Some people have only a little thinning; other people lose all their hair—including eyebrows and body hair. The rate of hair loss also varies tremendously —some people have a gradual thinning over a period of weeks; others have one shot and wake up the next morning to find all their hair on the pillow. There is no way to predict your reaction.

If you do lose your hair, you should know that it will come back in two phases. The first phase starts very shortly after you lose it: Very fine, baby-type hair begins to grow. When chemotherapy is completely over, your regular hair will come back—at least as thick as before, and sometimes thicker. This is something you just have to get through; after the initial shock is over, wigs and scarves make it fairly easy.

Bone-marrow depression is a more subtle and more serious concern. Your bone marrow produces certain essential parts of your blood and immune system. Some drugs used in chemotherapy can slow down, or depress, that production, making you more susceptible to infection, among other things. If the depression is too severe, you will be put in the hospital and given antibiotics until your own immune system recovers. If the recovery takes too long, you may be switched to other drugs.

Sometimes a switch in drugs is a planned part of the treatment. Changes may also be made if other side effects are too severe, or if a patient "fails" a treatment plan, i.e., the tumor has continued to grow. If this happens, you may be switched to a different combination of drugs or possibly a single drug. Sometimes as many as five different programs may be tried until the right combination is found for your cancer.

Besides these drug-related effects, and the ones listed at the end of this chapter, problems can arise from the injections themselves, particularly fluid drips.

An IV needle goes into the vein at an angle and should rest in the center of the vein, lying parallel to the sides. If it goes through the vein and comes out the other side, it is said to have "infiltrated." This means that the drugs are not going into the bloodstream—which is where they have to be to kill the cancer cells—and could cause harm if they get into the soft tissue that surrounds the vein. The chemotherapy nurse will be very careful when she administers the IV, and she will also ask you to keep an eye out for any signs of infiltration while chemotherapy is in progress. Since many of the drugs take a long time to drip and you will move during that time, the needle position could shift.

A general problem for patients who receive much chemotherapy by IV is "blowing veins." Although the human body is filled with veins, only a limited number can be used for chemotherapy. These are the veins that are close to the surface and large enough to take the needle. The "first choice" veins are those in the lower arm and hand. It is possible to use the veins in the lower leg and foot, but these veins are inconvenient, especially for the patient (if the IV is in your arm, you can move around fairly freely; if it is in your leg, you can't), and are usually saved to be used if necessary.

Because of the number of blood tests, the number of times the IV must be used during treatment, and the possible irritating effects of the drugs, some of the veins become hard and cordlike (it feels like there is rope under your skin). Those veins have been "blown." They cannot be used again because no blood is flowing through them. The body will grow a new network of veins around the one that no longer works, but this takes time. If many veins have been blown, or if the patient's veins are normally quite deep beneath the surface, the arm

119

may be wrapped in a hot pack before chemotherapy begins, to bring deeper veins to the surface, or make small, but usable, veins stand out so the IV is easier to insert.

There may be a temporary local reaction to any shots—soreness, a burning sensation, etc. Your doctor or chemotherapy nurse will tell you what to expect and what to watch out for, depending upon what drug you are getting.

Specific Drugs and Their Side Effects

In the list that follows, side effects are divided into two main groups: common side effects, which are temporary and are not serious (life-threatening) from a medical point of view; and more serious and/or delayed side effects. There is no direct relationship between how severe the side effects are and how effectively the drugs are killing your cancer. NOTE: If sterility is mentioned as a side effect, it may be either temporary or permanent. Ask your doctor.

Actinomycin-D

See DACTINOMYCIN.

Adriamycin

Common Side Effects: nausea and vomiting; red/orange urine; lack of appetite; diarrhea; local reaction if drug leaks out of IV.
Other Side Effects: bone-marrow depression; hair loss; mouth sores; damage to liver, heart, kidneys; skin pigmentation; fever; chills; can bring about skin reactions from past radiation.
Given intravenously.

Adrucil

See 5-FLUOROURACIL.

Alkeran

See MELPHALAN.

Amethopterin

See METHOTREXATE.

ARA-C

See CYTARABINE.

5-Azacytidine

Investigational drug.
Common Side Effects: nausea and vomiting; fever; diarrhea.

Other Side Effects: liver damage; blood-count depression; muscle weakness.

Given intravenously.

Bacillus Calmette Guérin

See BCG.

BCG

(Bacillus Calmette Guérin; immunotherapy drug)
Common Side Effects: 24-hour fatigue; local reaction.
Other Side Effects: fever, chills, lymph-node swelling; rare problems with ulcers, liver functioning, systemic BCG infection.

Given in the form of a vaccination or by IV.

BCNU

See CARMUSTINE.

Bischlorethyl nitrosourea

See CARMUSTINE.

Bleomycin

Common Side Effects: nausea and vomiting; loss of appetite; fever; chills.
Other Side Effects: skin reactions; lung problems; swelling and pain in the joints; mouth sores; hair loss; headaches; affects sense of taste and appetite.

Given intravenously, intramuscularly, subcutaneously, or by regional arterial infusion.

Blenoxane

See BLEOMYCIN.

Busulfan

Common Side Effects: nausea and vomiting; diarrhea.
Other Side Effects: bone-marrow depression; breast enlargement; hair loss; impotence; lack of menstruation; lung problems; skin darkening; sterility.

Given orally.

Calusterone

Common Side Effects: nausea and vomiting.
Other Side Effects: fluid retention; lowered blood calcium; masculinization.

Given orally.

Carmustine

Common Side Effects: nausea and vomiting; vein swelling.
Other Side Effects: blood-count depression.
Given intravenously.

CCNU

See LOMUSTINE.

CDDP

See CIS-PLATINUM.

CeeNU

See LOMUSTINE.

Chlorambucil

Common Side Effects: none.
Other Side Effects: bone-marrow depression.
Given orally.

cis-Diamminedichloroplatinum

See CIS-PLATINUM.

cis-Platinum

Common Side Effects: severe nausea and vomiting.
Other Side Effects: bone-marrow depression; hearing problems; kidney damage; immunosuppression.
Given by IV.

Cortisone acetate

Common Side Effects: fluid retention; weight gain.
Other Side Effects: risk of infection; high blood pressure; potassium loss; diabetes.
Given orally.

Corynebacterium parvum

See C. PARVUM.

C. parvum

(Corynebacterium parvum; immunotherapy drug)
Common Side Effects: local reaction at injection site; flulike symptoms (fever, chills, headache).
Other Side Effects: nausea and vomiting; joint pain; elevated blood pressure.
Given by IV or injected subcutaneously.

Cosmegen

See DACTINOMYCIN.

Cyclohexylchloroethyl nitrosourea

See LOMUSTINE.

Cyclophosphamide

Common Side Effects: nausea and vomiting.
Other Side Effects: bone-marrow depression; immunosuppression; bloody urine; hair loss; liver, bladder, and lung problems; skin darkening and sterility (may be temporary); lack of menstruation.
Given both intravenously and orally.

122

Cytarabine

Common Side Effects: nausea and vomiting; diarrhea.
Other Side Effects: bone-marrow depression; liver damage; mouth sores.
Given by intravenous, intrathecal, or subcutaneous injection.

Cytosar-U

See CYTARABINE.

Cytosine arabinoside

See CYTARABINE.

Cytoxan

See CYCLOPHOSPHAMIDE.

Dacarbazine

Common Side Effects: severe nausea and vomiting.
Other Side Effects: bone-marrow depression; hair loss; kidney and liver problems; flulike symptoms.
　Given by IV.

Dactinomycin

Common Side Effects: nausea and vomiting; vein swelling.
Other Side Effects: bone-marrow depression; hair loss; mouth sores; skin rash.
　Given by IV.

Daunomycin

Investigational drug.
Common Side Effects: nausea and vomiting; fever; red urine.
Other Side Effects: bone-marrow depression; hair loss; heart problems.
　Given by IV.

Daunorubicin

See DAUNOMYCIN.

Decadron

See DEXAMETHASONE.

Delalutin

See HYDROXYPROGESTERONE CAPROATE.

Depo-Provera

See DEDROXYPROGESTERONE ACETATE.

DES

See DIETHYLSTILBESTROL.

Dexamethasone

Common Side Effects: fluid retention and weight gain.

Other Side Effects: high blood pressure; increased risk of infection and diabetes; loss of potassium.
Given orally.

Diethylstilbestrol

Common Side Effects: nausea and vomiting; cramps.
Other Side Effects: feminization; fluid retention; lowered blood calcium; uterine bleeding.
Given orally.

Doxorubicin Hydrochloride

See ADRIAMYCIN.

Drolban

See DROMOSTANOLONE PROPIONATE.

Dromostanolone Propionate

Common Side Effects: none.
Other Side Effects: fluid retention; lowered blood calcium; masculinization.
Given by intramuscular injection.

DTIC

See DACARBAZINE.

Elspar

See L-ASPARAGINASE.

Endoxan

See CYCLOPHOSPHAMIDE.

Epipodophyllotoxin

See VP16-213.

Estinyl

See ETHYNYL ESTRADIOL.

Ethynyl Estradiol

Common Side Effects: none.
Other Side Effects: fluid retention; feminization; lowered blood calcium; uterine bleeding.
Given orally.

5-Fluorouracil

Common Side Effects: nausea and vomiting; diarrhea.
Other Side Effects: bone-marrow depression; hair loss; mouth sores; poor muscle coordination; brittle nails or nail loss; skin reactions (pigmentation and sensitivity to sun).
Given by IV push, orally, or as a surface cream (for basal-cell skin cancer).

Fluorouracil

See 5-FLUOROURACIL.

Fluoxymesterone

Common Side Effects: none.
Other Side Effects: fluid retention; jaundice; lowered blood calcium; masculinization.
Given orally.

Ftorafur

Investigational drug.
Common Side Effects: nausea and vomiting.
Other Side Effects: gastrointestinal problems; mouth sores; loss of muscle coordination; skin pigmentation.
Given by IV.

5-FU

See 5-FLUOROURACIL.

Halotestin

See FLUOXYMESTERONE.

Hexamethylmelamine

Investigational drug.
Common Side Effects: loss of appetite; nausea and vomiting.
Other Side Effects: bone-marrow depression; mental depression; abdominal cramps; diarrhea; reversible neurotoxicity; skin rash.
Given orally (capsules).

HN2

See MECHLORETHAMINE.

Hydrea

See HYDROXYUREA.

Hydroxyprogesterone Caproate

Common Side Effects: local abscess; pain.
Other Side Effects: jaundice and lowered blood calcium.
Given by intramuscular injection.

Hydroxyurea

Common Side Effects: nausea and vomiting.
Other Side Effects: bone-marrow depression; mouth sores; skin reactions (rashes, pigmentation).

ICRF-159

Investigational drug.
Common Side Effects: mild nausea.

Other Side Effects: bone-marrow depression; hair loss; mouth sores; skin problems; flulike syndrome.
Given orally.

Imidazole Carboxamide

See DACARBAZINE.

L-Asparaginase

Investigational drug.
Common Side Effects: abdominal pain; allergic response; diabetes; fever; nausea.
Other Side Effects: problems with the liver and pancreas; mental depression; problems with blood-clotting.
Given by intravenous or intramuscular injection.

Leukeran

See CHLORAMBUCIL.

Levamisole

Immunotherapy drug.
Common Side Effects: nausea and vomiting; fatigue; loss of appetite—all usually mild and of short duration.
Other Side Effects: none.
Given orally.

Lomustine

Common Side Effects: nausea and vomiting.
Other Side Effects: blood-count depression; hair loss; mouth sores; problems with kidneys.
Given orally.

L-PAM

See MELPHALAN.

Matulane

See PROCARBAZINE.

Mechlorethamine

Common Side Effects: severe nausea and vomiting; vein irritation.
Other Side Effects: bone-marrow depression; hair loss.
Given by IV, local instillation, and surface application.

Medroxyprogesterone Acetate

Common Side Effects: local abscess and pain (when given IM).
Other Side Effects: fluid retention; lowered blood calcium; nausea (when taken orally).
Given by intramuscular injection and orally.

Megace

See MEGESTROL ACETATE.

Megestrol Acetate

No side effects reported.
Given orally.

Melphalan

Common Side Effects: mild nausea.
Other Side Effects: bone-marrow depression.
Given orally.

MER

(Methanol extract residue; immunotherapy drug)
Common Side Effects: local reaction and pain.
Other Side Effects: local reaction; nausea; vomiting; abdominal cramps.
Given subcutaneously in several locations at once.

6-Mercaptopurine

Common Side Effects: nausea and vomiting.
Other Side Effects: bone-marrow depression; mouth sores; skin rash; liver damage.
Given orally.

Methanol extract residue

See MER.

Methosarb

See CALUSTERONE.

Methotrexate

Common Side Effects: nausea and diarrhea.
Other Side Effects: bone-marrow depression; hair loss; liver and kidney problems; mouth sores; gastrointestinal problems; fever; cough.
Given by intravenous, intramuscular, subcutaneous, intra-arterial, and intrathecal injection and orally.

Methyl-CCNU

See SEMUSTINE.

Meticorten

See PREDNISONE.

Mithracin

See MITHRAMYCIN.

Mithramycin

Common Side Effects: severe nausea and vomiting.
Other Side Effects: bone-marrow depression; bleeding; kidney and liver problems; mouth sores.
Given intravenously.

Mitomycin

Common Side Effects: nausea and vomiting.
Other Side Effects: bone-marrow depression; hair loss; kidney problems; mouth sores.
Given intravenously.

Mitotane

Common Side Effects: nausea and vomiting; diarrhea.
Other Side Effects: drowsiness; lethargy; mental depression; tremors; visual disturbances; and skin rash.
Given orally.

6-MP

See 6-MERCAPTOPURINE.

MTX

See METHOTREXATE.

Mustargen

See MECHLORETHAMINE.

Mutacin

See MITOMYCIN.

Myleran

See BUSULFAN.

Neo-hombreol

See TESTOSTERONE PROPIONATE.

Nitrogen Mustard

See MECHLORETHAMINE.

Nolvadex

See TAMOXIFEN.

Oncovin

See VINCRISTINE.

o,p¹-DDD Lysodren

See MITOTANE.

Ora-Testryl

See FLUOXYMESTERONE.

Oreton

See TESTOSTERONE PROPIONATE.

Phenylalanine Mustard

See MELPHALAN.

Platinol

See CIS-PLATINUM.

Prednisolone

See PREDNISONE.

Prednisone

Common Side Effects: fluid retention; weight gain.
Other Side Effects: diabetes; high blood pressure; increased risk of infection; potassium loss.
Given orally.

Procarbazine

Common Side Effects: nausea and vomiting; mental depression.
Other Side Effects: bone-marrow depression; mouth sores; skin rashes.
Given orally.

Provera

See MEDROXYPROGESTERONE ACETATE.

Purinethol

See 6-MERCAPTOPURINE.

Razoxane

See ICRF-159.

Razoxin

See ICRF-159.

Rubidomycin

See DAUNORUBICIN.

Semustine

Investigational drug.
Common Side Effects: nausea and vomiting.
Other Side Effects: lowered blood count.
Given orally.

Streptozotocin

Investigational drug.
Common Side Effects: nausea and vomiting; local pain.
Other Side Effects: damage to kidneys, liver, and blood (usually anemia).
Given intravenously or intra-arterially.

129

Tabloid

See 6-THIOGUANINE.

Tamoxifen

Common Side Effects: nausea.
Other Side Effects: none.
Given orally.

Teslac

See TESTOLACTONE.

Testolactone

Common Side Effects: none.
Other Side Effects: lowered blood calcium.
Given by intramuscular injection.

Testosterone Propionate

Common Side Effects: none.
Other Side Effects: fluid retention; lowered blood calcium; masculinization.
Given by intramuscular injection.

6-Thioguanine

Common Side Effects: nausea and vomiting.
Other Side Effects: bone-marrow depression; liver problems.
Given orally.

Thioguanine

See 6-THIOGUANINE.

Thio-TEPA

Common Side Effects: nausea and vomiting; local pain.
Other Side Effects: bone-marrow depression; loss of appetite.
Given by intravenous or intracavity injection; local instillation for bladder cancer.

Triethylenethiophosphoramide

See THIO-TEPA.

Velban

See VINBLASTINE.

Vinblastine

Common Side Effects: nausea and vomiting; local reaction if drug leaks from IV.
Other Side Effects: bone-marrow depression; hair loss; loss of reflexes; mouth sores; constipation.
Given intravenously.

Vincristine

Common Side Effects: local reaction if drug leaks from IV.
Other Side Effects: bone-marrow depression; constipation; hair loss; neurological effects (pain in arms, legs, jaw, stomach; numbness or tingling in hands or feet; foot drop).
Given intravenously.

VP16-213

Common Side Effects: nausea and vomiting.
Other Side Effects: bone-marrow depression and hair loss.
Given intravenously and orally.

Living with Chemotherapy

The extent to which chemotherapy will affect your normal life depends on the type of chemotherapy you receive and your reaction to the drugs. Most chemotherapy is scheduled on an outpatient basis, and most cancer-treatment centers try, whenever possible, to schedule treatments so they do not interfere with your normal life (for example, having the treatments on a Friday afternoon so that if you are sick for a day or so you can work comfortably on Monday morning). There is a tremendous range of individual reactions to chemotherapy: Some people find they can continue their normal routines and activities with a minimum of discomfort and disruption; on the other end of the spectrum, a few patients find that their whole life is disrupted for the entire time of treatment. Most people get sick for a few hours, feel fatigued for a day, and then are able to resume normal activities.

You might have to change some habits, and you will be called upon to be a front-line observer in monitoring your own side effects. Your oncologist will give you a complete list of dos, don'ts, and what-to-watch-out-fors, but there are some general rules of thumb for chemotherapy patients:

- Many over-the-counter, nonprescription drugs can interfere with your chemotherapy—even aspirin. Medicine that other doctors have prescribed for you for other medical problems can also be harmful (like anticonvulsant drugs, antibiotics, blood-pressure pills, diabetes pills). *Don't take any medicine, or drink alcoholic beverages, without checking with your doctor.*
- Don't have dental work done without checking with your doctor.
- Don't begin any unusual diets, exercise programs, etc., without checking with your doctor.

Keep your doctor informed about your side effects. Don't feel that telling him is complaining, or a sign of weakness. Sometimes the "little

131

things" are the most important pieces of information: fatigue, red spots on your skin, etc. You should also inform your doctor if you are exposed to illness or injury. Due to bone-marrow depression and immunosuppression, the drugs may affect your ability to fight off disease and infections, and your general ability to heal. In certain cases there are specific diseases that can be particularly dangerous: For example, lymphoma patients can have serious problems if they get a herpes infection (chicken pox or shingles). Your doctor will tell you.

Chapter Eleven

EXPERIMENTAL TREATMENTS

Introduction

Improvements in treatment techniques come out of experimental programs. They are carried out under the stringent rules described in chapter 7. Experimental programs involve refinements in the areas we have described as standard treatments (surgery, radiation, and chemotherapy) and the development of entirely new approaches to healing the patient: immunotherapy, hormone therapy, hyperthermia, and bone-marrow transplants. In this chapter we will explain what the experimental process is, what these new approaches are and where you can find out about specific treatments that may be applicable to you.

The Experimental Process: Chemotherapy

More patients become involved in experimental chemotherapy programs than any other kind of experimental program. These chemotherapy experiments are conducted in five basic areas: the testing of completely new drugs that have never been used to treat any kind of cancer; trying out new combinations of drugs, each of which has proven effective alone against a particular type of cancer, in the hope

133

that the combination will prove dramatically more effective than single-drug therapy; the application of a proven chemotherapy treatment (single-drug or combination), which was developed for treating one type of cancer, to other forms of cancer; trying new ways of combining chemotherapy with radiation and/or surgery to produce better results; and doing comparison studies of standard treatments currently in use (combination or separate standard treatments) to establish which is the most effective. The easiest way to understand the experimental process in all areas is to look at how new cancer drugs are tested.

New drugs are tested in four stages. First are the animal trials, in which a drug is shown to be effective against tumors in animals. This testing begins with small animals (mice and rats) and, if successful, goes on to larger animals whose physiology is closer to that of human beings. If a drug is effective in treating animal cancers, human testing is the next step, after approval is granted from the Food and Drug Administration.

There are three phases of human testing. *Phase I testing* is done to determine the proper dosage for humans and to see what types of cancers will respond to the treatment. In Phase I testing, the new drug is given in gradually increasing doses. The unfortunate thing about chemotherapy is that there is a very fine line between the amount of the drug necessary to kill cancer cells in sufficient numbers to stop the growth and/or kill the tumor, and the amount of the drug that will have very harmful effects on the healthy cells necessary to keep the patient alive. In Phase I, the object is to establish the maximum dose (enough to kill the cancer but not the patient) and determine the drug's side effects.

Volunteers for this type of testing are limited to patients with advanced cancers that have not responded to standard treatments, and who are thought to have virtually no chance of survival. Patients volunteer for these programs because there is a glimmer of hope, however slight, that the new drug may help them, but also because they feel that even if their cancer cannot be successfully treated, their participation in this kind of experiment may lead to successful treatment for patients in the future.

Once this phase of testing is completed, *Phase II testing* is set up to determine which types of tumors respond to the drug; the differences in their degree of response (if tumor A responds to the drug 80% of the time, but tumor B only 10% of the time, it is likely that this drug would become a regular part of treatment for type A cancers but not for type B cancers); and how often to give the drug for maximum tumor-kill (see the chapter on chemotherapy for why this is important).

Like Phase I testing, this is a very experimental level of testing, with many unknowns, so volunteers are limited to seriously ill patients, and the reasons for becoming involved in Phase II trials are the same as for Phase I.

Phase III testing is the final phase of the experiment. By this time the doctors know what kinds of cancer the drug works on, what the side effects are, what the maximum dosage is, and what the schedule of treatment should be. At this point, they are working on the assumption that, with the evidence accumulated so far, this drug is theoretically at least as effective as standard drugs, and that there is a good possibility that it is more effective. The objective in Phase III is to find out whether it is indeed more effective. It is this phase of testing which patients may want to think of as an advanced treatment program, particularly if their cancer has had a fairly low cure rate with standard treatments.

It can take two to five years to complete all three phases of human testing.

The experimental programs being coordinated by the National Cancer Institute involving chemotherapy, radiation, surgery, and the other areas described below are indicated at the end of each site discussion in part II.

Immunotherapy

The body's maintenance-and-repair department is called the "immune system." It is made up of the white-blood-cell-producing tissues in the bone marrow, lymphatic system, and spleen; and the glands that produce hormones—adrenals, pituitary, thyroid, parathyroid, thymus, ovaries, testes, and pancreas. There are also chemicals produced in every cell—like Interferon—that help the body ward off intruders and repair damage.

The experimental field of immunotherapy is based on the premise that all people regularly develop the abnormal cells that we call cancer, but that most bodies identify the abnormal cell as something foreign, and attack and destroy it. It is thought that people who actually develop the disease do so either because they have a malfunctioning immune system or because the cancer cells have found ways to confuse the normal process of cell communication so that the immune mechanisms are not triggered.

Attempts to develop techniques in immunotherapy have two purposes: to develop immunotherapy primary treatments (to be used alone or in conjunction with chemotherapy), and to use immunotherapy as a supportive treatment to help repair the damage done either by the cancer itself or by chemotherapy or radiation treatments. This becomes particularly important in cancers that directly affect part of the immune system—like leukemia—where death often comes not from the cancer itself but from the body's inability to fight off infection.

Immunologists talk about several different types of immunity. *Congenital* immunity is a temporary immunity given to an infant by its mother; due to the interaction of the two bloodstreams across the placenta, the baby will have the same immunities as its mother during the first few months of life. *Natural* immunities are also ones that we are born with, but they are permanent. They are generally thought to be part of our genetic makeup, but they may also be influenced by things such as diet. Most of our immunities are *acquired:* As our body has to deal with disease and infections of various types, there is a *general* immune response that marshals all our disease-fighting forces; if this general response is successful, the individual is left with a *specific* immunity against that particular form of infection. The intruders are called antigens; antibodies produced in response to specific antigens confer specific immunities.

Acquired immunities are either *active* or *passive.* Active immunity is developed by actually having had a particular disease—either a full-strength bout with a disease you happened to catch, or a very low-grade infection artificially induced by inoculation (vaccination) with a weakened version to stimulate the immune system. Doctors can also induce passive immunity: If a patient's own immune system cannot be made to produce the proper disease-fighting cells and chemicals, antibodies developed by another person with the same disease can be injected into the patient.

Immunologists have also discovered that besides our own cells and chemicals, we also act as hosts to microorganisms that are beneficial to us. In chapter 1 we talked about the mitochondria and lysosomes that provide energy and breathe for our cells; it has also been found that bacteria are used by the body to fight disease by stimulating and activating white blood cells called macrophages. Lucien Israel describes the situation this way:

There are . . . in nature bacteria that help the organism to rid itself of a cancer. I do not think this is accidental, for the list of such bacteria is too long. The chemical constituents of the membranes of certain microorganisms provide not only a specific immune response, a "vaccination," but also a reinforcement of the natural defenses against other aggressions. That is probably what has made it possible for complex organisms to survive in an environment dominated by microbes. . . . Activated microphages do not like tumor cells. When they come into contact with them, they kill them.

136

The various types of immunotherapy techniques are linked to what we know about the differing types of immunities and how they can be induced.

Active immunotherapy is directed at inducing the generalized, non-specific response—most commonly by injecting different strains of bacteria, usually combined with chemotherapy. The bacteria most widely used include BCG (bacillus Calmette-Guérin) and C. parvum (Corynebacterium parvum). Also used are MER (methanol extract residue—a derivative of BCG) and the chemical levamisole. Experiments are also under way in attempts to create vaccines, either from a patient's own tumor or from a similar tumor in other patients. Vaccines may be created to produce either a specific or general response.

Passive immunotherapy involves taking antibodies from a healthy person and administering them to patients who have deficient immune systems. In adoptive immunotherapy, the lymphocytes of a "cured" cancer patient are transferred to a patient with the same type of cancer in hopes that this transfer will enable the patient to hold on to the newly acquired immunity. Bone-marrow transplants, described below, may be thought of as a type of adoptive technique.

Immunotherapy resources are listed at the end of each section in part II. More-specific information can be obtained by writing to: Coordinator, International Registry of Tumor Immunotherapy, National Institutes of Health, Bethesda, Maryland 20014, or by calling your local Cancer Information Service (see part III).

Hormone Therapy

Hormones are substances originating in a gland or organ and carried through the blood to chemically stimulate another part of the body into increased activity and secretion. It has been found that for many cancers of the reproductive system (male and female) or cancers affecting any of the parts of the hormone (endocrine) system, altering the balance of hormones in the body can aid in destroying the cancer or preventing its recurrence. This is achieved either with *additive therapy* (giving doses of hormones in addition to the ones normally produced by the body) or with *ablative therapy* (removing the natural sources of hormones in the body). Hormones are frequently given along with chemotherapy.

In *additive therapy*, steroid hormones and nonsteroid hormones may be used, although the steroid hormones have thus far proved the most effective against cancer. Estrogens (female hormones) are steroids

137

that have been used to treat cancer of the prostate and breast cancer. Progestins are hormones produced by the ovaries, placenta, and, in small amounts, by the adrenal glands; they are used to treat cancers of the uterus, kidney, and breast. Androgens (male hormones) are used in the treatment of breast cancer. Androgens, when administered to female patients, may produce temporary masculinizing side effects, such as the growth of facial hair or deepening of the voice. When estrogens are administered to males, there may be a temporary decrease in sex drive and the breasts may swell. Corticoids are hormones of the adrenal cortex, the outer layer of the adrenal glands. These are used in treating leukemias, lymphomas, myelomas, and breast cancer.

The side effects of the most commonly used hormones, and the method of administering them (IV or pills), are listed in chapter 10 along with the other drugs. The most commonly used steroid hormones are:

Estrogens	DES; ethynyl estradiol
Antiestrogens	tamoxifen
Progestins	medroxyprogesterone acetate (Depo-Provera); hydroxyprogesterone caproate (Delalutin); megestrol acetate (Megace)
Androgens	Fluoxymesterone (Halotestin, Ora-Testryl); testosterone propionate (Oreton, Neo-hombreol); dromostanolone propionate (Drolban); testolactone (Teslac)
Corticoids	prednisone; prednisolone

Nonsteroid hormones are most commonly used in conjunction with the cancers of the glands that produce them. For example, thyroid hormone is given to prevent the recurrence of thyroid cancer.

Ablative therapy removes the source of a hormone that is linked to a particular cancer growth. Castration by surgery or irradiation may be indicated in certain men with breast or prostate cancer. Other surgical procedures used in ablative treatment may include an adrenalectomy (excision of one or both of the adrenal glands) or a hypophysectomy (surgical removal of the pituitary gland).

Hormone therapy is generally considered a part of the chemotherapy arsenal, so these treatments are supervised by a medical oncologist. Although the whole field of hormone therapy is considered technically experimental, many of the hormones are part of standard treatment. Contact the resources listed at the end of each section in part II for more information.

NOTE: It is fairly easy for patients to become confused about the differences between chemotherapy, immunotherapy, and even some aspects of nuclear medicine: All of these techniques may involve drugs given by IV or pills, and it is not obvious if the drug is designed to kill cancer cells by direct toxic action (chemotherapy); by stimulating the patient's own immune system (immunotherapy); by adjusting the patient's hormone system (hormone therapy), which is a part of the immune system; or by internal radiation (nuclear medicine). It becomes more confusing because all of these experimental fields have component parts that are part of "standard" treatments, and a medical oncologist may be the specialist who supervises all of them (a therapeutic radiologist or nuclear-medicine specialist would be involved in internal radiation treatments). This is why all drugs, regardless of classification, have been listed in chapter 10 and in part III.

Hyperthermia

Hyperthermia is the inducement of an abnormally high body temperature for therapeutic purposes. In theory, the heat is used to kill cancer cells by activating the immune system, or as a cellular sensitizer to make other treatments (chemotherapy or radiation) more potent. It may be administered either to the entire body or to a specific body site.

In whole-body hyperthermia, the patient is anesthetized, placed in a heat suit, and the temperature of the body is raised to 40–41° C. In local hyperthermia, the temperature is raised in a specific site by means of ultrasound, radiofrequency waves, microwaves, or perfusion. In the perfusion method, the blood itself is heated.

Hyperthermia is experimental and potentially dangerous; it is used only at a very few cancer centers throughout the country. For further general information, contact Dr. Joan Bull at the National Cancer Institute (301/496-4000). For information on whole-body hyperthermia, contact Dr. Sacki at the University of New Mexico (505/227-4951). Microwave hyperthermia is being studied at Roswell Park Memorial Institute (Buffalo, N.Y.); Stanford University; University of California at San Francisco; Washington University (St. Louis, Mo.); and Thomas Jefferson University in Philadelphia.

Bone-Marrow Transplants

High doses of radiation and chemotherapy can destroy the bone marrow's ability to produce substances necessary to the immune system, and certain types of cancer actually destroy the bone marrow directly. Healthy bone marrow can be transplanted from the brother or sister of a cancer patient, although there is no guarantee of success. This technique is used primarily in patients with leukemia.

The National Cancer Institute is supporting programs in bone-marrow transplantation at the University of California at Los Angeles School of Medicine; Fred Hutchinson Cancer Research Center (Seattle); Baylor College of Medicine (Houston); University of Washington (Seattle); Mercy Catholic Medical Center (Darby, Pa.); Children's Hospital (Boston); Johns Hopkins University (Baltimore); Memorial Sloan-Kettering Cancer Center (New York); and the University of Pennsylvania (Philadelphia).

Further Reading

Mark Renneker and Steven Leib, eds., *Understanding Cancer* (Palo Alto: Bull Publishing, 1979).
 See part II, the section on immunology, including "Fantastic Voyage (Through the Immune System)" by Isaac Asimov and "Introduction to Immunology" by William R. Clark; and part IV, in the section on therapies, the article by Yosef Pilch, "Research in Cancer Immunotherapy."
Lucien Israel, *Conquering Cancer* (New York: Vintage, 1978).
 See chapter 8, "Hormone Therapy," and chapter 10, "Immunotherapy."

Chapter Twelve

SUPPORTIVE
THERAPIES

There is a wide range of therapies available whose aim is not to kill the cancer but to alleviate some of the adverse effects that the cancer—and treatments—may have upon the body and mind. These are often incorporated into the general treatment plans or are services which should be coordinated with the cancer specialists. Some of these therapies are the subject of experimental protocols being conducted by the National Cancer Institute. In this chapter we will briefly summarize supportive therapies used to treat pain and nutritional problems and to aid in rehabilitation, and tell you where to get more information about them.

Pain

One of the main fears that cancer patients have is that of living (or dying) in great pain. In fact, the vast majority of cancers are painless. This area, however, has been the subject of intense research in the last ten years, and those patients who have to deal with high levels of pain should understand that there are many options open to them.

Several facts and theories are the basis for the various pain-controlling techniques. These will be explained more fully in the "Further Reading" section at the end of the chapter, but they can be summarized very quickly. Although the source of pain can be anywhere in the body, pain is something that is perceived by the brain. At times where the pain is "felt" has nothing to do with the actual physical location of its source—this is called referred pain. For example, when a peritoneoscopy is done—in which several tiny slits are made in the abdomen (see chapter 5, "Diagnostic Procedures and Tests"), the most intense pain afterward is usually felt in the shoulder. It is well known that when people have amputations, they often "feel" sensations, even severe pain, in the missing limb. The perceived pain is a product of very complicated electrical and chemical messages sent to the brain. How this actually works is not yet completely understood. What *is* known is that pain can be controlled, not only by treating the source of the pain but by dealing in various ways with the mind's ability to perceive the pain.

Techniques Used in Controlling Pain

Surgery

Surgical techniques used to control pain can be divided into two types. The first type, *palliative surgery* (discussed in the chapter on surgery) is aimed at removing the sources of pain—like large tumors that are causing pressure or blockages—even though the surgery itself cannot cure the cancer. The second type is neurosurgery, which in this situation can be employed to interfere with the ability of the pain message to reach the brain by severing nerves. These procedures include cordotomies, in which nerve bundles in the spinal cord are cut; nerve-root clipping, in which the roots of nerves are snipped high up in the neck; and rhizotomies, in which the nerve relaying the specific pain is cut where it enters the spinal cord. These neurosurgical techniques are dangerous and are usually not done unless other techniques have not worked.

Medication

Drugs are the most common way to alleviate pain, but problems can arise if pain is severe and long-term. Drugs that control pain are administered in ever-increasing doses, and are rotated so the patient does not build up a tolerance for or addiction to any specific drug.

The question of addiction has been partially resolved in recent years: There is general agreement that if a patient is terminal and in great pain, addiction should not be considered a problem. When severe pain is considered to be short-term (it is felt that the treatment for the cancer will be successful and that within weeks or months the source of the pain will be gone), and if the physician perceives that much of the intensity of the felt pain is due not to the physical problem but to severe anxiety (a problem common to cancer patients), the doctor may be reluctant to administer high doses of addictive drugs.

Many doctors have found, however, that if the drug dose is carefully controlled and gradually withdrawn as the physical condition improves, accompanied by supportive counseling by doctors and nurses, the patient can be kept free of both pain and addiction—even though the dosage was sufficient to have caused addiction. This matter is still being debated, but patients should be aware that there are two sides to the argument.

If pain is going to be a chronic problem, however, many patients do not want to be dependent on drugs and do not want to feel "doped up" all the time. Other techniques for controlling pain involve neither drugs nor surgery and have been used with greater and greater success.

External Electrical Stimulation

Because pain is a product of electrical impulses sent over the nerve pathways, it is possible to "jam" these messages with other kinds of electrical stimulation. One of these devices, *TENS* (transcutaneous electrical nerve stimulations), sends electric impulses through the skin. Another device, called the epidural dorsal column stimulator, utilizes electrodes that are surgically implanted in the patient's spinal cord. The mechanism is operated by the patient (much like a remote-control TV switch) when he feels there is need to control pain.

Acupuncture and Acupressure

Using an ancient Chinese form of medicine, pain is often relieved by inserting needles into the skin and either rotating them or using low-voltage electrical stimulation. Acupuncture must be administered by a trained acupuncture therapist, and the relief may last much longer than the treatment itself.

Patients who have found relief using acupuncture are taught to give themselves acupressure—a type of massage in which pressure is applied to the same places where the needles were inserted—whenever the need arises.

Mind Control

Also products of Oriental culture are a number of techniques based on their knowledge that the mind can directly control many of the physical processes that Western medicine has traditionally thought to be involuntary, or completely free of control by the conscious mind. Scientists do not know exactly how this works—just as we do not as yet know how acupuncture works—but the following techniques have been effective:

Hypnosis. At first the hypnotic suggestion is controlled by a trained hypnotherapist. If the techniques are effective, the patient is taught self-hypnosis.

Guided Imagery. The patient visualizes certain pictures in his mind that have been found to relieve pain and tension. At the start, the patient is taught the images and guided through the process by a trained therapist. If effective, the patient is taught to use the technique on his own. Guided imagery has also been used to increase the effectiveness of standard treatments. (See *Getting Well Again* in "Further Readings.")

Relaxation and Meditation. It is known that a body in a state of stress (tension) feels more pain than a relaxed body. These techniques are taught to promote general relaxation.

Biofeedback. The patient is taught to control certain body functions (heart rate, blood pressure, temperature, respiration, etc.) at will. At first, the patient gets feedback from monitoring machines so he can see how he's doing. After the techniques are learned, the patient can use them on his own. Again, the biofeedback techniques are based on the relationship between tension and perceived pain.

Where to Get Help with Pain Control

Many of these techniques have become a part of treatment at various hospitals, but patients may need to seek out these services if they are not available at their treatment centers.

A list of pain-control clinics is available from the Committee on Pain Therapy and Acupuncture, American Society of Anesthesiologists, 515 Busse Highway, Park Ridge, Illinois 60068. You can get similar information by calling the National Committee on the Treatment of Intractable Pain, in Washington, D.C., at (202) 983-1710. Information on biofeedback can be obtained from the Biofeedback Research Society, University of Colorado Medical Center, Denver, Colorado 80262.

The National Cancer Institute is conducting studies on pain control. General studies are being done under the chairmanship of:

Dr. Hubert Tosomoff
Department of Neurological Surgery
University of Miami School of Medicine
P.O. Box 520875, Biscayne Annex
Miami, Florida 33152

Dr. Berthod Wolff
New York University Medical Center
550 First Avenue
New York, New York 10016

Dr. Wolff Kirsch
University of Colorado Medical Center
4200 East Ninth Avenue
Denver, Colorado 80220

Drug studies are being done by a group headed by Dr. William Regelson, MCV Station, Box 273, Medical College of Virginia, Richmond, Virginia 23928.

Electrical stimulation studies are being done under the chairmanship of Dr. Ronald Ignelzi, Department of Psychiatry, University of California at San Diego, La Jolla, California 92093.

For biofeedback and hypnosis studies, contact Dr. Charles Graham, Midwest Research Institute, Behavioral Sciences Laboratory, 425 Volker Laboratory, Kansas City, Kansas 64110.

A special study using hypnosis with children who have cancer is chaired by Dr. Ernest Hilgard, Stanford University, Department of Psychology, Stanford, California 14305.

Nutrition and Vitamins

Of great concern to many cancer patients is the frequently acute weight loss. With this comes a general concern about proper diet and whether vitamins will help the condition, or even help prevent cancer, and whether diet can be used as a primary treatment. We spoke about the various theoretical links between diet and cancer in chapter 3, and about the problems of research in this area. In the next chapter we will briefly discuss primary diet treatments.

At this point, no major cancer center is offering diet treatment or nutritional therapy as a form of primary treatment. However, the supportive role of nutrition in increasing the effectiveness of standard treatments is presently being studied.

Total Parenteral Nutrition (TPN), also called *hyperalimentation,* is a therapy that is available generally and is also being studied experimentally. Designed to counteract severe weight loss and to aid the effectiveness of difficult treatments, this technique uses a special type of IV to get large amount of calories, vitamins, and nutrients into a cancer patient.

The reason a special kind of IV is needed is that the small veins in the arms, usually used for IV's, can handle only a limited amount of nutritional material; and if the nutritional concentrate is diluted to accommodate these small veins, there is too much fluid for the circulatory system. If the concentrate can be put into a large vein (usually the subclavian, right near your collarbone), the high volume of blood flowing through a vein of that size will dilute the concentrate to the proper level. This is done by a minor surgical procedure, in which a catheter is inserted into the vein, and the nutrients are pumped by a robot machine attached to the IV pole.

145

Experimental TPN protocols are coordinated by William DeWys, M.D., Project Office, Landow Building, Room 406B, National Cancer Institute, NIH, Bethesda, Maryland 20205. Phone 301/986-0030.

In addition, there is a nutritional-support research program for cancer treatment chaired by Dr. Thomas Nealon, Jr., St. Vincent's Hospital and Medical Center of New York, 153 West 11th Street, New York, New York 10011. Phone 212/260-1234.

Several vitamin studies are being done by NCI. Vitamin A is being studied in connection with treatment for breast cancer (contact Dr. Singhakowinta, Wayne State University, United Hospitals of Detroit, Department of Oncology, 5160 John R. Street, Detroit, Michigan 48235; phone 313/494-6422) and chronic nonlymphocytic leukemia (contact J. R. Durant, Southeastern Cancer Study Group, U.A.B. Medical Center, Birmingham, Alabama 35294; phone 205/934-5077).

Vitamin C is being used in studies involving children with advanced cancers (contact A. Cangir, University of Texas Health Science Center at Houston, M. D. Anderston Hospital and Tumor Institute, P.O. Box 20036, Houston, Texas 77025). It is also being studied in relation to acute lymphocytic leukemia (contact B. Hoogstraten at 913/588-5996), lung tumors, solid tumors, and general advanced (terminal) cancers. Vitamin D is being studied in relation to breast cancer and myeloma. See site discussions in part II for locations of these studies.

Rehabilitation Therapy

Certain types of cancers and their treatments can cause both physical and psychological adjustment problems for patients. In the chapter on surgery we talked about several of the support services available for cancer patients who have similar difficulties as a result of surgical treatment. We will discuss other such support services in chapter 15, "Living with Cancer," including hospice services.

Further Reading

David Bresler, *Free Yourself from Pain* (New York: Simon and Schuster, 1979).
    A book by the head of the University of California at Los Angeles Pain Control Unit, describing the techniques used by them and the rationale behind the techniques.
    Although there are several books on the market written for people who suffer from chronic pain, this one has been recommended because of the thoroughness with which it details all the various factors associated with pain and how to alleviate pain. It includes discussions of everything that may con-

tribute to pain: emotional stress; pollutants in the air, water and food; general nutrition; electromagnetic forces. It also discusses traditional medical approaches, unconventional approaches, and the role of laughter. In addition, there is an excellent bibliography. It is an open-minded book written by a responsible and qualified practitioner.

O. Carl Simonton, Stephanie Matthews-Simonton, and James L. Creighton, *Getting Well Again* (New York: Bantam Books, 1978).

Chapter Thirteen

CHILDREN WITH CANCER

Many books on cancer—both for the professional and for the layman—list childhood cancers as a separate "type" of cancer. We have chosen to give the more technical information about these kinds of cancers in the regular listings of specific cancers in part II, just as we have done with the "adult" cancers—partly because many of these cancers affect adults as well as children. Children who have cancer do have different needs than the adult patients, and cancer-treatment centers acknowledge these differences by having separate facilities and programs for children, and by having subspecialties of oncology that deal primarily with children: pediatric oncology, pediatric radiology, etc.

Childhood Cancers: What Are They?

Childhood cancers are generally divided into two groups. The first is called *pediatric solid tumors,* and includes Wilms's tumor (kidney); neuroblastoma (central nervous system—see "Brain" in part II); rhabdomyosarcoma (a soft-tissue sarcoma); Ewing's sarcoma (bone); and retinoblastoma (eye). One may also find in children such solid tumors as testicular tumors, osteosarcomas, carcinomas, embryonal carcinomas, and teratomas.

The second group is comprised of the *systemic cancers,* including

148

leukemias—particularly acute lymphocytic leukemia (ALL)—and lymphomas, both Hodgkin's and non-Hodgkin's.

Incidence

In children under fifteen years of age, the leading forms of cancer are leukemias. Of these, ALL affects the most children, followed by acute (not otherwise specified) leukemia, acute granulocytic, chronic granulocytic, and acute monocytic (the last two being extremely rare). In descending order, the other cancers affecting children are central-nervous-system tumors, lymphomas (Hodgkin's and non-Hodgkin's), soft-tissue sarcomas, sympathetic-nervous-system tumors, kidney and bone tumors, and retinoblastomas.

Half of all childhood cancers appear in children under four years old.

Childhood cancers follow different patterns than adult cancers. The most common malignant tumors in adults are carcinomas, whereas in children they are blastomas. They develop from the blastoma tissue

TABLE 5

Leading Causes of Death Among Children Aged 1–14,
United States, 1977

Rank	Causes of Death	Number of Deaths	Percent of Deaths	Death Rate Per 100,000 Population Age 1–14
1.	Accidents	9,502	45.5	19.6
2.	Cancer	2,364	11.3	4.9
3.	Congenital Anomalies	1,470	7.0	3.0
4.	Homicide	766	3.7	1.6
5.	Pneumonia & Influenza	718	3.4	1.5
6.	Heart Diseases	540	2.6	1.1
7.	Meningitis	454	2.2	0.9
8.	Cerebrovascular Diseases	274	1.3	0.6
9.	Cystic Fibrosis	249	1.2	0.5
10.	Cerebral Palsy	239	1.1	0.5
11.	Suicide	190	0.9	0.4
12.	Anemias	149	0.7	0.3
13.	Bronchitis	126	0.6	0.3
14.	Benign Neoplasms	124	0.6	0.3
15.	Septicemia & Pyemia	113	0.5	0.2
	All Others	3,608	17.3	7.4
	TOTAL: ALL CAUSES	20,866	100.0	43.1

Source: Vital Statistics of the United States, 1977.

149

TABLE 6

Cancer Incidence by Site for Children Under 15

Rank	Site	Number of Cases	Percent of Total	Rate Per 1,000,000 Children
1.	Leukemia	664	30.2	33.6
2.	Central Nervous System	409	18.6	20.7
3.	Lymphomas	298	13.6	15.1
4.	Sympathetic Nervous System	170	7.7	8.6
5.	Soft Tissue	141	6.5	7.1
6.	Kidney	135	6.1	6.8
7.	Bone	101	4.6	5.1
8.	Retinoblastoma	58	2.6	3.0
9.	Liver	26	1.2	1.3
	All Others	195	8.9	9.9
TOTAL: ALL SITES		2,197	100.0	111.1

SOURCE: SEER Program, 1973–76, National Cancer Institute.

present in all children. Blastoma tissue produces adult organs, which is one of the reasons why childhood cancers can show up in so many different places in the body. For older children, sarcomas are a common type of cancer, although rare in adults. Leukemias and lymphomas make up about 40% of the cancers in children, while they only account for about 9% of adult cancers.

Support Services

Childhood cancers create special problems for the child, his parents, and his siblings, particularly psychological ones. There are the normal fears associated with hospitalization, treatments (which are the same kinds used on adults), and diagnostic procedures. There are the possibilities of being away from home and the disruption of normal family life; and there are the adjustments to having cancer, to having treatments, and to the debilitating effects of the treatments. Childhood is a difficult enough time under the best of circumstances; these problems require special support systems.

One of the most serious (and wonderful) psychological problems that people now have comes from the very success achieved by medical treatments for childhood cancer. In the past, childhood cancer was a death sentence; the child became the center of attention and was completely catered to. Now that such a large proportion of childhood cancers are completely curable, great care has to be taken to keep perspective, see the cancer as an intensive but temporary experience, and make sure that the child will be psychologically ready to resume normal life.

There are many support services available for children and their parents. The Candlelighters is a national organization for parents of children with cancer and has over 110 chapters in forty states. It is a source of all types of information (including *The Oncology Handbook for Parents*), but most important, it has family-support groups that help families deal with common problems. Such groups provide all family members, including the patients, with outlets for venting frustrations, offer a social outlet for parents and siblings who are often isolated by the cancer experience, and disseminate technical information on cancer, insurance, and professional counseling. Some groups maintain a toll-free hot line; others provide the personal help of hospital visits to newly diagnosed families by experienced parents and patients.

For more information about the Candlelighters, contact:

Candlelighters Foundation
123 C Street, S.E.
Washington, D.C. 20003
Phone: (203) 483-9100, or 544-1696.

One serious problem confronting many families is the expense of hospital treatment, particularly when the hospital is not close to home. Many of the children's hospitals allow parents to "room in" with their child. There are also Ronald McDonald Houses (presently in Chicago and Washington, with one planned for Atlanta, Boston, Denver, San Diego, Palo Alto, New York, and Houston) where families of seriously ill children can stay at minimal cost. For further information, contact:

Mr. A. L. (Bud) Jones
Ronald McDonald House Coordinator
c/o Golin Communications, Inc.
500 North Michigan Avenue
Chicago, Illinois 60614
Phone: (312) 836-7100.

The most comprehensive source of help will be found at the children's hospitals and special pediatric oncology departments of major cancer centers.

About a third of the National Cancer Institute's *Coping with Cancer: A Resource for Health Professionals* (see "Further Reading") is devoted to the problems of children with cancer. They summarize the situation as follows:

> Once coping with childhood cancer involved the acceptance of a poor prognosis and the feelings that accompanied seeing a child rapidly deteriorate and die. Today, childhood cancer in general can be viewed as a chronic illness with an uncertain outcome—the child may be cured or may die. Treatment may extend over years. Remissions are common, but so are recurrences. Although the child has a life-threatening illness, he is still growing and developing, and has needs similar to his healthy age mates. The physical and psychological demands on the patient and family are great and disruptive on many levels. The child, family, caregivers and community must cope with a host of factors.

The book focuses on helping the family during the major times of emotional stress: diagnosis; major treatment episodes; hospitalization; the onset of side effects; relapse; serious infection; and death. The reader is directed to professional teams who are prepared to intervene with additional support at these times. Great emphasis is placed on preserving as much normalcy as possible: resisting the natural tendency to overprotectiveness once the child has gone into remission and returned home; maintaining the child's academic progress in hospital schools and homebound programs; and preparing the child and his parents for return to regular school.

A special set of problems confront the adolescent: The normal urge for independence conflicts with the dependency of being a patient; the normal need for privacy conflicts with the necessary lack of privacy; and so on. The frustration these circumstances create can be enormous: "It is not uncommon for them to refuse treatment, break hospital rules, miss outpatient appointments, or undertake activities they have been advised against." Normal rebellion against authority at this age creates special problems in relationships with parents and caregivers. At the same time, adolescents are often very concerned about the burdens their illnesses have imposed on their families. There are also problems with body image and peer relations, and many questions are raised about the future: Will there be any future? And if there is, what effect will the cancer and the treatments have on education, career, marriage, and having children?

Because coping with cancer in children is so complex, parents are strongly urged to avail themselves of the special services provided at children's hospitals and pediatric oncology departments, and make full use of the support groups.

Further Reading

Oncology Handbook for Parents. Prepared by the Candlelighters (South Florida Chapter), April 1976.

Milton H. Donaldson, "The Multidisciplinary Team Approach to the Care of Children with Cancer," in *Cancer Review*, January 1977, pp. 1–9.

Shirley B. Lansky, et al., *A Team Approach to Coping with Cancer* (Lawrence, Kansas: University of Kansas Medical Center, 1975).

Eugenia Wild Schweers, *Parents' Handbook on Leukemia.* American Cancer Society, 1977.

William M. Easson, *The Dying Child* (Springfield, Illinois: Charles C. Thomas, 1970).

Coping with Cancer: A Resource for the Health Professional. U.S. Department of Health, Education & Welfare, Public Health Service, National Institutes of Health, National Cancer Institute, May 1979.

> Although this is a professional book, it deals with human problems we all face, and is thus very understandable by the layman. The book summarizes what is known about coping with cancer and is an excellent source of information, including the bibliography.

The National Cancer Institute puts out several publications (listed below) for parents and children. They can be ordered free of charge from:

Publications Order
Office of Cancer Communications
National Cancer Institute
Building 31, Room 10A18
Bethesda, Maryland 20205
Phone: 800-638-6694 (toll-free)

"Hospital Days, Treatment Ways." A coloring book to help the child orient himself to the hospital and treatment procedures. It was originally produced by the Ohio State University Comprehensive Cancer Center and Children's Hospital, Columbus, Ohio.

"Eating Hints: Recipes and Tips for Better Nutrition During Treatment." Originally produced by the Yale–New Haven Medical Center. Written like a cookbook.

"Diet and Nutrition: A Resource for Parents of Children with Cancer."

"The Leukemic Child." A mother tells her story of coping with the problems of having a leukemic child and gives advice to parents in the same situation.

"Feeding the Sick Child." Nutritional information and recipes designed to appeal to children.

The Childhood Cancer Resource Directory, published by the American Cancer Society, New Jersey Division Childhood Cancer Committee, contains information on how to manage a child's education and where to get practical assistance: lists and descriptions of available counseling services; home-care and information resources; possible sources of blood and of blood donors. Available from the ACS Service and Rehabilitation Department, phone (201) 297-8000.

Chapter Fourteen

UNORTHODOX THERAPIES

Introduction

Another group of cancer treatments is called "alternative," "non-standard," "unorthodox," or "nontoxic" therapy. These therapies can be divided into four groups: nutritional/metabolic therapies; "natural" drug therapies; psychological therapies; and holistic therapies. What distinguishes most of them is not so much their techniques, or even a theoretical acceptance of these techniques, but the use of these techniques as *primary* treatment and the exclusion of any standard treatment.

As you read through this chapter, and should you decide to explore any of these therapies, several things should be kept in mind:

· We have not attempted to deal with these treatments in the same detail as we have discussed standard, experimental, and supportive treatments. The purpose of this book is to explain standard cancer therapies by board-certified oncologists and licensed hospitals. Most practitioners of unorthodox therapies are not part of this group.

· It is impossible to give you bottom-line information about the effectiveness of these therapies. The information is almost completely descriptive; there are no statistics available.

· The information comes from two different directions—which we will call Group One and Group Two. These two groups are virtually at

154

war with each other, and there are enough substantiated charges of "bias" on the information produced by both groups on any single topic to make it difficult to even summarize the situation objectively.

· The qualifications of the people who give these therapies vary enormously. Most practitioners are not M.D.s, let alone highly trained cancer specialists. There is a high percentage of true "quacks"—totally unqualified, often ruthless people who prey on the fears of cancer patients and will promise you anything if you will only give them your money.

· The real problem for the cancer patient is that the situation is not totally black and white. Not all the people who practice or support these therapies are quacks, and not all the theories are scientifically invalid. How do you sort it out?

In this chapter we will attempt to describe these other therapies and will give you labeled sources of information about them (sources labeled "Group One" are fundamentally opposed to these therapies; sources labeled "Group Two" are for them). We will also explain the problems that create the "gray areas" in which you may be able to find treatment that combines Group One and Group Two therapies, and talk about the side effects of choosing an unorthodox therapy.

Group One

Group One is represented by the National Cancer Institute, the American Cancer Society, and the major cancer centers. This group has developed the standard and experimental treatments that we have been describing in this book.

What really defines this group is the carefully gathered, reliable information about the treatments that are offered. Proven treatments are known quantities: We know the odds for successful response in a given type of cancer, the process, the side effects, etc. Even those involved in experimental programs must be fully informed about the phase of the experiment and the doctors' expectations for this treatment. And treatment takes place under very controlled conditions. All of this does not mean that a patient has any guarantees, but he does have a good idea of what he is getting involved in.

Group One used to call Group Two approaches "quackery" and all the practitioners "quacks." The language has been softened in recent years to "unproven methods," and there has been acknowledgment that some practitioners may be qualified M.D.s. However, the criteria used by the American Cancer Society to put doctors on the Unproven Methods list, and the reasoning behind the appearance and disappearance of certain names from the list, have been questioned. (See *The Cancer Syndrome* in "Further Reading" at the end of this chapter.)

155

Group Two

This group is represented by such organizations as the International Association of Cancer Victors and Friends, and the Cancer Control Society. Their criteria for supporting treatment methods is that they be nontoxic and "natural." Since the standard cancer treatments kill cancer cells and, at least for a limited time, also damage some of the healthy, normal cells, they are considered toxic. The feeling against standard treatment is very intense: The IACV calls surgery, radiation, and chemotherapy "cutting," "burning," and "poisoning." They are also highly critical of how Group One has suppressed natural and/or inexpensive cancer cures.

Obviously feelings run high on both sides, and the exercise in name-calling is not very helpful to the cancer victim and those who care about him. How do you cut through the emotions and evaluate what is best for you? The answer, unfortunately, is that at this stage it is extraordinarily difficult, if not impossible.

There are some Group Two information sources that will supply books, articles, lists of practitioners, and lists of patients who say they have been successfully treated. These general sources are:

International Association of Cancer
   Victors and Friends
7740 Manchester Avenue,
Suite 110
Playa del Rey, California 90291
Phone: (213) 822-5032

Cancer Control Society
2043 North Berendo Street
Los Angeles, California 90027
Phone: (213) 663-7801

Second Opinion
P.O. Box 548
Bronx, New York 10468

Arlin J. Brown Information Center
P.O. Box 251
Fort Belvoir, Virginia 22060
Phone: (703) 451-8638

National Health Federation
P.O. Box 688
212 West Foothill Boulevard
Monrovia, California 91016
Phone: (213) 357-2181

Foundation for Alternate Cancer
   Therapies
Box HH
Old Chelsea Station
New York, N.Y. 10011
Phone: (212) 741-2790

Nutritional Therapies

Nutritional, or metabolic, therapies are generally based on the premise that the traditional American diet (which is high in sugars, fats, and animal proteins), combined with the chemicals used to produce, process, and commercially prepare our foods, is fundamentally unhealthy. Diet and the usual American life-style (high stress, low exercise) results in the stress-reaction breakdown described in chapter 1. Although nutritional therapies focus on the dietary aspect of health, almost all of them are holistic approaches that involve a total change in life-style.

A wide variety of diets are recommended: some therapies offering one blanket diet to treat all forms of cancer; others recommending more specific programs, depending on the patient. They are all "natural-food" diets and strongly vegetarian, although some may include fish or lamb.

In general, many of these diets conform to the nutritional recommendations of the U.S. government. What is truly unorthodox is the use of such diets as primary treatments to bring about cancer cures. While nutritional components are being integrated more and more into standard and experimental treatments, and are being studied as a part of cancer prevention, at this time no clinical oncologist uses nutrition as a primary treatment for cancer.

The two most famous cancer-cure diets used by Group Two people are the Gerson diet and the Kelley diet. Each of these men have written books about their particular approach: *A Cancer Therapy: Results of Fifty Cases,* by Max Gerson (Del Mar, California: Totality Books, 1977), and *One Answer to Cancer,* by William D. Kelley (Beverly Hills, California: International Association of Cancer Victors and Friends, Inc., 1974). The most comprehensive source of information about nutritional information is Ruth Yale Long, Ph.D., president of the Nutrition Education Association, Inc., P.O. Box 20301, Houston, Texas 77025; Phone: (713) 665-2946. She has written "Nutrition and Cancer Update 1980," and "No More Cancer: A Review of Non-Toxic Cancer Therapies Plus a Diet and Supplements for Cancer Prevention." In the latter she talks about many nutritional therapies, such as those developed by Warburg, Wang, Davison, Stickle, Issels, Wigmore, Hunsberger, Chiu-Nan Lai, Krebs, Richardson, Manner, and Oden, as well as Gerson and Kelley. She also discusses laetrile as well as vitamins and other nontoxic therapies.

It is important to underscore a disclaimer that Dr. Long includes in her material: "Persons seeking unorthodox and orthodox help for cancer are urged to investigate carefully the doctor, the product, and the price before deciding on a course of action. Please remember that the Nutrition Education Association, Inc., *does not recommend or endorse* in this instance, *nor does it assume any responsibility* [italics ours]."

Vitamin therapies are usually considered a part of nutritional therapies—they are the "nutritional supplements." They are also incorporated into various types of experimental therapies being tested by Group One, particularly in conjunction with hormone and immunotherapy protocols. Vitamin A is used in protocols for breast cancer and chronic nonlymphocytic leukemia. Vitamin C is used in treatments of general hematologic (blood) malignancy, acute lymphocytic leukemia, lung tumors, melanoma, and general solid tumors. Vitamin D is being tested for use with breast cancer and myeloma.

Vitamin C's most prominent advocate has been Linus Pauling, who along with Ewan Cameron, M.D., of Vale of Leven Hospital, Loch Lomondside, Scotland, has written numerous articles and books for professional and lay audiences. They published a comprehensive summary of all their work in *Cancer and Vitamin C: A Discussion of the Nature, Causes, Prevention and Treatment of Cancer, with Special Reference to the Value of Vitamin C* (available from the Linus Pauling Institute, Menlo Park, California 14025, at $9.95).

The use of vitamins and minerals in medical treatment is also called "orthomolecular medicine," and more information can be gotten from the Orthomolecular Medicine Society, 2340 Parker Street, Berkeley, California 94704.

Imagery Therapy, Biofeedback, and Other Psychological Approaches

The great split between Group One and Group Two occurs in the application of the psychological approach. The basis for this approach is the theory that there is a much stronger link between mind and body than Western medicine has traditionally accepted, and that the mind can be trained as a powerful force in healing.

As we explained in chapter 12 on supportive therapies, psychological approaches are being incorporated more and more into Group One treatments, primarily as a way to relieve stress, anxiety, and pain. But no Group One cancer specialist is using this approach as a primary treatment for cancer, although the most widely known technique, the Simonton method, was developed by a certified radiation oncologist. In fact, the Simonton approach offers a good example of a technique that is currently being used both responsibly and irresponsibly.

Part of the Simonton approach is an imagery technique designed to help fight cancer directly: In your mind you visualize the cancer cells, your own armies of white blood cells, the chemotherapy drugs and/or radiation that have been sent in to war against the cancer cells. By mentally visualizing and controlling the battle, you help the anticancer forces win. The Simontons state many times in their book, *Getting*

Well Again, * that their point is to describe "what you can do *in conjunction with medical treatment* [italics ours]."

Because we will be emphasizing the psychological processes used in our approach, we may appear to be neglecting or excluding physical treatment. This is by no means our intention. Although we believe medicine has developed too narrow a focus, concentrating primarily on the physical symptoms, it has made monumental strides in developing and refining physical therapies. We encourage all cancer patients to obtain the best medical treatment they can find from a physician or health team they feel cares about them. . . . *We are particularly concerned that the patient not decide to substitute a psychological technique for appropriate medical treatment.* Thus, we cannot emphasize too strongly the importance of pursuing *both* physical treatment and emotional intervention [italics ours]."

The Simontons are not the only people using their techniques—they have trained over 5000 "therapists." But, as pointed out in an excellent article by Gina Kolata, they do not keep informed about, or exercise any control over, how their techniques are actually used. As Ms. Kolata's small-scale investigation showed, some practitioners of the "Simonton Method" are promoting it as a primary treatment, using it as a way to defraud cancer victims.* *

Holistic Medicine

This is another difficult area to sort out because of the wide range of people who claim to practice it. Very simply, holistic medicine takes the same general view that the Simontons take: The health of the human body does not depend simply on the availability of medical treatments, but involves the whole person—what he eats, his life-style, and his psychological and emotional status. The field developed outside traditional medicine, and therefore the largest group of practitioners are not M.D.s but people whose primary approaches to health have been nutritional, herbal, psychological, etc. These people do not incorporate standard medical treatment into their concept of holistic medicine.

More and more M.D.s have been quietly incorporating this total-person approach as they treat patients, and it is obviously the basis for treatment at such places as the University of California at Los Angeles

---

* O. Carl Simonton, Stephanie Matthews-Simonton, and James L. Creighton, *Getting Well Again* (New York: Bantam Books, 1978), pp. 84–85.

* * Gina Kolata, "Texas Counselors Use Psychology in Cancer Therapy," *Smithsonian*, vol. 11, no. 5 (Washington, D.C.: Smithsonian Associates, August 1980), pp. 48–59.

Pain Clinic. However, because the field has developed outside the mainstream of American medicine and still has a fairly bad reputation because of the medically unqualified people associated with it, even the M.D.s who use this approach will not use the words "holistic medicine" to describe what they practice (it is sometimes called the "Wellness movement"). The only way a patient can find out if his doctor favors the holistic approach to health care is to talk to him about the nuts and bolts of his approach to treatment.

"Natural" Drug Therapies

Quotation marks have been placed around the word "natural" here because many of the drugs used in standard chemotherapy, hormone therapy, and immunotherapy are also natural (not man-made), but when Group Two talks about drug therapies, they are talking about a specific set of drugs not used in standard treatments. The most widely known of these drugs is laetrile.

Laetrile has undergone some testing at the National Cancer Institute, but the results of the tests have not been accepted by those who support its use, primarily because of the way the tests were set up. The major laetrile treatment centers—which are in Mexico (run by Dr. Ernesto Contreras in Tijuana) and in Germany (run by Dr. Hans Nieper at the Silbersee Clinic in Hanover)—use laetrile as part of a holistic treatment plan. They maintain that what should be evaluated is the whole treatment, not just the anticancer effects of laetrile alone (which is what was done at NCI). A detailed examination of laetrile and many of the other treatments can be found in *The Cancer Syndrome* (see "Further Reading").

Gray Areas of Cancer Treatment and Research

In the past few years, many areas of cancer treatment and research have been the subject of investigative exposés. Some of them have been published under the auspices of Group Two—such as the *Cancer News Journal*'s article entitled "The Suppression of Cancer Cures" (see "Further Reading"). Others have been written by Group One people who disagree with the direction of cancer-research funding and its emphasis on cures rather than prevention. Samuel Epstein's *The Politics of Cancer* (San Francisco: Sierra Club Books, 1978; revised edition, Garden City, New York: Anchor Press/Doubleday 1979) is one example. Others, like Ralph Moss's *The Cancer Syndrome* (see "Further Reading"), were written by people who began as part of Group One but have become so critical of it that despite their research, one must carefully weigh their conclusions. Whether or not you agree with their bottom line, the information they present is worth reading.

In general, the gray area of thinking results from overlap of the approaches favored by the two groups: For example, several treatment components are accepted by both groups but used in different ways. For some components, like the Simontons' method, this difference can be described as *responsible* vs. *irresponsible* use of the method: Responsibly used, the Simontons' method is a supportive therapy; irresponsibly used, it is offered as a primary therapy. To a certain extent, the use of vitamin C in treating cancer also falls into this category, but the debates going on about vitamin C are actually a better example of a second type of gray area: promising lines of thinking that are not being pursued to the fullest at this time.

This includes the lack of conclusive testing of many approaches that Group Two advocates (nutritional therapies, herbal therapies, holistic medicine), some of which may have originated outside of Group One. It also includes areas of research that began in Group One but got sidetracked before there was conclusive evidence one way or the other: research into vitamin C, for example, as well as the work of Lawrence W. Burton, who has a clinic in Freeport, Bahamas, and Dr. Stanislaw Burzynski of Houston, Texas, and his antineoplastons or Coley's toxins (which no one is using at the moment). Questions have been raised as to why hydrazine sulfate, a chemotherapy drug, has not been pursued more actively in the research.

In these gray areas, the main differences between Group One and Group Two lie in the use of treatments as primary or supplemental, and in the amount of testing each group considers necessary before a treatment is given to a patient: Group One oncologists will not use little-tested therapies as primary treatments; Group Two practitioners will.

Evaluating Group Two Information: A Serious Problem

The problem in evaluating the nontoxic methods which are not a part of Group One programs is that there is no reliable information. However, there are certain guidelines that a layman can use to at least sort out the complete quacks from other unorthodox practitioners:

· They have unusual degrees after their names.
· They do not publish the results of their treatments in scientific or medical journals, but use testimonials from patients who state that they have been cured.

161

- They usually have just one treatment, which they claim works for all cancers. The treatment is often the practitioner's secret, personal medicine.
- They often claim to be persecuted by the government or by doctors.
- They offer sure success with no side effects.
- They are often flamboyant, charismatic people.
- They often claim to have special tests to evaluate your cancer that are different from the tests that doctors normally use.
- They are willing to treat you without a biopsy confirming that you have cancer.*

"Side Effects" of Unorthodox Treatments

Unorthodox treatments, even if nontoxic, may have side effects that in the final analysis may prove devastating.

There is no proof that unorthodox treatments can help you. If your cancer is treatable by standard or experimental therapy and you do not use it, a side effect of nonstandard treatment may be death.

If nonstandard treatments are pursued before standard treatments, the time lost may mean the continued growth and spread of the cancer, lowering your chances for cure.

The cruelest side effect of many nonstandard treatments is the placement of blame wholly on the patient for his illness and for the failure of the proposed cure: If the treatment does not work, it is because the patient did not eat correctly, or think correctly, or change his life-style sufficiently, etc. This is an unconscionable and totally unwarranted position for any "doctor" or "therapist" to assume, but many of them do. The situation is made even worse by the fact that the patient, having disassociated himself from Group One, may be ashamed to go back to a qualified cancer specialist for palliative care or pain relief if the nonstandard treatment has proven to be ineffective.

In short, the side effects of these treatments may be a shortened life; overwhelming guilt and depression; and unnecessary physical pain.

The only way to be assured that you are receiving the best known medical treatment for your type of cancer while incorporating the promising (though unproven) new theories on nutrition, mental health, biofeedback techniques, etc., is to do what Norman Cousins did (*Anatomy of an Illness*, New York: W. W. Norton, 1979): Find a medically qualified (Group One) cancer specialist who is sympathetic to

---

* Harold Glucksberg and Jack W. Singer, *Cancer Care: A Personal Guide* (Baltimore: The Johns Hopkins University Press, 1980).

the value of these other areas, and work out a treatment plan that is acceptable to both of you.

Further Reading

"Neutral" Evaluations

These sources have attempted some type of middle-ground, objective evaluation of both standard and nonstandard treatments and are intellectually accepting of the value of both.

"Cancer": Part I, "Cancer Politics," and parts II and III, "Cancer Therapies," in *Health Facts*, vol. II, No. 12, and vol. III, Nos. 13–14, November/December 1978, January/February/March/April 1979. Published by the Center for Medical Consumers and Health Care Information, Inc., 237 Thompson Street, New York, New York 10012. Phone: (212) 674-7105.

Ralph W. Moss, *The Cancer Syndrome* (New York: Grove Press, 1980).

Although not disapproving of standard treatments for the types of cancer where they have proven to be effective, Mr. Moss is highly critical of Group One and the way in which some possible treatments are pursued and others are not. There is a very extensive bibliography.

Group One Sources

Mark Renneker and Steven Leib, eds., *Understanding Cancer* (Palo Alto: Bull Publishing, 1979).

See especially the section entitled "Cancer Quackery," as well as articles in the "Special Topics" section entitled "The Simonton Approach to Cancer," "Vitamins and Cancer," "Supplemental Ascorbate (Vitamin C)," and "Laetrile."

Unproven Methods of Cancer Management (New York: American Cancer Society, 1976).

Group Two Sources

Gary Null, "Suppression of Cancer Cures" and "Alternative Cancer Therapies," in *Cancer News Journal*, vol. 14, No. 4, December 1979. Published by the International Association of Cancer Victors and Friends, Inc., 7740 West Manchester Avenue, Suite 110, Playa del Rey, California 90291. Phone: (213) 822-5032.

The following sources have been supplied by the Nutrition Education Association, Inc., and the Cancer Control Society for information on the major areas of nontoxic treatments:

Laetrile Research

Dean Burk, Ph.D.
Dean Burk Foundation
4719 44th Street
Washington, D.C. 20016

Ernst T. Krebs, Jr., D.Sc., L.L.D.
John Beard Memorial Foundation
P.O. Box 685
San Francisco, California 94101
Phone: (415) 824-1067

Harold Manner, Ph.D.
Loyola University
Department of Biology
6525 N. Sheridan Road
Chicago, Illinois 60626
Phone: (312) 274-3000

Andrew McNaughton
McNaughton Foundation
P.O. Box B 17
San Ysidro, California 92073
Phone: (714) 428-2248/2249
(Tues., Wed., Thurs. only)

163

Nutritional Programming

Ruth Yale Long, Ph.D.
3647 Glen Haven
Houston, Texas 77025
Phone: (713) 665-2946

Bob Gibson, M.D.
215 N. 3rd Street
Ponca City, Oklahoma 74601
Phone: (405) 765-4414

The Kelley Foundation of Life
P.O. Box 354
Winthrop, Washington 98862
Phone: (509) 996-2214

James Privitera, M.D.
629 S. Eremland Drive
Covina, California 91723
Phone: (213) 966-1618

Metabolic Therapy

Bruce Halstead, M.D.
Richard Welch, M.D.
511 Brookside Avenue
Redlands, California 92373
Phone: (714) 824-1750

Dan Dotson, M.D.
805 Cherry
Graham, Texas 76046
Phone: (817) 549-3663

John Richardson Center
514 Kains Avenue
Albany, California 94706
Phone: (415) 527-3020

Owen Robins, M.D.
6565 DeMoss
Houston, Texas 77074
Phone: (713) 981-7500

Keith S. Lowell, D.O.
3429 W. Holcombe Boulevard
Houston, Texas 77025
Phone: (713) 668-1135

James LaRose, D.O.
8300 Homestead
Houston, Texas 77028
Phone: (713) 631-4474

Laetrile (also known as vitamin B-17 or amygdalin) Therapy

Ernesto Contreras, M.D.
Central Medico Del Mar
Paseo de Tijuana 1-A
Playas de Tijuana
Tijuana, B.C., Mexico

Phone: (903) 387-1540/1850/1788
(Mailing address)
P.O. Box 3793
San Ysidro, California 92073
Phone: (714) 239-1939 (24 hrs.)

Wheatgrass Therapy

Hippocrates Health Institute
Ann Wigmore, D.D., Founder
25 Exeter Street
Boston, Massachusetts 02116
Phone: (617) 267-9525

Hippocrates Health Institute of
San Diego
6970 Central Avenue
Lemon Grove, California 92045
Phone: (714) 464-3346

Amygdalin (B-17), Enzymes, Vitamin B-15, etc.

Texas Metabolics
610 4th Street
Graham, Texas 76046
Phone: (817) 549-6141/6053

Omega Pacific
P.O. Box 6765
Modesto, California 95355

Gerson Therapy

Charlotte Gerson Straus
P.O. Box 535
Imperial Beach, California 92032

Phone: (714) 575-0967
(Eves. or before 10:00 A.M.)

Legal Service

Laetrile Information Service
P.O. Box 844

Graham, Texas 76046
Phone: (817) 549-6141/6053

Literature

Nutrition Education Association, Inc.
Ruth Yale Long, Ph.D.
P.O. Box 20301

Houston, Texas 77025
Phone: (713) 665-2946

Chapter Fifteen

LIVING WITH CANCER

Introduction

Once cancer has been diagnosed, life is never quite the same for the patient or the family. Most cancer patients need to learn how to live with cancer; some need to find out the best way of dealing with the terminal part of a terminal illness. In this chapter we will show you how to get the information you need to make those adjustments.

The problems of adjustment to cancer are really of two types. One type is the concrete problems; the other type concerns the very real emotional difficulties encountered by the patient and the family. Mila Tecala, the director of a counseling center for people with life-threatening diseases, has summarized the emotional reactions of cancer patients around four issues:

Alienation. The cancer patient feels that having cancer has made him unacceptable to his friends, family, and close associates. This feeling is often more powerful than the fear of death.

Mutilation. The fear of disfigurement can arise from both the surgical removal of a part of one's body and from such temporary conditions as hair loss after radiation or chemotherapy.

Mortality. This issue includes not only the fear of death but also the fear of having to live with an uncertain future.

Vulnerability. There is a feeling of loss of control over one's life.

Fatigue and debility may make it difficult or impossible to lead one's life "as usual," and any crisis is perceived as life-threatening. Certain things specific to dealing with cancer make this sense of vulnerability even more acute:

> Uncertainty about the type and extent of treatment, as well as the duration of the disease, create an atmosphere of unending sickness. Further, there seems to be little the patient can do to stop the onslaught of cancer. Other diseases have concrete courses of action that, if followed, hasten recovery and prevent future illness. Heart disease, for example, can be controlled by medication, proper diet, regular exercise, and cessation of smoking. Cancer offers no comparable courses of action. *

Elisabeth Kübler-Ross, in her book *On Death and Dying* (New York: Macmillan, 1969), identifies five stages that people go through when faced with the fact that they are dying. They apply equally well, however, to the emotional stages people go through when faced with the *possibility* that they, or a loved one, may be dying.

The first stage in the coping process is denial: "This can't be happening! The diagnosis is wrong, the tests are wrong, the doctor's opinion is wrong," etc. The second stage is anger: "I don't deserve this, I've led a responsible and good life, I'll be damned if I'm going to let the cancer get me. . . ." This gives way to the bargaining stage, where promises are made—to God, to doctors, to your spouse, children, or yourself—that you will mend your ways if you are cured: "I'll spend all my time with my family if I get through this, and stop fooling around with that worthless boat. . . ." This stage gives way to depression, which is followed by acceptance, finally, of the situation.

It is very valuable for patients and especially their loved ones (who are the emotional support) to know these are only stages, and to realize that patients and families repeat this cycle when a new situation or unpleasant piece of information presents itself. Once the diagnosis has been accepted, the cycle may begin again when the patient has to deal with the hospital; the side effects of treatment or complications, convalescence, and, most surprisingly, even when dealing with remission, cure, and the resumption of a normal life: One does adjust to being a cancer patient, and, after the adjustment is made, there can be as difficult an adjustment to being normal.

Communicating needs, wants, fears, hopes, and concerns is terribly important not only for the cancer patient but for those who care about him. It is strongly urged that you become acquainted with the coping

---

* *Coping with Cancer: A Resource for Health Professionals,* U.S. Department of Health, Education, and Welfare, Public Health Service, National Institutes of Health, National Cancer Institute, September 1980, p. 24.

167

books listed in "Further Reading" at the end of this chapter, and that you make use of the supportive services discussed below.

Concrete Problems

Being a cancer patient also presents one with some practical, "concrete" problems—such as deciding where to go for treatment, coming to terms with the world of doctors and hospitals, working out financial problems, problems concerning child care or other household help, and organizing time around the schedule of treatment and reactions to treatment.

Since virtually all cancer patients have to deal with hospitals, let's take a look at them first.

The Hospital

Hospitals are often very intimidating and not very supportive places, thus we strongly advise that you arrange to have a friend or relative who is trustworthy and fairly assertive with you throughout your hospital stay. You should also read a paperback called *The Hospital Experience* by Judith Nierenberg and Florence Janovic (New York: Bobbs-Merrill, 1978, $7.95). Of particular value is part I ("The Hospital: What Kind of Place Is This?" "You're Admitted: What Happens Now?" "Patients' Rights, or Don't Just Lie There!" "A Guide to Language, or Why Your CC Is Important to Your Px" and "Drugs: What You Should Know, Ask and Tell"), and part V, "Times of Crisis," which discusses the intensive-care unit, the emergency room, and dying.

Hospital Staffs

We have talked about the various specialists who may be called in on your case; a complete list of specialists can be found in part III, and the discussions of specific cancers in part II indicate what specialties may be involved in any particular type of cancer. Specialists will supervise your case and see you from time to time, but during the diagnosis and treatment you will have most contact with other members of the hospital staff.

House Staff: Residents and Interns. These are not medical students—they have already graduated from medical school and are in various phases of advanced training. Everything they do is supervised by specialists.

The house staff rotates through the different "services" (special sections) of the hospital. The schedule of rotation varies from hospital to hospital but is usually three months in each service for the interns. The intern is a rank beneath the resident, and each resident has interns who report to him daily.

The house staff participates in cancer clinics and in reviews of laboratory smears and examinations; participates in or observes surgery; and, in many hospitals, spends a month or more being trained in the management of cancer patients. They participate in "rounds" (going around to all the patients, checking on present conditions, talking about each case) with the senior physician. They observe patients, assist in their care, and take part in the diagnosis and treatment process.

Nurses. Several levels of nurses work in a hospital. An R.N. (registered nurse) has graduated from an accredited school of nursing, received a degree, passed boards, and is legally licensed as a professional nurse. R.N.s can be general-duty nurses, have supervisory positions (in charge of a floor or a special unit), or may specialize (with further advanced training) as surgical nurses, oncology nurses, or anesthetists. Acting on the physician's orders, the R.N.s design a plan of treatment and nursing care for patients. The nurse must have a working knowledge of cancer therapy and diagnosis in order to evaluate a cancer patient, and is relied on to observe changes in his physical and mental condition.

Licensed practical nurses have had a year of training and have passed an examination. Their training is not as extensive as that of the R.N., and the type of care they can give is limited: For example, they cannot give medications or start an IV. The L.P.N. works under the supervision of an R.N. who assigns her duties.

Nurses' aides are trained on the job and usually have passed registration examinations. Their specific jobs have been discussed in the appropriate sections on diagnosis and treatment.

Therapists. Therapists are highly trained people who specialize in a wide variety of areas. Inhalation and respiratory therapists usually work in the hospital, but make home visits if necessary. Their job is to help patients to breathe, and they generally work with patients with chronic respiratory diseases as well as those with pulmonary cancer. They operate breathing machines and may administer drugs as well as oxygen.

Speech and hearing therapists may help patients after head-and-neck or brain surgery if either speech, hearing, or language have been

169

affected by the surgery or by the cancer itself. Speech and hearing therapists are usually a part of a department of Rehabilitation and Physical Medicine, which seeks to help patients resume normal lives after treatment. Within this department you will also find physical therapists, who help patients regain as much normal functioning of their bodies as possible and who teach patients how to use prosthetic devices, such as an artificial leg; and occupational therapists, who teach patients a variety of applied skills. The team may also include social workers and vocational counselors.

Social workers. These people often have key roles in helping cancer patients and their families adjust to living with cancer. They can help identify sources of financial help, obtain and fill out the endless forms necessary for such help, and arrange for housekeepers, transportation, housing, and hospice services. Besides this practical help, they often have the greatest experience and expertise in helping patients and their families cope with the cancer experience. They often run individual and group-therapy support groups and can put you in touch with other support groups in your area.

Rights of the Hospital Patient

Being a hospital patient makes most people feel helpless, and they often tolerate situations that, under normal conditions, they would find totally unacceptable. The American Hospital Association has developed a patient's bill of rights which every hospital patient should know. They are both ethical and legal rights that have been agreed to by the medical professions and the courts.

Patient's Bill of Rights*

I.   The patient has the right to considerate and respectful care.

II.   The patient has the right to obtain, from his physician, complete current information concerning his diagnosis, treatment, and prognosis in terms the patient can be reasonably expected to understand. (When it is not medically advisable to give such information to the patient, the information should be made available to an appropriate person on his behalf. He has the right to know by name the physician responsible for coordinating his care.)

III.   The patient has the right to receive from his physician informa-

---

* Reprinted by permission of the American Hospital Association, 840 North Lake Shore Drive, Chicago, Illinois 60611.

tion necessary to give informed consent prior to the start of any procedure and/or treatment. Except in emergencies, such information or informed consent should include, but not be limited to, the specific procedure and/or treatment, the medically significant risks involved, and the probable duration of incapacitation. Where medically significant alternatives for care or treatment exist, the patient has the right to such information. The patient also has the right to know the name of the person responsible for the procedures and/or treatment.

IV. The patient has the right to refuse treatment to the extent permitted by law, and to be informed of the medical consequences of his action.

V. The patient has the right to every consideration of his privacy concerning his own medical care program, case discussion and consultation.

VI. The patient has the right to expect that all communications and records pertaining to his care should be treated as confidential.

VII. The patient has the right to expect that within its capacity a hospital must make reasonable response to the request of a patient for services. The hospital must provide evaluation, service and/or referral as indicated by the urgency of the case. When medically permissible, a patient may be transferred to another facility only after he has received complete information and explanation concerning the needs for and alternatives to such a transfer. The institution to which the patient is to be transferred must first have accepted the patient transfer.

VIII. The patient has the right to obtain information as to any relationship of his hospital and other health-care and educational institutions insofar as his care is concerned. The patient has the right to obtain information as to the existence of any professional relationships among individuals, by name, who are treating him.

IX. The patient has the right to be advised if the hospital proposes to engage in or perform human experimentation affecting his care or treatment. The patient has the right to refuse to participate in such research projects.

X. The patient has the right to expect reasonable continuity of care. He has the right to know in advance what appointment times and physicians are available and where. The patient has the right to expect that the hospital will provide a mechanism whereby he is informed by his physician, or a delegate of the physician, of the patient's continuing health-care requirements following discharge.

XI. The patient has the right to examine and receive an explanation of his bill regardless of source of payment.

XII. The patient has the right to know what hospital rules and regulations apply to his conduct as a patient.

171

Financial Considerations

Cancer is an expensive disease. Even a "simple" Stage I cancer curable by surgery can cost thousands of dollars. More-complicated treatments can cost as much as $100,000. If the patient is a husband/wife/parent, additional expenses may arise because of the time away from work and the need for housekeepers or child care. What resources are available to cancer patients?

Health Insurance

Check your health insurance to see what kinds of services it includes. The general types of insurance are: hospital insurance, which pays for some or all hospital costs; surgical insurance; medical insurance, which pays doctors' costs other than surgery; major medical, designed to cover the costs of serious, expensive illnesses and accidents; and Medicare. Health-insurance plans, even ones in the same general category, vary widely in terms of payment, types of inpatient and outpatient services covered, number of hospital days covered, etc.

You cannot assume that your insurance will cover all your treatment, rehabilitation, and convalescence costs; many policies do not pay for drugs or outpatient treatment, which can have disastrous consequences for people being treated by chemotherapy. This is also true if you have purchased "cancer insurance," which is an area of the insurance business that has been under intense governmental investigation because people have had severe problems in collecting on these policies.

Free Treatment

We have already discussed the free cancer treatments available from the National Cancer Institute if you become involved in their experimental programs. Free care is also available at many of the major cancer centers, Veterans Administration, and public-health hospitals.

Financial Assistance for Medical Bills

Limited financial aid is available from the American Cancer Society and the Leukemia Society of America; the amount varies from community to community. The largest source of help is the federal, state, and local government through the various Medicare, Medicaid, and public-assistance programs. Cancer patients may qualify for Social Security Disability or Social Security Supplemental Income, which can help ease the financial burden caused by absence from work. If you need financial assistance, contact a social worker in your hospital to see if you qualify for any of these programs.

You should check over other insurance policies you have, particularly life insurance, to see if they have disability clauses. You may also have purchased disability insurance directly or through your place of employment. Many employers will also give advances on sick leave.

Many communities have a "welfare fund" that was specifically set up to deal with emergencies and differs enormously from the regular state and federal welfare programs. Some communities feel it their responsibility to make sure local residents do not lose their homes during a long-term disability, and will pick up mortgage payments on the patient's home.

As a last resort, it may be realistic to consider such extreme measures as welfare or declaring bankruptcy. Although both of these alternatives are abhorred by people used to being self-sufficient, you should explore these options without feeling guilty. Most working people have already paid more into welfare than they will receive in benefits, so it is not exactly a situation of trying to bum a free ride.

Other Types of Assistance

Your hospital social worker can put you in touch with organizations that offer other types of help. We briefly list these groups below. If no phone number is given, call your local chapter of the American Cancer Society or the Cancer Information Service number for local chapters of these organizations.

LEUKEMIA SOCIETY OF AMERICA, INC. Financial assistance and consultation services for leukemia and lymphoma patients. 211 East 43rd Street, New York, New York 10017. Phone: (212) 573-8484.

MAKE TODAY COUNT. Assists patients and families in resolving personal and emotional problems through group self-help programs. P.O. Box 303, Burlington, Iowa 52601. Phone: (319) 754-7266 or 8977.

UNITED OSTOMY ASSOCIATION. Emotional support and rehabilitation for people who have had ostomies. It is basically a self-help group, but the organization has an active advisory board of medical experts. Members of the association are also eligible for UOA insurance programs. Services are offered both in the hospital and at home. 1111 Wilshire Boulevard, Los Angeles, California 90071. Phone: (213) 481-2811.

CANSURMOUNT. Emotional and educational support for cancer patients and their families. There is a "therapeutic community" formed of the patient, family members, the CanSurmount volunteer (a cancer patient himself), and a health professional. Contact the American Cancer Society.

INTERNATIONAL ASSOCIATION OF LARYNGECTOMIES. A program sponsored by the American Cancer Society designed for the total rehabilitation of people who have had laryngectomies.

173

REACH TO RECOVERY. A program to meet the physical, psychological, and cosmetic needs of women who have undergone mastectomies. A program of the American Cancer Society.

AMERICAN CANCER SOCIETY. Services vary from community to community. Besides counseling services, they can provide concrete help for patients and their families: rehabilitation; equipment loans for care of the homebound patient; surgical dressings; transportation to and from treatment; home health care; blood programs; assistance with employment problems; social-work assistance; medications; and rehabilitation programs.

Practical help can often be forthcoming from organizations not directly linked to cancer patients: the Red Cross; Salvation Army; your church; social and fraternal organizations; and your union.

The following regional and local organizations also provide special services:

Illinois—*Cancer Call-PAC.* An emotional-support telephone service of the American Cancer Society. Phone: (312) 372-0471.

California—*UCLA Psychosocial Telephone Counseling Service.* Provides direct counseling or refers you to other qualified professionals. Callers from area codes 213, 714, and 805 can use a toll-free number: 1-800-352-7422. Others should call (213) 824-6017.

New York/New Jersey/Connecticut—*Cancer Care, Inc.,* and the *National Cancer Foundation.* Professional counseling for advanced cancer patients, covering home nursing care, homemaker home-health aides, housekeepers, etc. Phone: (212) 679-5700.

Alabama—*TOUCH* (Today Our Understanding of Cancer is Hope). The program's goal is to provide assistance in forming realistic, positive attitudes in regard to work, social and leisure activities, and locating community resources. Phone: (205) 934-2248.

Minnesota—*"I Can Cope."* A course designed to meet the educational and psychological needs of people with cancer. Contact: Judi Johnson, Ph.D., Cancer Education Coordinator, North Memorial Medical Center, 3220 Lowry Avenue North, Minneapolis, Minnesota 55422. Phone: (612) 588-0616, Ext. 541.

Nutrition

Nutrition has already been touched on in our discussions of prevention, unorthodox therapies, supportive therapies, and cancer in children. In this section we are addressing the problem of weight loss due to cancer or as a side effect of radiation or chemotherapy.

Weight loss is often the most prominent worry a patient has (especially if the cancer is otherwise painless), and a frequently voiced complaint is that doctors and health teams do not treat this aspect of patient care in a manner satisfactory to the patient. If you find yourself in this situation, press the point with your team: All hospitals have nutritionists on their staffs.

The National Cancer Institute and many of the major cancer centers have published booklets of recipes and nutritional information which are available free or at minimal cost—these are listed in "Further Reading" at the end of this chapter. The recipes and special diets focus on getting enough calories and nutrients into a patient who has no appetite, or may have an incompletely functioning or highly sensitive digestive tract. They stress high-protein, high-liquid diets with vitamin and nutrient supplements. Often they are blenderized and have low fiber content. For those who take solids but simply have no appetite, there are suggestions for making food appetizing and for making each bite count, getting as many calories and nutrients per mouthful as possible.

You should always discuss any special diet with your cancer specialist to make sure it is compatible with your physical condition and your therapy.

The Terminal Cancer Patient and the Hospice Movement: Living and Dying With Dignity

Our society has been particularly inept at dealing with people who are dying. Because we are a youth-oriented, future-oriented society that avoids any "unpleasantness," dying with dignity has been, until recently, a real problem in the United States. One solution has come in the form of the hospice movement: an organized system of home-care programs and special facilities with professional teams who provide dying patients with the highest quality of life and the opportunity to die on their own terms, surrounded by those who love them.

The hospice movement was actually begun over a century ago by the Sisters of Charity in England. In the 1960s the idea began to take hold in the United States, and began to flower in the mid-Seventies. At the moment, more than 170 health organizations in 39 states are planning or developing hospice services.

The best way to describe hospice programs is to say they are organized to fulfill the rights expressed in "The Dying Person's Bill of Rights," reprinted from the *American Journal of Nursing* (January 1975):

I have the right to be treated as a living human being until I die.

I have the right to maintain a sense of hopefulness however changing its focus may be.

I have the right to be cared for by those who can maintain a sense of hopefulness, however changing this might be.

I have the right to express my feelings and emotions about approaching death in my own way.

I have the right to participate in decisions concerning my care.

I have the right to expect continuing medical and nursing attention even though "cure" goals must be changed to "comfort" goals.

I have the right not to die alone.

I have the right to be free from pain.

I have the right to have my questions answered honestly.

I have the right not to be deceived.

I have the right to have help from and for my family in accepting my death.

I have the right to die in peace and dignity.

I have the right to retain my individuality and not be judged for my decisions which may be contrary to beliefs of others.

I have the right to discuss and enlarge my religious and/or spiritual experiences, whatever they may mean to others.

I have the right to expect that the sanctity of the human body will be respected after death.

I have the right to be cared for by caring, sensitive, knowledgeable people who will attempt to understand my needs and will be able to gain some satisfaction in helping me face my death.

Hospice teams, whether in institutions or home-care programs, are trained to deliver any necessary services to patients and their families as the needs arise, on a twenty-four-hour basis. A typical home-care program includes work with a physician to establish the optimum program of symptom and pain control; weekly meetings with the family; instruction for family members in patient care; family counseling and frequent telephone contact; and, after death, support for the family via phone calls, visits, and monthly gathering.*

Two books are recommended: *Hospice* by Parker Rossman (New

---

* C. Carter, "Hospice Home Care Nursing: A New-Old Challenge" (Presented at the Oncology Nursing Society Third Annual Congress, Washington, D.C., April 6, 1978).

York: Fawcett Columbine, 1977; $4.95) and *The Hospice Movement* by Sandol Stoddard (New York: Vintage, 1978; $3.75). You can get more information about hospice services by contacting the National Hospice Organization, 765 Prospect Street, New Haven, Connecticut.

Once a patient is certain that death is imminent, some very practical matters must be considered.

If the patient docs not have a will, one should be drawn up. If he does have a will, it should be checked with a lawyer to make sure that it is up-to-date and will leave the maximum amount to survivors, not the government. A relative or the executor of the estate should be made aware of any existing life-insurance policies, and the patient and his family should discuss any funeral arrangements. The patient may also want to draw up a *living* will expressing his feelings about the use of heroic measures to keep him alive and about the disposition of his body for scientific purposes.

Although facing the details of death and dying is not pleasant, most patients find that once these things are taken care of, and once death has been discussed in an open way with the people they care about, they gain great peace of mind.

Further Reading

Coping with Cancer

Ernest H. Rosenbaum, *Living with Cancer* (New York: Praeger, 1975).
A general book.

Robert Chernin Cantor, *And a Time to Live* (New York: Harper & Row, 1978).
A general book about maximizing the quality of life.

Orville E. Kelly, *Until Tomorrow Comes* (New York: Everest House, 1979).
This book discusses patients, doctors, and hospitals; support needs of family and friends; readjusting to life (work, sex); the emotional roller coaster; financial aid; religion and cancer; children and cancer; etc.

O. Carl Simonton, Stephanie Matthews-Simonton, and James L. Creighton, *Getting Well Again* (New York: Bantam Books, 1978).
We have recommended this book before in relation to supportive therapies, but it also discusses what the patient can do to promote his own health: It identifies types of thinking that are helpful or harmful to recovery; talks about the role of exercise; offers advice on

dealing with pain and fear, and on how to activate a family support system.

Concrete Problem Solving

Hospitals

Judith Nierenberg and Florence Janovic, *The Hospital Experience* (New York: Bobbs-Merrill, 1978).

Nutrition

Two publications available free (from the Publications Order Department, Office of Communications, National Cancer Institute, Building 31, Room 10A18, Bethesda, Maryland 10105) are particularly useful for both adults and children: *Eating Hints: Recipes and Tips for Better Nutrition During Treatment*, and *Diet and Nutrition, A Resource for Parents of Children with Cancer*.

Other sources for diets and recipes include the American Cancer Society and some of the major cancer centers. Unless otherwise stated, these booklets are free.

"Nutrition for Patients Receiving Chemotherapy and Radiation Treatment." Available from local chapters of the American Cancer Society.
"A Diet Guide for Chemotherapy Patients." Ellis Fischel State Cancer Hospital
Business 70 and Garth Avenue
Columbia, Missouri 65201.
Phone: (314) 449-2711.
"A Guide to Good Nutrition During and After Chemotherapy and Radiation." ($2.00)
Fred Hutchinson Cancer Research Center, Research Kitchen
1124 Columbia Street
Seattle, Washington 98104.
Phone: (206) 292-6301.
"Soft and Blended Foods (for Head and Neck Radiation Patients)." ($1.00)
Mountain States Tumor Institute
Department of Patient and Family Support
151 East Bannock
Boise, Idaho 83702.
Phone: (208) 345-1780.

"Nutritional Guide for Patients Receiving Upper and Lower Abdominal
Radiation Therapy." ($1.00)
Mountain States Tumor Institute (see above).
"Progressive Blenderized Diet." (50¢)
Shands Teaching Hospital and Clinics
Department of Food and Nutrition Services
University of Florida
Gainesville, Florida 32610.
Phone: (904) 392-3575.
"Blenderized Diet."
University of Wisconsin Clinical Cancer Center
Public Affairs Office
1900 University Avenue
Madison, Wisconsin 53705.
Phone: (608) 262-0046.
"Restricted Fiber Diet: High Protein Liquid Diet."
Also available from the University of Wisconsin (above).

Information on how to maximize nutritional intake can be found in
Choices by Marion Morra and Eve Potts (New York: Avon, 1980),
pages 601–11. ($8.95)

Terminality

Parker Rossman, *Hospice* (New York: Fawcett Columbine, 1977).
Sandol Stoddard, *The Hospice Movement* (New York: Vintage, 1978).
Elisabeth Kübler-Ross, *On Death and Dying* (New York: Macmillan,
1978).

Conclusion: Part I

This book was written primarily as a guide to the medical world of
diagnosis and treatment. It is meant to be the starting point of your
search for proper treatment and of your becoming an integral part of
your recovery program. It is not a replacement for discussions with
your oncologist. By this time you have read enough to understand
that "meaningful information" for a cancer patient is very detailed
information: You can only get that from your own treatment team.

We have purposely not discussed in depth those topics that have
already been handled well in other books. We have referred you to
many sources throughout part I, and more will be given in part II
(but these are books and articles that deal only with specific types of

179

cancer). Because we realize that most people will not have the time or opportunity to read all the material recommended, we will conclude part I with a list of books that, read in conjunction with this one, will make you a rather well-informed nonprofessional.

Basic Cancer Library for the Layman

Cancer Biology, Epidemiology, Research, and
Nonstandard Treatments

Mark Renneker and Steven Leib, eds., *Understanding Cancer* (Palo Alto: Bull Publishing, 1979). $12.95

Lucien Israel, *Conquering Cancer* (New York: Vintage, 1978). $2.95

Samuel S. Epstein, *The Politics of Cancer* (San Francisco: Sierra Club Books, 1978). $6.95

Ralph W. Moss, *The Cancer Syndrome* (New York: Grove Press, 1980). $12.95

Hospitals and Surgery

Judith Nierenberg and Florence Janovic, *The Hospital Experience: A Complete Guide to Understanding and Participating in Your Own Care* (New York: Bobbs-Merrill, 1978). $7.95

Lawrence Galton, *The Patient's Guide to Surgery* (New York: Avon, 1976). $2.50

Paul J. Melluzzo and Eleanor Nealson, *Living with Surgery* (New York: Lorenz Press, 1979). $9.95

Living with Cancer

O. Carl Simonton, Stephanie Matthews-Simonton, and James L. Creighton, *Getting Well Again* (New York: Bantam, 1978). $2.75

David Bresler, *Free Yourself from Pain* (New York: Simon and Schuster, 1978). $12.95

Orville E. Kelly, *Until Tomorrow Comes* (New York: Everest House, 1979). $9.95

Parker Rossman, *Hospice* (New York: Fawcett Columbine, 1979). $4.95.

PART II

Specific Cancers

Ampulla of Vater
(Papilla of Vater, Hepatopancreatica)

The ampulla of Vater is the bottom end of the common bile duct, which comes out of the liver, gallbladder, and pancreas, carrying bile and other secretions to the small intestines. Cancers of this site are very rare and causes are unknown. They may be considered cancers of the **pancreas.**

Symptoms
Jaundice (caused by obstruction of the bile ducts); abdominal pain; weight loss; nausea; chills; and anemia.

Diagnosis
After taking a **medical history** and doing a complete **physical examination,** the patient will have **X-rays** taken, particularly a special X-ray called a hypotonic duodenography, which looks at the muscle tone of the duodenum. A special type of **cholangiogram** called a transhepatic percutaneous cholangiogram will examine the bile ducts (see "Pancreas" for an explanation of the procedure), and an **upper G.I. endoscopy** (duodenoscopy) will be done.

Types of Cancers
Papillary cancer is the most common type; *adenocarcinomas* may also be found. These tumors are of low-grade malignancy and are often confused with benign tumors. The cancer spreads locally to the walls of the common bile ducts and the head of the pancreas, and may spread to nearby lymph nodes.

Treatment
The standard treatment is **surgery,** using a procedure called a pancreaticoduodenectomy. See "Pancreas" for details.

Experimental Treatments
Experimental treatments are being conducted using **radiation** and **chemotherapy** in addition to surgery. This cancer is often not diagnosed until after it has spread, so the outlook for patients is poor. Contact: EST, MDA, MSKCC, NCOG, NCCTG, RPMI, RTOG, SEG, SWOG, SFCC, UCLA, CAN-UICC (see appendix H).

Doctors Who May Be Involved in Treatment
Abdominal surgeon, gastroenterologist, medical oncologist, therapeutic radiologist.

Anus

See "Large Intestine."

Bladder, Ureters, and Urethra

Urine is manufactured in the kidneys and travels through tubes called ureters to the bladder, which acts as a reservoir. The urine is discharged through the urethra, a tube that runs from the bladder to the outside of the body. Cancers of the bladder account for 3% of all cancers; cancers of the ureters and urethra are quite rare. Bladder cancers are more common in men than women, and particularly affect the 50–70 age group.

The prognosis for bladder cancers varies enormously, depending on the type of cancer, how early it is detected, and where it is located. Superficial, early tumors have the best prognosis; long-term survival after metastasis has occurred is very rare. With endoscopic removal of superficial tumors, 80% of patients examined in a recent study survived five years or longer. Advanced bladder cancer, cancers of the urethra, and cancers that have spread to the lymphatic system have a much poorer prognosis, and in these cases experimental treatment programs should be considered.

In certain occupations, exposure to various chemicals can cause bladder cancer. These include: aniline dye, used in rubber and cable industries; aromatic amines, used by rubber workers, textile workers, paint manufacturers, and dyestuff users; coal soot, coal tar, and other products of coal combustion encountered by gashouse workers, stokers, and producers; asphalt, coal tar, and pitch workers; leather used by leather and shoe workers.

Schistosoma, a parasitic infection common in the tropics, has been implicated as a cause of bladder cancer. It enters the body through the foot and then buries itself in the wall of the bladder.

There is also conclusive proof that cigarettes are a cause of bladder cancer, particularly when used with coffee, which may also be carcinogenic to the bladder.

There has been a great deal of controversy about the use of saccharin, an artificial sweetener. It, too, may be a carcinogen in bladder cancer, but its effects are far less severe than the effects of industrial exposure.

Chronic bladder infections and congenital abnormalities of the urinary organs may also predispose a patient to bladder cancer, although this has not been conclusively proven.

Symptoms

Blood in the urine; fever; sharp, cramplike pain in the back; painful, difficult, and/or frequent urination.

Diagnosis and Staging

In the doctor's office a complete **medical history** will be taken, with emphasis on problems within the urinary tract. A physical examination will follow, during which the doctor, using rubber gloves, will feel the urinary tract by inserting one hand into the vagina or rectum while pressing on the outside of the abdomen with the other hand. This manual (digital) examination is done without anesthetic and is uncomfortable but not painful. Samples of blood and urine may be taken in the office. Laboratory tests on these samples include urinalysis, CBC, and a urine sediment smear, serum chloride and blood-urea nitrogen test. A catheterization (insertion of a slender tube into the urethra) may be performed to get a clean urine sample. Again, this procedure is uncomfortable but not painful.

Numerous tests will take place in the hospital to find out what cell type of cancer is involved and how far it has spread. The tests and procedures may include **X-rays** of the chest and abdomen; **IVP; cystoscopy;** cystogram (a catheter is inserted into the bladder, dye is injected, and X-rays are taken to watch the bladder fill up under controlled conditions; it is done in the radiology department without anesthesia); **bone scan; liver scan; ultrasound; lymphangiogram;** and cystourethrogram (similar to the cystogram, except both the urethra and the bladder are watched during urination; the test is usually done on an outpatient basis in the Radiology Department without anesthesia).

There are several methods of staging bladder cancers. Some are very complex. The easiest method uses a three-stage system: (1) superficial stage (no invasion): low-grade cancer; (2) deep stage (invasion of bladder muscles and/or wall): high-grade cancer; (3) metastatic stage (spread outside the bladder): high-grade cancer.

Types of Cancers

Some tumors are slow-growing, localized, and easy to treat; others are fast-growing, hard to treat, and spread rapidly by invasion and through the bloodstream and lymph system to such sites as the liver, lung, and bones. Sometimes bladder-tumor symptoms are mistaken for prostatic disease since they are very similar. Bladder tumors may be single or multiple. The most important factor in diagnosis is how far the tumor has invaded the bladder wall: Deep invasion usually means the tumor is highly malignant.

The bladder consists of the epithelium, which is the covering (or lining); the muscles of the bladder wall; and the bladder itself. Most bladder tumors are epithelial.

Papillomas may be benign or malignant and may remain localized in the bladder for a long time. *Polyps*, or *"balloon" tumors*, grow like balloons in the lining of the bladder. They do not invade the muscles of the bladder and are fairly easy to remove by surgery. *"Lava" tumors* tend to invade and, since they destroy the bladder wall, require the removal of the entire bladder.

Transitional-cell carcinomas are common, fast-growing, invasive cancers that often involve the lymph nodes in the pelvis. *Adeno-carcinomas* are rare and at times inoperable. *Squamous-cell carcinomas* are also rare, and very invasive.

The bladder may also become a site for the spread of cancers originating in the colon, uterus, and cervix.

Treatment

Surgery. Depending on the type and stage of the cancer, surgical procedures may involve removal of the tumor alone, or part of the bladder, or all of the bladder.

Certain procedures use a **cystoscope** (a type of endoscope—see chapter 5) to remove superficial tumors by cutting or burning (fulguration) after a small flexible tube has been inserted either through the urethra (this technique is also used to control bleeding in advanced cases) or through a small slit in the abdominal wall. The first procedure is called transurethral resection; the second, endoscopic resection. Both can be done on an outpatient basis using local anesthetic.

Removal of part of the bladder requires major surgery for which the patient must remain in the hospital for seven to ten days. For large localized tumors at the dome of bladder, a segmental bladder resection (also called segmental resection or partial cystectomy) may be done— which simply means removing part of the bladder. The patient can urinate normally after surgery.

Total, or radical, cystectomy is the removal of the entire bladder. This operation is performed when tests have proven that a very malignant tumor has spread beyond the confines of the bladder. Nearby organs are also removed: in men, the prostate and part of the urethra.

When the bladder is removed, the surgeon must create another way for the body to dispose of urine—an "artificial bladder." There are three methods of doing this. The first is called the ilial loop: A part of the small intestine is disconnected to be used as a natural tube; the ureters are attached to the loop, which runs to the abdominal wall and links up with a tube connected through a permanent slit in the abdomen. The tube empties into a disposable bag that the patient wears on the outside of his body, either strapped to the abdomen or leg.

The second method is the creation of a rectal bladder. A colostomy is performed (see "Large Intestine") so that solid wastes drain through the abdomen into an external disposable plastic bag. The ureters are run into the rectum itself, and the patient urinates through his rectum.

The last, and perhaps least desirable, method is the ureterocutaneous bladder, wherein the ureters are connected directly to a bag on the outside of the body.

All three methods usually require hospitalization for two to three weeks. The creation of an artificial bladder means a change in lifestyle for the patient and a period of adjustment. In the hospital, the patient will be taught by nurses and volunteers from the United Ostomy Association how to use and clean the ostomy bag, and how to care for the skin.

Although it may take a little time to get used to wearing a bag and caring for it, most people are able to lead perfectly normal lives. The bag does not emit odors and is not visible under clothes. Women are still able to have children. Removal of the bladder can cause impotence in men, however, and both men and women become very susceptible to urinary infections.

Since there may be a period of psychological adjustment following this surgery, it often helps if patients are able to talk to others who have had similar surgery. The United Ostomy Association has branches nationwide, and is of tremendous help in counseling patients and introducing them to other patients with ostomy devices.

Radiation may be used prior to surgery to destroy deeply invasive tumors or retard tumor growth. Early localized or superficial tumors can be treated successfully with external radiation, and radiation has been used alone to treat tumors that have not extensively invaded the bladder wall. But it can produce side effects, such as damage to the bowel and a hemorrhagic bladder. When radiation is used instead of surgery, it is usually only because the tumor's location makes it inaccessible, or because the patient's general health is too poor for surgery. Radiation therapy may also be used when surgical measures have failed, or when the lesion changes and becomes more invasive. Radiation therapy is used to treat pelvic-node metastases and in metastatic cancers if there is pain and bleeding. Cancer of the ureter has also been treated with radiation therapy, particularly in advanced cases.

The type of radiation used depends on the type of cancer. The intracavitary method has been successfully used for superficial lesions. Gold radon seeds are implanted in the bladder or ureter, left in place for approximately seventy-two hours, and then removed. Since the treatment uses radioactive material, this treatment involves a hospital stay of about a week. Temporary side effects may include diarrhea and the urge to urinate frequently at night.

For larger tumors that invade the bladder wall, surgery may be performed, followed by the implantation described above.

For deep lesions, supervoltage radiation is used in addition to surgery. The treatment regimen and dosage depend on the tumor, but the radiation may begin five to six weeks after surgery in a fairly high dosage, followed by a much smaller dose some weeks later. The dosage will include radiation to the pelvic nodes.

Side effects from radiation may occur a few days after treatment has stopped or may develop anywhere from six months to a year after treatment. Diarrhea, painful and frequent urination, and nocturia are common problems soon after radiation; late side effects may include persistent cystitis, colitis, hemorrhage of the bladder, and possible bleeding and obstruction of the bowel.

Chemotherapy is not used as a primary treatment for bladder cancer, and has had only limited standard use, mainly in the form of adjuvant therapy following surgery for superficial lesions. This consists of local instillation of a drug called thio-TEPA, given weekly for about six weeks (it may be repeated) in order to lessen the chance of recurrence. There are many experimental treatment plans, however, that make use of chemotherapy (see below).

Experimental Treatments

Surgery, radiation, and **chemotherapy** (both single-agent and combination) are being tried in various combined-treatment plans. Contact: EST, MDA, MSKCC, SFCC, NBCCGA, NBCP, NCOG, RTOG, SEG, SWOG, UROG (see appendix H).

Doctors Who May Be Involved in Treatment

Gastroenterologist, abdominal surgeon, therapeutic radiologist, medical oncologist.

Resources

See "Large Intestine" for support services if an ostomy is part of treatment.

Bone Cancers

"Bone cancer" is a term that refers to a wide range of cancers that affect all of the musculoskeletal system: not only the bones, bone marrow, and cartilage, but also the soft and fibrous tissue found in muscles and fat, and the various types of blood and lymph cells manufactured in the bone. Reticulum-cell sarcoma, although originating in the bone marrow, is usually classified as a type of lymphoma and will be discussed under "Lymphomas (Non-Hodgkin's)."

In this discussion we will divide the broad group of "bone cancers" into three groups: cancers of the bone, bone-marrow, and cartilage; soft-tissue sarcomas; and myelomas. Myelomas are also classified as blood tumors, but originate in bone marrow, so will be discussed here.

These cancers tend to spread easily, and usually are not diagnosed until they are well advanced. Different types of bone cancers appear to favor different age groups. Primary bone cancers make up less than 1% of known cancers, although it is common for other types of cancer to spread to the bone.

Cancers of the Bone, Bone Marrow, and Cartilage

Symptoms

Bone or joint pain is the most common symptom, although the specific description of the pain varies from individual to individual: Sometimes it is worse at night; sometimes it is relieved by exercise; sometimes it is aggravated by exercise; sometimes swelling and fever come before, during, or after the pain. Bone cancers are difficult to diagnose because the symptoms are easily confused with arthritis, bursitis, or benign tumors.

Diagnostic Procedures

Although specific tests vary, the following procedures are common: **chest X-ray; skeletal survey (X-rays); bone scan; blood and urine tests,** including **alkaline** and **acid phosphatase tests, serum calcium tests;** and **bone biopsy (aspiration** or **open).**

Types of Cancers and Treatments

Osteogenic sarcoma (osteosarcoma) is the most common type of bone cancer found in children and young adults (most commonly in taller-than-average adolescents). The cause is as yet not known, but studies indicate possible involvement of an increased production of a growth chemical and a virus or other infectious agent. It starts in the bone and cartilage, and spreads into the bone marrow, muscles, lungs, and liver. Because of the pattern of spread, lung **tomograms** and **liver scans** are used in diagnosis in addition to the other procedures.

189

Standard treatment of osteogenic sarcoma involves **surgery** (amputation of the involved limb) as well as external **radiation** and **chemotherapy** to stop the development of metastases. (Radiation cannot be used alone on the primary tumor because it is radioresistant.) Experimental treatments include refinements in chemotherapy and radiotherapy techniques and immunotherapy. Combinations are being tried to eliminate the need for amputation.

Although osteogenic sarcoma has had a poor survival rate (15–20%), the interim reports coming from experimental programs are showing dramatic improvements. The data are not complete, but it is thought that the new generation of treatments may change the survival rate to 60+%. There has recently been some question as to whether the increased survival rates are due to the effects of the new treatment or are the results of technological advances in diagnostic techniques which permit a greater percentage of cases to be diagnosed in the early stages.

For information on Experimental Treatments, contact: CCG, CLB, RTOG, SWOG, MAYO, MDAR, SFCC, CHOC, CAN-NCIC, CAN-UICC (see appendix H).

Ewing's sarcoma is a common childhood cancer (although it can occur to age 30) that starts in the marrow of the long bones. It affects males more often than females. It spreads rapidly to other bones and to the lungs and brain, making the **liver scan** and **brain scan** a usual part of the diagnostic procedure.

Standard treatment uses external **radiation** and **chemotherapy**. Recent advances in experimental treatments have made the prognosis quite hopeful (50% survive). Often long-term chemotherapy is used, and at times **surgery** is used to remove the tumor. Experimental programs are being conducted by SWOG and SJCRH.

Chondrosarcoma is a slow-growing tumor that starts in the cartilage at the end of the large bones. It tends to occur in middle-aged individuals, the most common symptom being joint swelling accompanied by pain. At times **arteriograms** are used in diagnosis. Since the tumor does not respond to radiation or chemicals, **surgery** is the standard treatment, often involving amputation of the limb.

Chordomas are very rare tumors arising at the end of the spinal cord or near the base of the skull. Pain in the region at the end of the spinal cord is most typical for those tumors growing in that region; tumors growing at the base of the skull produce symptoms that involve the cranial nerves, most commonly the nerves of the eyes. Symptoms may last for months. These tumors grow slowly and spread by invasion. Because of their location and the fact that they are relatively radiosensitive, they are generally treated by **radiation**. Experimental treatment plans using **chemotherapy** are showing some promise.

Experimental treatments on a wide range of bone sarcomas are being conducted by: EST, MAYO, MDA, MSKCC, SFCC, CHOP, SEG, SWOG, WCCC, and WFU (see appendix H).

Soft-Tissue Sarcomas

These tumors are rare and have some very frustrating characteristics. Although treatable by **surgery, radiation,** and **chemotherapy,** and combinations of these, they have an annoying tendency to come back. Because they arise in the muscle and fat that is found throughout the body, they can occur almost anywhere and spread easily and quickly. The prognosis for patients varies tremendously not only with the type of soft-tissue sarcoma but also with the chances of recurrence: The general five-year survival rate is 60% after surgery if it doesn't recur, but only 30% if the tumors recur and have to be removed again.

Symptoms

These are often first noticed as firm, painless lumps that grow in a muscle or under the skin, resembling benign tumors. At times weight loss, fever, and hypoglycemia (a blood-sugar disorder) may be symptoms. Some fibrosarcomas can cause endocrine disorders such as goiter, or, depending on the location of the tumor, can cause numbness and pain if there is pressure on nerves or reduction of blood supply.

Diagnosis

Diagnostic procedures include **skeletal survey (X-ray); CBC; SMA-12; X-ray (chest); bone scan; biopsy (excisional); arteriograms; and liver scan.**

Types of Soft-Tissue Sarcomas

Soft-tissue sarcomas are divided into groups named for the types of tissue in which they develop: *Fibrosarcomas* come from the fibrous tissue: *liposarcomas* grow from fatty tissues; *rhabdomyosarcomas* and *leiomyosarcomas* come from muscle tissue; *angiosarcomas* and *lymphangiosarcomas* come from the vascular tissue that our veins, arteries, and lymph channels are made from; *synovial sarcomas* come from the cells that form the sheathing around tendons and the fluid around joints.

Fibrosarcomas are most frequently found in patients between the ages of fifty and seventy, but may also occur in children. Standard

191

treatment is **surgery** followed by **radiation** and/or **chemotherapy** for metastases.

Liposarcomas are fairly large tumors that tend to spread to the lungs. They are most common in patients between the ages of 40 and 60. They are removed by **surgery** followed by **radiation.**

Rhabdomyosarcomas are the most common soft-tissue sarcoma of childhood (2–6) and spread very quickly; the swelling, bleeding, and lumps can be found anywhere in the body. In addition to the general diagnostic procedures, a **brain scan, IVP,** and/or **cystoscopy** may be done, depending on the location of the tumor. Treatment usually consists of radical **surgery, radiation,** and **chemotherapy,** possibly extending over two years. Rhabdomyosarcomas are divided into three types: *adult pleomorphic,* which occurs in older patients in the muscles of the arms and legs; *embryonal alveolar,* affecting children and young adults, also in the arms and legs; and *embryonal botryoid,* again found in children but occurring in the head and neck, the eye, and the genitourinary tract. The prognosis varies with the stage of the disease, the size and location of the tumor, the extent of spread, and the age of the patient, adults having a better prognosis.

Experimental treatments: CLB, EST, SEG, SWOG, MDAR, MSKCC, SFCC, MAYO, CHOP, WCCC, and WFU (see appendix H).

Myelomas

Myelomas grow from the bone marrow, affecting both bone and plasma cells. Because they involve components of both blood and bone, they may be classified as either hematologic tumors or bone tumors.

Multiple myeloma is an adult disease usually seen in patients over 50 years of age. The disease is characterized by widespread bone destruction, with cancer cells replacing normal bone cells. The disease spreads rapidly, causing multiple fractures, particularly of the vertebrae, and leaving the patient open to infections, possible kidney failure, and an excess of calcium in the blood (hypercalcemia).

Symptoms include severe bone pain, especially in the back; fatigue; anemia; improperly functioning kidneys; broken bones (ribs, vertebrae, pelvis, or skull).

Diagnostic procedures may include laboratory analysis of blood and urine (including the Bence-Jones protein test, CBC, paper electrophoresis, and immunoelectrophoresis tests); **bone marrow** aspiration for **biopsy;** and a myelogram, in which dye is injected into the fluid around the spinal cord, followed by an **X-ray.**

Standard treatment is palliative rather than curative. External radiation may be given for bone pain. **Chemotherapy** may be used on a long-term basis, either in low doses or intermittent high doses. This is a rapidly progressing disease with a poor prognosis for cure. With treatment, patients can live as long as five years; without treatment, life expectancy is about a year.

Other myelomas include *plasmacytoma* (caused by abnormal protein metabolism) and *plasma-cell myelomas*. Both are primarily older-adult diseases and are similar in diagnostic and treatment details to the description of multiple myeloma.

Experimental Treatments

CLB, EST, SEG, SWOG, WCG, MDA, MSKCC, WCCC, CAN-NCIC (see appendix H).

Doctors Who May Be Involved in Treatment

Orthopedic surgeon, hematologist, medical oncologist, therapeutic radiologist.

Further Reading and Resources

In addition to the supportive services listed in the chapters "Children with Cancer," "Living with Cancer," and "Surgery," the National Cancer Institute is sponsoring a program on sensory-feedback leg prostheses for cancer patients. Contact:

Dr. Frank Clippinger, Principal Investigator
Duke University Medical Center
Department of Surgery
P.O. Box 2919
Durham, North Carolina 27710

Besides the rehabilitation programs available in large hospital centers for amputees—programs that include physical rehabilitation, training in the use of prosthetic devices, and psychological rehabilitation—each state has a department of rehabilitation that offers extensive support services, many of them free. If you are a veteran, contact the Veterans Administration for rehabilitation and support services in your area.

Brain and Central Nervous System (CNS)

Cancers of the brain and CNS account for only 3% of all cancers; 85% appear in adults, particularly in the 50–60 age range, with the remainder found in children. Males are more commonly affected than females. Because they grow in an enclosed space, often unreachable by surgery or radiation, and because chemotherapy has only been minimally effective (although experimental combined treatments are being conducted), the mortality rate with brain tumors in high—over 50%.

The brain is a complex, compact organ that is usually mapped out by regions. Viewed from the top, the first thing one encounters is the cerebrum. This takes up the most space in the brain, and is divided into two halves—the left and right hemispheres. Each of these is divided into lobes (frontal, parietal, occipital, and temporal). The functions of the cerebrum include thought, judgment, memory, and speech. The lower, back part of the brain is called the cerebellum; it functions as a center for the coordination of muscle movements and balance. Toward the center of each hemisphere of the brain are the ventricles, which are spaces filled with fluid that act as shock absorbers for the nerve tissue.

At the very base of the brain is the brainstem—actually the top end of the spinal cord—which contains the nerve fibers that regulate heartbeat, breathing, and sleep. The spinal cord is a column of nerve tissues and carries all the nerves that affect the limbs and lower part of the body. It is also the pathway that carries the impulses going to and from the brain.

Tumors in the brain and CNS are not uncommon, but most are benign. However, because of the problems caused by their location, benign tumors must be treated as seriously as malignant ones. Since tumors of this "site" can vary so much in location, depth, and rate of growth, you should ask your doctor for the details of how the grading and staging classifications described in chapter 2 relate specifically to the type of cancer you are concerned about. Also, most malignant brain tumors are metastatic: The brain is a common site of metastases that originate in tumors of the breast, lung, and kidney, and from Hodgkin's disease. These are generally treated with **radiation** and **chemotherapy**, rather than surgery.

Many brain tumors cannot be removed because of their location within the brain, and therefore have a very poor prognosis. The prognosis varies with the location of the tumor—deep tumors are much more difficult to treat than surface tumors. Patients have been known to live for many years with a surface or low-grade tumor. Advanced malignant tumors are usually not treatable and grow rapidly, with a survival rate of about two years. In children, astrocytomas completely removed surgically are curable, while brainstem gliomas that cannot be completely removed are not.

194

Symptoms

The symptoms of these tumors vary enormously, depending on where they are located. They may include personality changes; loss of memory; confusion; severe headaches; nausea and vomiting; seizures; visual disturbances; muscle weakness; loss of balance; poor coordination; loss of the sense of smell; partial hearing loss; ringing in the ears; pressure on the brain; fluid accumulation; paralysis of nerves in face, teeth, etc.; pain in the back. In children, the most common symptoms include nausea and vomiting, frequent falling and difficulty walking, vision problems, and hydrocephalus (an enlarged head caused by fluid accumulation).

Diagnostic Procedures

A complete medical history and physical examination will be done, including examination of the eyes and ears. In addition, the following procedures may be done: **X-rays**—a chest X-ray to make sure the suspected tumor has not metastasized from the lung; skull X-rays to check for enlargement of the brain, increased intracranial pressure, or the presence of calcification; and spinal cord X-rays. A **mammogram** will be done to check for breast cancer as the primary site. **CAT scans** have proven effective in diagnosing brain tumors with 98% accuracy. A **brain scan, electroencephalogram, cerebral angiogram, ventriculogram, pneumoencephalogram, spinal puncture,** and **myelogram** may be done. Laboratory tests will be done on blood, urine, and spinal-fluid protein (for spinal-cord tumors).

Types of Cancers

Approximately half of all brain tumors are *gliomas,* which grow from the brain tissue itself. These are broken down further into four groups:

Glioblastoma multiforme accounts for half of all gliomas, is very fast-growing and malignant, affects adults and children, and may be found in the cerebrum, cerebellum, brainstem, and spinal cord. It results in swelling, hemorrhaging, and the death of brain tissue itself, and has the ability to spread from one side of the brain to the other.

Astrocytomas are slow-growing, can be either benign or malignant, recur rapidly, and are found in the cerebellum and brainstem, most often in children. These tumors are curable in children.

Ependymomas are also found most frequently in children, but are located in the ventricles, are fast-growing, invasive, highly malignant, have a rapid recurrence rate, and cannot be removed surgically.

Oligodendrogliomas grow in the white matter of the frontal lobe of the brain, are found in adults and children, and are slow-growing, but

195

they can become very large and they have a tendency to recur. They can be either benign or malignant and are extremely rare.

Medulloblastomas are childhood gliomas that are very malignant and spread to other parts of the brain and central nervous system from the cerebellum.

Other fast-growing, malignant gliomas found mainly in children include gliomas of the brainstem and optic nerve, and *pinealomas (germinomas)* which are found in the pineal body and spinal columns.

Twenty percent of brain tumors are *meningiomas,* which grow from the meninges—the membrane covering the brain and spinal cord. These are slow-growing tumors, benign or malignant, but may grow quite large and can cause bone destruction.

Pituitary adenomas comprise another 15% of brain tumors. As they grow they tend to affect the optic nerve (causing vision problems) and compress the hypothalamus, which can lead to diabetes. As gland tissues become destroyed, growth-hormone production is affected. These tumors are found in both adults and children.

There is a grab bag of other tumor types that arise in the brain and central nervous system. *Ganglioneuroblastomas* affect the nerve cells in both adults and children, are fast-growing and malignant. *Neurofibrosarcomas* are similar to ganglioneuroblastomas but are found in nerves located in the peripheral nervous system. The most common form is *acoustic neuroma,* affecting the acoustical nerve (see also **ear**). *Schwannomas* and *glioblastomas* are usually found in adults. *Neuroblastomas* are the second most common childhood cancer, usually found in children under 3 years of age. It is a nerve cancer and can originate in, or spread to, many parts of the body—most commonly the abdomen, chest, eye, adrenal gland, neck, and lower back. It is most effectively treated in children under 2. Congenital tumors appear to be linked to genetic malfunctions. Although the "program" for the growth of these tumors is present at birth, they can remain undetected until adulthood.

Nearly 15% of all brain tumors are metastatic—they have spread to the brain from another site.

Treatment

Surgery. The treatment of central-nervous-system tumors is largely surgical when possible. If a tumor cannot be completely removed by surgery, it usually means it is incurable. Surgery is sometimes followed by postoperative radiation, but it is not always successful. Chemotherapy is sometimes used in combination with surgery and radiation, but with very little success. Chemotherapy used alone thus far has not been successful. Radiation therapy can relieve the symptoms of malignant tumors and can retard the growth of recurrent tumors. Radiation also provides palliative relief from the pain of symptoms.

Tumors of the brain are extremely difficult to remove completely by surgery without damaging the brain. The operation—called a craniotomy—must be performed by a board-certified neurosurgeon, and usually requires a two- to three-week hospital stay. It may be performed under a local anesthetic, but is usually done with a general. It involves cutting the scalp and removing a section of the skull so that the surgeon can see the tumor and the extent of its growth. The tumor is removed with as much normal tissue around it as possible to minimize recurrence. The piece of skull is put back in place and the scalp sutured. After surgery, radiation is used to retard the growth of any remaining tumor.

Radiation. In some cases when the tumor is too deep-seated for surgery, radiation is used alone. Brainstem tumors, for example, are usually located deep within the brain on the top of the brainstem. Since the brainstem controls breathing and heartbeat, and the only way to get to the tumors is to cut this vital tissue, it is an inoperable tumor.

Radiation therapy is the only form of therapy capable of curing medulloblastoma after surgery. The treatment of medulloblastoma may take as long as four to five months since radiation therapy is also given to the spinal cord. Ependymomas are also radiosensitive.

Radiation therapy is usually indicated if a tumor is centrally located; if surgery cannot be attempted due to the tumor's location and involvement with vital structures; for metastases; and for tumors such as medulloblastomas and pituitary tumors.

The dose is determined by the tumor type, the site of the tumor, and the level of tolerance. Sometimes the dosage is increased gradually.

Complications of radiation therapy include immediate postoperative brain swelling, which is temporary. Since radiation interferes with bone growth, there may be permanent damage to the spinal cord in children. Occasionally, vascular changes may lead to infarction or necrosis within the brain, resembling a stroke.

Hormone Therapy. Steroids, such as Decadron, are sometimes given orally before and after surgery to relieve some of the symptoms and to decrease the amount of swelling in the brain; this swelling can be fatal if the brain presses too tightly against the skull. Steroids may also be used to treat metastatic brain tumors, and cortisone may be given upon diagnosis of a secondary brain tumor.

The administration of steroids results in almost immediate relief of brain swelling. The dose is gradually reduced, and the patient may then be maintained on a drug such as prednisone for the rest of his

197

life. Prednisone, which is an adrenocorticosteroid, may be given intravenously or intramuscularly. Dexamethasone may also be given via the same methods or by mouth on alternate days. The therapy may produce improvement not only in intracranial metastases but also in spinal-cord compression. Sometimes these drugs are used concurrently with radiation therapy.

Other forms of treatment. Radiosensitizers, which make the tumor more responsive to radiation, are currently being tested. Cryosurgery (freezing) is being used on pituitary tumors in addition to radiation therapy. After treatment, the patient may be maintained on hormone therapy indefinitely since the pituitary gland has probably been destroyed by the radiation treatment. Lowering the temperature of the body or brain (hypothermia) during brain surgery has also been tried. This method is still under investigation and not widely used.

Experimental Treatments

Although surgery and radiation techniques are constantly being refined and are a part of many experimental treatment plans, the major effort is a search for chemotherapy treatments that can prevent recurrence and get at cancers that cannot be reached by surgery and radiation. Until recently, these efforts had not shown promising results. This was due to the effect of the "blood-brain barrier"—a special defense system in the brain's capillary walls that does not allow substances circulating in the bloodstream to enter the brain. This blood-brain barrier has prevented chemotherapy drugs from entering the brain tissues, and therefore from reaching brain tumors.

A new group of drugs, called nitrosoureas, can penetrate this barrier. These investigational drugs are CCNU (or Lomustine) and BCNU. At this time, the most success has been reported using BCNU plus radiation to treat spinal-cord tumors.

The most exciting news involves the drug cis-Platinum. In September 1980, researchers at Georgetown University in Washington, D.C., announced very dramatic preliminary results in treating children with recurrent brain cancer. Currently, researchers at Yale and the Mayo Clinic are using the drug experimentally with adults. Besides the direct cancer-killing effect on the tumor itself, cis-Platinum also appears to make the cancer cells more radiosensitive. Readers should be cautioned that these are very preliminary results, and it will be five or six years before researchers have detailed information on the effectiveness and best use of the drug, not only in terms of dosage but also how and when to combine it with other forms of treatment.

Clinical cooperative groups: BTSG, CCG, EST, NCOG, RTOG, SWOG, MAYO, MDA, BTRC, CCSF, CHOC, YALE, CAN-UCIC (see appendix H).

Resources and Support

For children with brain and central-nervous-system cancers, see chapter 13, "Children with Cancer." NOTE: It is particularly important that children with medulloblastoma and neuroblastoma be treated at a major cancer center or children's hospital with a large, experienced pediatric-oncology treatment team. These cancers are very fast-growing and malignant, but they do respond to complex combination treatments with surgical, radiological, and chemotherapeutic components.

Breast

Breasts (also called mammary glands) frequently develop lumps. Eighty percent of these lumps are not cancerous; but the 20% that are make breast cancer the leading form of cancer among women aged thirty-five to seventy-four, and the number-two cancer among women aged fifteen to thirty-four. (Breast cancer is also found in men, but in far fewer numbers.) There appears to be a link between breast cancer and the activity of a female hormone called estrogen: first, because the course of breast cancer before and after menopause (when hormone production slows down) is quite different (and different types of treatment will be prescribed depending on which group the patient falls into); and second, because some of the specific cancers respond to the presence or absence of estrogen; those that are called estrogen-dependent need estrogen in order to live.

Women at highest risk of developing breast cancer are over 54, with a previous history of breast cancer and/or a history of breast cancer in the family (mother or sister). Women in the following groups have a higher than average risk of developing breast cancer: history of breast cancer in a maternal or paternal grandmother, father's sister, or mother's sister; history of cystic disease in the breasts; birth of first baby after age 30; never have had children; early onset of menstruation and late menopause; excessive exposure to ionizing radiation (either work with radiation or have had radiation treatments); history of cancer of the uterus, ovary, or colon; those who are obese; those who have undergone estrogen-replacement therapy.

Breast cancers affect 6% of all women in the United States. They appear more often in the left breast than in the right. More than half of all patients develop metastases or have metastases present at the time of diagnosis. Breast cancers metastasize most frequently to the lymph nodes, lungs, bone, and brain.

Different types of breast cancer have a wide range of growth rates: Some are extremely slow-growing and take over a year to double in size; others grow so quickly that they can double in a week. Because it is possible that a breast-cancer patient has a fast-growing kind that has already spread at the time of diagnosis (or may spread in a short time), breast-cancer patients should confirm diagnosis and begin treatment quickly—within a few weeks of spotting the lump. This will not be an easy task, because the patient will need to consult at least two surgeons, a therapeutic radiologist, and a medical oncologist. As we will explain below, the choices a patient must make regarding which doctors to go to and what treatment to get are broader and more serious than for many other types of cancer.

To help you understand what choices are involved and what specific questions to ask, we strongly recommend two books. The first is *Breast Cancer Digest: A Guide to Medical Care, Emotional Support, Educational Programs and Resources* put out by the National Cancer Institute in 1979. It is available free from the Communications Office, National Cancer Institute, Building 31, Room 10A18, Bethesda, Maryland 20205. You may also be able to get it at your local library, in hospital or medical libraries, or through a hospital social worker or your local chapter of the American Cancer Society. The second book is *Why Me?* by Rose Cushner (New York: Signet, 1977; $2.50). It is available at most bookstores and supermarkets and is an even more complete book than *Breast Cancer Digest.* You should get these books at the point when you *suspect* you may have cancer: Although we will cover the main points of diagnosis and treatment in this section, it is clear from the length of these books (*Why Me?* is 350+ pages) that the subject cannot be covered completely in a volume of this kind.

Symptoms

The first symptoms of breast cancer are usually a painless movable lump in the breast or under the arm, unusual discharge from the nipple, or retraction of the nipple. Sometimes the skin over the lump resembles an orange peel in texture (rough and thickened); this is called "peau d'orange."

As the tumor grows, the symptoms become more obvious: There may be pain and redness, and sometimes the mass becomes immobile. If the mass has been present for a while and is malignant, the axillary lymph nodes—between the upper part of the chest and the armpit—are already positive (there is cancer present) in 50% of all cases. If the lump has been present for some months, the lymph nodes will be positive in over 68% of the cases diagnosed.

The symptoms of breast cancer may vary according to the type of cancer involved: For instance, in inflammatory carcinoma, the skin of the breast is red, warm, swollen, and painful; and in Paget's disease, the nipple becomes crusted.

After a patient has had surgery for breast cancer, she should be carefully followed by her physician for any evidence of recurrence. Even when there are no symptoms, evidence of new growth may be found via **physical examination, X-rays,** and **scans.** Bone pain may be symptomatic of recurrent breast cancer that has metastasized to the bones. Chest pain and shortness of breath may indicate lung metastases, and anorexia or weight loss may mean there has been liver involvement.

Diagnosis and Staging

Ninety percent of all breast cancers are discovered by the patient (or her husband or lover) feeling (palpating) the tumor. The doctor will also palpate the breast and the axilla (armpit area, where the lymph nodes are located). As a rule, lumps that are movable and rubbery are benign; hard, immovable lumps are usually cancerous. All lumps should be explored immediately. After palpating the breasts, doing a thorough **physical examination,** and taking a **medical history,** the physician may ask you to go through a series of procedures.

The first group of procedures examines the whole breast. A **mammogram** is a soft tissue X-ray which is highly reliable (98%) in detecting breast cancer. A similar procedure called xeromammography (**xerography**) may also be scheduled. A **thermogram** also takes a picture of the breast, but uses the natural heat-producing differences in various types of tissues to produce a picture on infrared film. It is not 100% accurate and is usually used in conjunction with a mammogram.

A definitive diagnosis cannot be made until a **biopsy** is taken. A **needle biopsy** is used to distinguish between a cyst and a tumor. If the doctor uses a fine needle, only fluid can be withdrawn (a cyst is filled with fluid). A wide-needle biopsy can take tissue samples, but they are usually not definitive and a surgical biopsy may be needed to confirm the results of the needle biopsy. Only the needle biopsy may be done if the patient is to start treatment immediately, but surgical biopsy is the preferred type: **excisional biopsies** will be done on small tumors; **incisional** or **wedge biopsies** may be done on larger tumors.

Because of the way breast cancer spreads, the following procedures may also be done: **X-rays** of the chest and skeleton; **bone marrow aspiration** and **biopsy; gallium scan; liver scan; bone scan.**

Laboratory tests will be done on blood and urine samples, and in addition, the estrogen-receptor assay and progesterone receptor assay, to detect whether or not the tumor is responsive to endocrine (hormonal) therapy. These two tests require special equipment and specially trained personnel and are done on tissue samples obtained during the biopsy. Not every hospital is equipped to do these tests. Since half the breast-cancer patients do not respond to endocrine therapy, it

201

is important that these tests be done before embarking on this form of treatment. The patient should make sure these tests have been scheduled.

There are several classification systems used in breast-cancer staging (all can be found in *Breast Cancer Digest*). In summary, they are:

Stage I: A tumor less than 5 cm in diameter with minor skin involvement and confined to one breast.
Stage II: Cancer in one breast, with possible lymph-node involvement.
Stage III: Cancer present in the breast with extensive involvement of lymph nodes but no metastasis to other organs.
Stage IV: Cancer in the breast, lymph-node involvement, and metastasis to other parts of the body.

Types of Cancers

The various cancers that begin in the breast are all *carcinomas,* but they differ enormously in terms of their growth rates, how they spread, and their tendency to recur. *Papillary, medullary,* and *scirrhous* are slow-growing, painless tumors that are very apt to metastasize. *Inflammatory carcinoma* is characterized by rapid growth and rapid recurrence (the symptoms of this type of tumor resemble those of an infection, since the breast skin becomes warm and red). *Lobular carcinoma in situ* usually does not metastasize to the lymph nodes but spreads by invasion. *Paget's disease* is a deeply situated tumor in the breast that progresses to the ducts of the nipple and then to the skin. In this type of cancer the nipple becomes crusted and a biopsy of the nipple itself is necessary.

Benign, noncancerous lumps in the breast include intraductal papilloma, adenofibroma, cystosarcoma phyllodes, mammary fat necrosis, plasma-cell mastitis or mammary duct ectasia.

Treatment

Treatment for breast cancer may include **surgery, radiation, chemotherapy,** and **hormone therapy.** Surgery is usually the first step, which may be followed by one or more of the other types of therapy.

Surgery. The type of operation most often used on breast cancer is called *mastectomy.* Several different types of mastectomies are currently being used; which type is appropriate for any single case depends on a number of factors: type and stage of the cancer, general health and age of the patient, and also (unfortunately) a genuine difference of opinion on the part of surgeons who specialize in this field.

This last factor puts a great burden on the patient and is the reason you must inform yourself fully before deciding what type of operation is appropriate for you. Also, because the range of possible operations is very large, and because all these operations are done under general anesthesia, you must have complete confidence that you and your surgeon see eye to eye on what is going to be done. As with any other form of surgery, you should get a second opinion on the surgery itself as well as on the overall treatment plan. The surgical options are listed below, beginning with those that remove the least amount of tissue.

(NOTE: Many surgeons routinely perform one "cancer operation" during which the biopsy is taken and, if it is positive, the mastectomy performed at the same time. The patient may want some space between the diagnostic procedure and the treatment procedure, although this may involve some risk. This should be discussed at length with your surgeon prior to any surgery.)

Lumpectomy (tylectomy, wedge incision, local wide excision). The lump and a small amount of surrounding tissue are removed, usually followed by radiation and/or chemotherapy. It is only performed on small tumors and is a controversial procedure at the moment, some surgeons considering it very risky: It could leave tiny tumors behind and it does not address possible problems in the lymph nodes.

Subcutaneous mastectomy. In cases of lobular cancer *in situ* or other noninvasive cancers that are not located close to the nipple, the internal breast tissue is removed while leaving the skin intact. The tissue is carefully examined by a pathologist. If it is not an invasive cancer, a silicone implant may be put inside the remaining skin to restore normal breast contours. This procedure is called *mammoplasty,* and may be done either at the same time as the mastectomy or in a second operation.

Partial or quadrant mastectomy. This involves removing the tumor and about a quarter part of the breast. Lymph nodes are not removed, and the procedure is generally followed by radiation.

Simple (total) mastectomy involves the removal of the whole breast and is frequently performed on elderly patients. It may be followed by radiation therapy.

Modified radical mastectomy. The breast and the axillary lymph nodes are removed. At times only part of the lymph nodes are removed and/or it may be necessary to remove the chest muscles.

Halsted radical mastectomy. This involves removal of the entire breast, as well as the fat and lymph nodes in the axilla (armpits), the muscles supporting the breasts, and the fat under the skin around the breasts. After recovering from surgery, the patient will have a flattened or sunken chest wall and the potential for developing lymphedema (swelling of the arm) and shoulder stiffness. This used to be the standard operation, but it has come under increasing fire for being unnecessarily mutilating without statistical evidence to support the position that this procedure produces a better outlook (in terms of longevity or lack of recurrence of disease) than the modified radical mastectomy or even the simple mastectomy.

Extended radical mastectomy.   This includes everything done in the Halsted mastectomy, but goes further in removing the thoracic nerve as well as the internal mammary lymph nodes (usually a section of the rib cage must be removed to reach these nodes). This procedure is rarely done and has not proven more effective than the Halsted mastectomy. It is a high-risk procedure and should only be done by an experienced surgeon at a major medical center.

In addition to those surgical procedures designed to remove the cancer itself, there are several other surgical procedures that might be performed. If the tumor has been typed as one of those whose growth is related to hormones, the glands that produce those hormones may be removed. *Adrenalectomy* is the removal of the adrenal glands; *hypophysectomy* is the surgical removal of the pituitary gland. In patients with recurrent disease and in premenopausal patients, a *bilateral oophorectomy or ovariectomy* (removal of both ovaries) may be performed. (See "Ovary.") The ovaries are also a source of hormone production.

All of the procedures described in this section are considered major surgery and are done under general anesthesia. The patient can expect to be hospitalized for ten to fourteen days. After surgery, there may be some swelling of the arm due to injury to the lymph canals. If the swelling is very uncomfortable, an elastic sleeve like those used for legs with varicose veins may be employed. Exercises for the arm and hand will be given with instructions from a physical therapist or nurse. Normal functions such as brushing hair and dressing oneself should be resumed as soon as possible to assure normal circulation in the arm and chest and aid in reducing edema (swelling).

Radiation.   Currently, radiation has four specific applications in breast-cancer treatment: (1) as a primary treatment for inflammatory breast cancer, for local control of inoperable breast cancer, or for patients who refuse surgery; (2) as an adjunct to mastectomy or lumpectomy; (3) to shrink a large tumor so that surgery can be more effective; and (4) as palliative treatment to relieve pain caused by metastases.

Radiation as a primary treatment is fairly limited; when combined with surgery, the results are better than either surgery or radiation alone. However, there is controversy about how radical the surgery should be. Most radiologists feel that a lumpectomy or partial mastectomy combined with the proper dose of radiation will do the job without removing the breast. A great many surgeons disagree. The statistics are not conclusive: There are problems with the studies themselves, but the five-year survival rates appear to be quite similar.

High-dose radiation plus chemotherapy after surgery has produced good results in patients with Stage III cancers: So far, 85% of those cancers have remained under control after four years. For patients who are inoperable, radiation plus chemotherapy has proven more effective (fewer recurrences) than radiation alone.

Chemotherapy. Chemotherapy is not used as a primary therapy for breast cancer, but as a way to control metastases and recurrence. Recent studies have shown that chemotherapy following surgery has been more effective in premenopausal women and in women whose tumors are linked to hormones than in postmenopausal women and women whose tumors are not dependent on estrogen. The use of chemotherapy varies enormously from low-dose, long-term maintenance therapy using one drug, to high-dose combination chemotherapy. At the moment, ninety-four different drugs are being used in standard and experimental treatments (see Appendix K) singly, in combination, and combined with **surgery, radiation, immunotherapy** and/or **hormone therapy.** The drugs most widely used include L-PAM, Cytoxan, methotrexate, 5-FU, Adriamycin.

Hormone Therapy. Whether or not hormone therapy (also called endocrine manipulation) is used depends on the menopausal status of the woman and whether or not the tumor is estrogen-dependent. For those whose tumors are estrogen-dependent, hormone therapy may be recommended in place of chemotherapy, or combined with chemotherapy drugs. We have already discussed ablative hormone treatment (the removal of adrenal and pituitary glands and the ovaries, all of which produce hormones that may cause tumor growth) in our discussion on surgery. In addition, certain hormones may be given to the patient on a long-term basis. These include five groups of hormones: estrogens (estradiol, ethynyl estradiol, and diethylstilbestrol—DES); antiestrogens (Tamoxifen, Nafoxidine); progestins (hydroxyprogesterone caproate, medroxyprogesterone acetate); androgens (testosterone propionate, fluoxymerterone); and adrenocortical steroids (prednisolone, prednisone). Hormone therapy is not used as a primary treatment.

Immunotherapy. This is only being used experimentally in combination with chemotherapy. Initial results show this area to be a promising line of research, but it is as yet unproven.

Experimental Treatments

There are 105 separate experimental treatment programs currently under way in the United States and Canada involving **surgery, radiation, chemotherapy, hormone therapy,** and **immunotherapy** for all

205

stages of breast cancer. Contact: CBCG, CLB, EST, NCOG, NSABP, RTOG, SEG, SWOG, WCG, MAYO, MDA, MSKCC, MTS, SFCC, WSU, BCTF, CCSF, UARIZ, UCLA, WCCC, WFU, YALE (see appendix H).

Doctors Who May Be Involved in Treatment

General surgeon, therapeutic radiologist, medical oncologist, plastic surgeon.

Further Reading and Resources

In addition to the two books mentioned in the introduction *(Breast Cancer Digest* and *Why Me?),* women who have early-stage breast cancer should read "Local Excision and Primary Radiation Therapy for Early Breast Cancer" by Martin B. Levine, M.D., in *Ca—A Cancer Journal for Clinicians* (vol. 31, No. 1, January/February 1981), available through your local chapter of the American Cancer Society. Summarizing and explaining the work done by the Joint Center for Radiation Therapy at Harvard Medical School and by other investigators, they have found that Stage I and Stage II tumors treated by lumpectomy plus radiation have had a local regional control exceeding 90%. The article describes clearly and in detail specific surgical and radiation techniques, and provides an excellent background for the patient who is seeking the proper treatment team for herself.

It has been found that making use of support services provided by the organizations listed below helps immeasurably in adjusting to having cancer, as well as to the long- and short-term side effects of treatment. Facing breast removal is a valid cause for depression, and some radiation and chemotherapy treatments may compound this "self-image problem" with temporary baldness and months of nausea. These support programs are staffed by women who have been through what you are going through, and they can make a remarkable difference in your ability to deal with your treatment and your life by providing both concrete help and emotional support. Nearly everyone who has successfully gone through this process recommends that you do not do it alone.

REACH TO RECOVERY
American Cancer Society
777 Third Avenue
New York, New York 10017
Phone: (202) 371-2900

ASK A FRIEND TO EXPLAIN RECONSTRUCTION (AFTER)
99 Park Avenue
New York, New York 10016
Phone: (212) 986-9099

ENCORE/YWCA
(local YWCA's have exercise and discussion groups for women who have
had breast cancer operations)

Bronchus

See "Lung."

Buccal Mucosa

See "Head and Neck."

Central Nervous System

See "Brain."

Cervix

Cancer of the cervix is the second most common type of cancer in
American women. At the same time it is one of the easiest to recognize
and cure in its very early stages because it can be spotted in regular
physical examinations using the Pap smear test. Carcinoma *in situ*
that has been treated surgically has a cure rate nearing 100% (it is not
even included in the "cancer statistics"). In Stage I cancers, the cure
rate is 80%.

Cervical cancer appears most often in women over forty. It is also
associated with high sexual activity with multiple partners, particularly
uncircumcised partners, and is more common among women who have
had multiple pregnancies, black women, poor white and Mexican-
American women. It is rare in celibate women, virgins, and Jewish
women. Cervical cancer may be linked to genital herpes (Herpes
type 2 virus) which is transmitted by intercourse and can cause sores
on the cervix and genitalia.

The cervix is the neck of the uterus (womb) which serves as a canal
between the uterus and the vagina. Most cervical cancer originates
within the internal tissue of the cervix and then spreads to involve

the entire cervix. As it metastasizes, it may reach into the vagina, into the uterus and ovaries, to nearby areas of the pelvis such as the rectum and bladder, with distant metastases to the liver, lungs, and bones. It can spread by either the lymph system or veins, but more commonly spreads through the lymph system.

The disease goes through three general stages: dysplasia (cellular abnormality that is precancerous) to carcinoma *in situ* (a true cancer growing on the surface of the cervix) to invasive cancer. It may take as long as thirty years for this progression to occur and for the disease to change from a curable to an advanced stage. Occasionally it happens more rapidly. Women who have undergone a total hysterectomy (see "Ovary") have no risk of developing cervical cancer.

Symptoms

There are no symptoms in the early stages. In the intermediate stages, there may be painful intercourse or bleeding after intercourse, pain in the pelvis, foul-smelling vaginal discharge, and bleeding or spotting between periods.

As the cancer advances, there may be urine leakage, weight loss, anorexia (loss of appetite), and fecal matter may come out of the vagina. Kidney failure is possible in very advanced stages due to obstruction of the ureters.

Diagnosis and Staging

After taking a **medical history** and doing a **physical examination,** diagnosis of the cancer is done via a **pelvic examination,** including a **Pap test.** If the Pap test is positive, or if the woman comes in with any of the symptoms listed above, the gynecologist will do a **cone biopsy** in the hospital under general anesthesia. This may be a therapeutic as well as diagnostic procedure, since the entire cancer may be removed in the process. A **colposcopy** may be performed in the doctor's office to make visual observations and get tissue samples. A **Schiller test** (see **colposcopy**) is usually done at the same time; it is a staining procedure (done with iodine) that makes the cancer cells black and leaves the normal cells untouched. A pelvic examination may be done in the hospital under anesthesia to determine the extent of the disease, palpate the rectum, inspect the vagina, and establish what is to be done in staging.

Procedures used to determine the spread of the disease may include the following: chest **X-ray** to check the lungs; **bone scan; liver scan; IVP** and/or **cystoscopy** to check the bladder wall and for evidence of obstruction of the ureters; **ultrasound** of the pelvis to detect additional masses; **lower GI** or **sigmoidoscopy** to check the rectum; **lymphangiogram** for checking the lymph system; **scalene-node biopsy,** particularly if the lymphangiogram is positive. A fractional D&C (dilation and curettage) may also be scheduled. This involves a hospital stay of twenty-four hours. While you are asleep, a little rake (curette) is inserted through the vagina to scrape the inside wall. All material scraped out is sent to the pathology laboratory for analysis.

The Pap smear reports its findings in five classes: (1) normal cells; (2) some atypical cells, no malignancy evident but should be re-checked; (3) abnormal cells, require further investigation; (4) early cancer cells, biopsy indicated; (5) malignant cells.

After the biopsy is done and the staging procedures completed, the cancer is formally "staged." There are several systems in use, some highly detailed. In general, they can be described as:

Stage 0   *in situ*, surface of cervix only (preinvasive)
Stage 1   cervix invaded but localized to cervix
Stage 2   spread beyond cervix, part of vagina involved but has not spread to the pelvic wall
Stage 3   spread to pelvic wall; involves lower third of vagina
Stage 4   spread beyond pelvis to adjacent and/or distant organs; may involve mucosa of bladder or rectum

Types of Cancers

Most cervical cancers are epidermoid *squamous-cell carcinomas*. About 10% are *adenocarcinomas*, which are harder to detect, invade earlier, and therefore have a poorer prognosis than squamous-cell. *Sarcomas* of the cervix have the poorest prognosis but are extremely rare. *Ulcerating carcinoma* destroys the cervical canal and infiltrates the entire cervix. *Exophytic* cervical cancer grows toward the vagina, filling half the vagina, and is associated with secondary infections.

Patients with cervical cancer risk developing another cancer in the rectum. It is not known at this time if this is a natural tendency of the cancer itself or is due to the carcinogenic properties of radiation treatment for the cervical cancer.

Treatment

The standard treatment for cervical cancer involves surgery alone in the earliest-stage cancers. For Stage I, surgery in the form of a **hysterectomy** (see "Ovary" for descriptions of the various types of hysterectomies) or **radiation** or a combination of both is used. In more advanced cases, surgery will be more extensive, and will be followed by radiation in higher doses than is used in Stage I. For even more advanced cases with metastases in the lymph and/or blood, chemotherapy may be added, but most chemotherapy is being used experimentally (see below).

Surgery. For preinvasive cancers, particularly in younger patients who want to have children, a *conization* may be performed. This is simply the removal of the cancerous tissue, although more tissue may be removed than with a biopsy. The procedure is done under general anesthesia, requiring hospitalization. It can be done as standard surgery or as **cryosurgery,** which kills the unwanted cells by freezing them with a gas like nitrous oxide or carbon dioxide. This is usually effective, but patients should be monitored closely after this form of treatment.

With carcinoma *in situ* (Stage o), surgery may be in the form of a *hysterectomy* (see "Ovary"). At times the fallopian tubes, lymph nodes, and ovaries are removed in addition to the uterus, but if the patient is a young woman and the type of cancer warrants it, the ovaries will be left intact so that she may continue to produce normal estrogens.

With Stage I cancers, the hysterectomy will be performed as above, but the pelvic lymph nodes and the upper half of the vagina will also be removed. (If this interferes with normal sex life, due to shortening of the vagina, plastic surgery can be performed later to restore the normal size and shape.) **Radiation** will also be delivered to the cervix and the rest of the pelvis. At times radiation is used without surgery to treat tumors of this stage.

With more advanced stages of cervical cancer, high-dose external radiation may be used as well as more extensive surgery like *pelvic exenteration,* which involves a total hysterectomy plus the removal of the bladder and rectum. This may involve a **colostomy** (see "Large Intestine") or an **iliostomy** (see "Bladder"), where the feces and/or urine are diverted through tubes to plastic bags on the outside of the body.

After any form of surgery, patients will be monitored closely for infections, which are common in this type of surgery.

Radiation. In many hospitals, radiation is used as the primary form of treatment in Stages I and II. This may be in the form of radium **implants,** which are put in place in the cervix (or vagina, or uterus, depending on the cancer) for seventy-two hours. The implants are done in the operating room (see the chapter on radiation for details). **External radiation** may be given to treat the pelvic lymph nodes and the general area around the cervix. This may involve a five-to-seven week treatment course. Radiation is often preferred to surgery since it can destroy both the tumor and any nearby cancer cells that may have been missed by surgery.

Radiation is also used with surgery: before surgery, to shrink large tumors; and after surgery, as a cleanup technique. Thus far, radiation has proven a more effective adjunct to surgery than has chemotherapy, which is usually used only in situations where the cancer has spread outside the pelvis and surgery and radiation are not effective.

Special Condition: Pregnancy

If cervical cancer is diagnosed after a patient has become pregnant, the standard treatment plan will be altered according to the stage of the cancer and the number of weeks of the pregnancy. With an invasive tumor and a pregnancy of less than twenty to twenty-four weeks, an abortion is usually performed. Past that point, the pregnancy will be allowed to continue until it is safe to deliver the baby. This will be done by cesarean section (C-section) and a hysterectomy may be performed at the same time, with lymph nodes removed. Radiation will be started as soon as healing is complete.

With *in situ* cervical cancers, the patient will usually be allowed to deliver normally (through the vagina) and treatment will be started two to three months after delivery.

Doctors Who May Be Involved in Treatment

Gynecologist, gynecological surgeon, therapeutic radiologist, medical oncologist.

Experimental Treatments

Experimental protocols are being carried out to examine the effectiveness of different surgical techniques, different radiation techniques, different chemotherapy drugs and combinations, immunotherapy, and combinations of all these therapeutic techniques. Contact: EST, GOG, NCOG, RTOG, SEG, SWOG, MDA, MSKCC (see appendix H).

Further Reading and Resources

If surgery is extensive, requiring removal of the bladder and/or rectum, the United Ostomy Association should be contacted. See "Large Intestine."

Cheek

See "Head and Neck."

Colon

See "Large Intestine."

Connective Tissue

See "Bone."

Ear

The ear is a complex mechanism composed of many small parts. It is generally divided into three sections: the external ear, which is the part that can be seen from outside and also includes the auditory canal that leads to the middle ear; the middle ear, which houses the eardrum and is the point of contact for the eustachian tube that runs to the nasal passages; and the inner ear, the innermost section, which is the point of contact for the acoustic nerve, which runs to the brain.

Cancers of the ear are extremely rare, and most can be treated easily and successfully. We will explain cancers of the acoustic nerve (acoustic neuromas) here, although they are technically **brain** and **central-nervous-system** cancers. Patients with this type of cancer should also read the section on brain and CNS tumors. Cancers that affect the bones around the ear, and the middle and inner ear, are dangerous because of their proximity to the brain.

Symptoms

Hearing loss; vertigo; severe pain in the ear; paralysis of part of the face; tinnitus (hearing sounds that are not there—ringing, buzzing, a roar).

Diagnosis

An extensive **medical history** will be taken and a thorough **physical examination** done, with particular attention given to the head and neck. Special procedures will include transillumination of the sinuses (shining a light up the nose for visual inspection); head **X-rays**, particularly of the mastoid process and temporal bone (the bones surrounding the ear); and hearing tests to see what type of loss has occurred, if any, since the type of loss can indicate where the problem is located. Patients will be tested for perception of sound, using a tuning fork and an audiometer (earphones attached to a machine that emits sounds of varying pitches and tones; the patient indicates what she hears), and will have speech tests. A parotid sialogram may also be done. The parotid gland is a major salivary gland located near the ear. In this test, a dye is injected into a vein in the arm, which highlights this gland so that a clear X-ray picture can be taken.

Types of Cancers

OUTER EAR: The skin on the outside of the ear may develop *basal-cell* and *squamous-cell carcinoma* (see "Skin" for more details). These can spread inward to the auditory canal, or can actually start there. *Ceruminomas* are tumors (usually benign) of the ceruminous glands, which produce earwax (cerumin). *Osteomas* are tumors composed of bone tissue.

MIDDLE EAR: *Chemodectomas* (also known as *nonchromaffin paragangliomas,* or *glomus jugulare,* or *glomus tympanicum* tumors) grow from structures in the jugular or the wall of the middle ear. In rare situations, *squamous-cell carcinoma* may begin here. *Adenocarcinomas* may also be found.

INNER EAR: *Acoustic neuromas* are actually **brain** and **central nervous system** tumors (they are also called *vestibular schwannomas* or *eighth-nerve* tumors) which affect the acoustic nerve. They are found in both adults and children and make up 7% of the tumors that are found inside the skull. As the tumor grows, it compresses the cerebellum and brainstem, and involves other nerves.

Treatments

EXTERNAL EAR: Basal-cell and squamous-cell carcinomas on the visible skin of the ear are easily treated in the early stages using cautery (destroying the cells by burning), curettage (scraping the lesion off), **radiation,** or simple **surgery** that can be done in the doctor's office. More advanced lesions require more extensive surgery. If bone is involved in this area or the middle part of the ear, perhaps due to spread of the cancer, a more complicated operation called a *radical mastoidectomy* will be performed. This involves removing the middle ear, exploring the eustachian tubes for involvement, and removing all or part of the facial nerve. (If only part of the nerve is removed, a nerve graft may be done to restore sensation.) This is a long and complicated operation (five to six hours) and requires several weeks of hospitalization. (NOTE: Ears can be reconstructed with plastic material and any disfigurement of the face can be corrected with plastic surgery at a later date.)

MIDDLE EAR: Chemodectomas and squamous-cell carcinomas may be removed with microsurgical techniques. Radiation may be used for tumors too large to remove surgically.

INNER EAR: Acoustic neuromas are removed surgically. If they are small and the patient still has hearing in the ear, microsurgery will be used, approaching from the outside through a slit in the skin behind the ear. If no useful hearing remains, they will be approached from the inside of the ear. Large tumors require both techniques.

213

Experimental Treatments

Depending on the exact type of cancer, its location, and the spread of the cancer, it might be advisable to explore the experimental treatments in radiation and chemotherapy that are listed under "Head and Neck" cancers and "Brain and Central Nervous System" cancers. Check with your doctor.

Doctors Who May Be Involved in Treatment

Otolaryngologist (ear, nose and throat specialist)—be sure the specialist has experience with cancers; neurologist; neurosurgeon; maxillofacial surgeon; plastic surgeon; therapeutic radiologist. It is suggested that for anything other than a simple skin cancer on the outside of the ear, a patient consult a major cancer center that has a large program in head and neck cancers or, if you are dealing with acoustic neuromas, a large program in treating brain and central nervous system cancers.

Further Reading and Resources

If major surgery is required, resulting in disfigurement and the need for subsequent reconstruction and rehabilitation, contact the resources listed under "Head and Neck" cancers in the chapter on surgery.

Endometrium

See "Uterus."

Esophagus

The esophagus is the upper part of the digestive (gastrointestinal) system. It joins the lower end of the pharynx (the tube through which food goes down your throat and air passes into the trachea). It is about ten inches long and is divided into two sections: the upper section, located in the neck, is called the cervical esophagus; the lower portion, running through the chest, is called the thoracic esophagus.

Persons at higher risk of developing cancers of the esophagus include: older white men; patients with a history of difficulty in swallowing; long-term smokers (including pipes and cigars as well as cigarettes); patients with bad teeth or no teeth; patients who have had head-and-neck or colon cancer; and patients with hiatus hernias.

Correlations have made between nutritional factors and esophageal cancer: malnutrition and vitamin deficiencies; long-term ingestion of certain alcoholic beverages that contain nitrosamines (smoking plus alcohol is a particularly bad combination); habitual, long-term ingestion of very hot (both temperature and spicy) foods and drinks. There is a higher incidence of this type of cancer among poor people who live in cities as well as among various occupational groups: laborers and construction workers; metal workers, particularly brass and bronze; plumbers; and people who make liquor.

Symptoms

Dysphagia (difficulty in swallowing) with pain is the most common symptom, and it is progressive—from difficulty swallowing foods such as meat and bread to eventual difficulty swallowing even liquids. Choking often accompanies dysphagia.

Weight loss, malaise, anorexia, vocal-cord paralysis, persistent cough, and anemia are also symptoms. As the disease progresses, there may be regurgitation and secondary perforation of the trachea and bronchi. Clinical exam may reveal lymph-node metastases in the neck or mediastinum.

Diagnosis and Staging

The process of swallowing will be watched and photographed using a fluoroscopic **upper GI** (a **lower GI** may also be done, to check for problems in the rest of the gastrointestinal system). During an **esophagoscopy**, the esophagus will be observed directly and tissue samples taken for **biopsy**. While this exam is in process, an *esophageal lavage* will be done, which is a washing of the lining of the esophagus in order to obtain cells for examination under a microscope. Biopsies will also be taken of the lymph nodes near the esophagus (scalene nodes and celiac nodes). Chest **X-rays** and **tomograms** will be taken to note any spread to other parts of the chest; **liver** and **bone scans** will be done to find evidence of spread to those sites; and a **bronchoscopy** will be done to see if there is any spread to the bronchial tubes. Evidence of this type of spread usually rules out surgery. Blood and urine analysis will be done in the laboratory, including CBC, SMA-12, and liver chemistries.

The staging classifications are fairly complex, as follow:

TIS   tumor *in situ*
T_1 a tumor involving 5 cm (1 inch) or less of the esophagus, that causes no obstruction and has not spread
T_2 a tumor larger than 5 cm without outside spread, or a tumor of any size that produces an obstruction or involves the entire circumference but without having spread
T_3 any tumor that has spread outside the esophagus

215

Cancer of the esophagus is usually not diagnosed until it has reached an advanced stage, although the cancer itself may have been present for as long as thirty years. This is because there may be no symptoms in the early stages, and because the esophagus, being an internal organ, is not easily checked during a regular physical examination.

Types of Cancers

The most common type is *epidermoid carcinoma,* which appears in the lower third of the esophagus. *Squamous-cell carcinoma* is also common. *Adenocarcinomas* are fairly rare, and doctors are not certain if these start in the esophagus or really begin in the stomach.

Carcinomas *in situ* are extremely rare; most carcinomas of the esophagus are invasive and encircle the esophagus before diagnosis is made.

The liver, lungs, and pleura (membranes surrounding the lungs) are common sites for metastases. The disease may spread to distant locations using both the lymphatic and circulatory systems.

Treatment

Surgery is usually necessary, although only 50% of the patients with esophageal cancer are good surgical risks. Many patients are in such poor general health (due to malnutrition, anemia, dehydration) that they must be "built up" before any surgery can take place. This generally entails *hyperalimentation:* feeding a high-calorie nutrient solution into the large vein under the collarbone. (See the chapter on supportive treatment for a detailed explanation.)

The procedures used depend on the type of cancer and where it is located: Tumors in the lower third of the esophagus are the easiest to treat surgically; tumors of the middle third are more difficult to treat; and those of the upper third are rarely treated this way (**radiation** is used instead). Surgery may involve removing only that part of the esophagus which is cancerous with a margin of healthy tissue and the regional lymph nodes. In this case, the remaining esophagus must be linked with the stomach. This is done in two ways: *Esophagogastric anastamosis* uses a segment of the large intestine as a substitute esophagus; *intubation* uses plastic tubes. Pulsion tubes are used for tumors of the upper esophagus and inserted through the mouth. Traction tubes are used in the lower esophagus and are inserted in a surgical procedure such as an **esophagoscopy.**

If the entire esophagus must be removed, the spleen and the tail of the pancreas will also be removed. Again, a link must be made between the remaining upper part of the esophagus and the stomach, using a portion of the intestine.

This is major surgery and requires two to four weeks' hospitalization.

Radiation. Some esophageal tumors are responsive to radiation, although treatment is usually for palliation of symptoms (obstruction and pain) rather than for cure.

Experimental Treatments

Experimental treatments are being conducted using **chemotherapy, radiation,** and **surgery** in various combinations to improve the cure and response rates, which are poor for most esophageal cancers. Contact: EST, NCOG, RTOG, SEG, SWOG, GTSG, MDA, MSKCC, VASAG (see appendix H).

Doctors Who May Be Involved in Treatment

Gastroenterologist; otolaryngologist (ear, nose, and throat specialist); thoracic surgeons; gastrointestinal surgeons; pulmonary specialists; therapeutic radiologist; medical oncologist.

Eye

The eye is a complex sensory organ made up of several structures. Cancers of the eye are grouped not only by the specific type of cancers but also by which part of the eye they affect: the lids; conjunctiva (the mucous membrane that lines the eyelids and front of the eyeball); the cornea (the clear, curved lens of the eye); the sclera (the white of the eye); the intraocular area (the iris or tinted part of the eye, the choroid or middle coat of the eyeball, the ciliary body, and the retina, which is the part of the eye that actually "sees"); and the orbit, or bony cavity, which contains the eye.

Cancers of the eye are quite rare, and tend to affect either the very young in the form of retinoblastoma (average age is 18 months) or patients in their sixties and seventies—malignant melanoma being the most common type among this age group. Other types of cancers can metastasize to the eye, particularly from the lung and breast. Neuroblastomas of childhood may metastasize to the orbit of the eye.

Symptoms

Symptoms will vary depending on the type of cancer and the part of the eye affected.

Malignant melanomas: In the early stages, or if located at the periphery of the visual structures, these may not cause symptoms. In later stages, or if the tumor is located near the center of the eye, there may be decreased visual acuity (inability to see clearly) or meta-

217

morphopsia (a visual disturbance in which objects are distorted in shape). Other symptoms may include detached retina, hemorrhage, pigmented lesions on the iris, possible second-degree glaucoma, a feeling of "floating spots" before the eyes, and/or cataracts. These can be difficult to diagnose.

Retinoblastomas: Early symptoms include a change in the look of the pupil of one eye. As the tumor grows, a white shine appears in that pupil, which is not a reflection of light but actually the tumor itself. Eventually the tumor fills the eye so that the eye looks yellowish-white (often referred to as "cat's eye") and pushes the eyeball out from its normal position in the socket. Other symptoms include squinting, red and painful eyes, visual difficulties, and a family history of retinoblastoma.

Eyelids and Conjunctiva: A persistent growth or sore that does not heal, or a solid, white, slow-growing nodule.

Orbit tumors: There may be changes in the contours of the eyelids (such changes are also symptomatic of other conditions besides cancer); double vision stemming from involvement of the intraocular muscles; and loss of visual field.

Diagnosis and Staging

Diagnosis begins with a **medical history** and **physical examination.** Direct examination of the structures of the eye will be done by an eye specialist (ophthalmologist). Most require dilation of the eye to keep the pupil open even when light shines directly on it. To achieve this, one drop of a solution is put in the eyes two times in a five-minute interval. The drops burn or sting slightly as they are applied and the patient may have a funny taste in the mouth. Both feelings pass quickly. The drops will keep the eye dilated for several hours, during which vision will be impaired (someone should take the patient home) and bright light will hurt the eyes (dark glasses help).

Transillumination of the eyes is a visual examination of the eye in which light from an outside source is used to illuminate the interior structures, which are observed by a simple hand-held viewer called an ophthalmoscope.

Slit lamp examination (biomicroscopy) uses a microscope with a special light source mounted on a table with extensions to support the patient's head. The patient is told to look straight ahead without blinking while the doctor moves the equipment in order to look at different parts of the eye. The pupils must be dilated during this examination. The test only takes ten to fifteen minutes.

Binocular indirect ophthalmoscopy is used to look at the back part of the inside of the eye. After the eyes have been dilated, the patient sits in a dentist-type chair and the ophthalmologist holds a special convex lens over one eye at a time. The lens projects an image seen through a small viewer strapped to the doctor's head, like a miner's cap. The patient will be asked to look in different directions so the doctor can examine different parts of the eye. The examination takes fifteen to thirty minutes. Children may be sedated before the examination.

Fluourescein angiography is a type of **angiogram** done to look at the circulation patterns in the eye. The patient's pupils are dilated, the patient is seated, and a dye is injected into a vein in the arm. The patient's head is placed in a frame to keep it steady while the doctor looks at the eyes through the binocular indirect ophthalmoscope (described above) and X-ray pictures are taken using a fundus camera, which looks like a standard 35-mm camera. Pictures can be taken seconds after the dye has been injected, but, because abnormalities may not immediately be apparent, they may continue to take pictures for up to an hour.

A *radiophosphorous uptake* may also be done. A radioactive isotope of phosphorus is injected into a vein in the arm and a picture is taken of the tumor: Whether or not the tumor absorbs the isotope indicates whether it is benign or malignant.

Ultrasound tests of the eye are usually taken since they are quite reliable for diagnosing this type of tumor. A **CAT scan** may also be done to see if there is involvement in the orbit. **Biopsies** of tumors of the eyelid and conjunctiva are essential, but they are not done for intraocular tumors since the biopsy might produce a spread of malignant cells, particularly with melanomas.

Procedures to check for metastases include: **X-rays** to detect bony invasion and evidence of calcification around the area of the eye; skeletal X-rays to check for bone metastases; blood tests and the **liver/spleen scan** for liver metastases; spinal-fluid studies; **lumbar puncture,** and **bone marrow aspirations** for retinoblastomas. They are repeated every few months until the tumor is destroyed.

Staging

There is no mechanism for grading and staging malignant melanomas and cancers of the orbit. Cancers of the skin in the eyelid and conjunctiva are staged as they are in **skin cancers**. Retinoblastoma patients are staged as follows, with groups linked to suitability for treatment:

Group I   Very favorable. Either one tumor or multiple, none more than 4 dd (optic disk diameter) in size, at or behind the equator (an imaginary line halfway between the front and back of the eye).

Group II   Favorable. One or multiple tumors, each 4–10 dd in size, behind the equator.

219

Group III Doubtful. Any lesion in front of the equator; single lesion larger than 10 dd behind the equator.

Group IV Unfavorable. Multiple tumors, some larger than 10 dd, or any lesion extending to the ora serrata.

Group V Very unfavorable. Massive tumors involving over half the retina, or vitreous (glassy) seeding of cancer cells throughout.

Types of Cancers

Malignant Melanomas: It is thought that a large percentage of these tumors start in preexisting nevi (colored spots, like moles) which grow in size until they become malignant. Many melanomas involve the uvea, which consists of the iris, the choroid (which is skinlike, contains a layer of blood vessels, and provides nutrition for the retina and lens), and the cilia. Melanomas of the iris are less malignant and grow more slowly than those of the choroid. There are two types of melanoma cells: spindle and epithelioid. Spindle are more benign than epithelioid, which are rare. Some melanomas of the eye have mixed cell types. The liver is the most common site of metastases for these tumors. They also may give rise to secondary glaucomas.

Retinoblastomas: These are the second most common malignant tumor of childhood. They affect the retina of the eye, which perceives and transmits the sensory impulses of light to the optic nerve. Six percent of these tumors are familial: If a parent has had retinoblastoma, there is a 50% chance that the child will also develop a tumor.

These tumors can grow in one or both eyes; 20 to 55% of retinoblastomas are bilateral (they affect both eyes), and these occur at a younger age than unilateral tumors. As the tumor grows it forms a large, ulcerating mass. It may spread along the optic nerve to the brain and orbit of the eye, and most frequently metastasize to the bones and to the liver. The tumor at times will outgrow its own blood supply and may destroy itself in rare cases; frequently areas within the tumor will die from lack of blood.

Tumors of the Eyelid and Conjunctiva: Cancers of the eyelid are obvious because of their location, but, by the same token, difficult to treat—often requiring reconstruction of the eyelid itself. Premalignant tumors or lesions include Bowen's disease and senile keratosis. Benign tumors of the skin of the eyelid are very common: nevi, papillomas, and hemangiomas. Malignant tumors are the same as those that appear at other locations on the skin: The most common is *basal-cell carcinoma*, which spreads by local invasion but does not metastasize; *squamous-cell carcinomas* are much less common, but do metastasize; *melanomas* are also found. In the conjunctiva, *carcinomas, melanomas,* and *lymphosarcomas* may be found, as well as *carcinomas in situ*. These tend to grow very slowly.

Tumors of the Orbit: There are a large number of different types of tumors that affect the orbit, but they are all extremely rare. They are difficult to diagnose because of their location deep within the eye. Benign tumors that may be found here include hemangiomas, aneurysms, and lymphangiomas. Malignant tumors that start in the orbit include *embryonal rhabdomyosarcomas* in children, and some very rare sarcomas, such as *lymphosarcomas.* Tumors may metastasize to the orbit from other sites: breast, neuroblastoma in children, and at times from the nasal sinuses.

Treatment

Treatment for eye cancers often involves **surgery,** using procedures and techniques that are unique to the eye. There are certain terms you should become familiar with:

Enucleation means the complete removal of the eyeball. This is a major operation, but painless. The patient will stay in bed for a few days and will leave the hospital in about a week. A patch will be worn for three or four weeks until the socket is healed, after which a false eye can be inserted that matches the remaining eye, both in color and ability to move. Enucleation is done under general anesthesia in children and general or local anesthesia in adults. During the procedure, the surgeon will cut the conjunctiva, the muscles attached to the outside of the eye, and the optic nerve. The muscles will be stitched in such a way that when a false eye is inserted, it will move normally.

Photocoagulation and *laser* techniques use intensive light to kill abnormal cells by heat. Photocoagulation using a xenon light is now used rarely, since the laser techniques are so exact (they can focus on areas that are only a hundredth of a millimeter in size) and much easier to use.

Heat may also be applied in the form of *diathermy.* With photocoagulation and laser surgery, the pupil is dilated and the light goes directly to the tumor. This can be done under local anesthesia (in which case the patient will sit on a stool, head in a chin rest) or general anesthesia, with the patient lying down. The treatment itself takes a fraction of a second. Diathermy treatments apply heat through the coats, or layers, of the eye (rather than through the dilated pupil), usually in the form of an electric needle. **Cryosurgery,** using cold instead of heat, may also be used to destroy cancer cells.

Malignant Melanomas: When the cancer affects the choroid, *enucleation* is the usual procedure. If one eye has already been removed, the remaining eye is treated conservatively in an attempt to save it. This may involve the use of internal or external **radiation,** photocoagulation, or surgical removal of the tumor along with only a small amount of

221

healthy tissue. If the melanoma is in the iris, often the eyeball is not removed. Some tumors may be treated by photocoagulation; others may be effectively treated with two operative procedures: an *iridectomy,* in which part of the iris is removed; or an *iridocyclectomy,* in which part of the iris is removed along with part of the ciliary body. Diathermy is also used. **Chemotherapy** is not yet a proven treatment, although some experimental work is going on in major cancer centers. See also "Skin."

Retinoblastomas: In early stages, **radiation** is used, since these tumors are radiosensitive and, in cases where only one eye is affected, this can cure the cancer while preserving the eye. Radiation "plaques" (small patches of radioactive material) are sewn to the sclera in the exact location of the tumor, like a compress. This is left in for three to five days and removed. There is some chance of damage to the lens, but in very early stages vision is maintained in 95% of the cases. Radiation may also be used for the remaining eye when one eye has been removed.

After the early stages, surgery is the treatment of choice. If one eye is involved, it is enucleated with as much of the optic nerve as possible (to prevent metastasis to the brain). If both eyes are involved, the most damaged eye is removed and the other is treated with photo-coagulation or **cryosurgery** or radiation combined with **chemotherapy.** As with all childhood cancers, treatment requires a highly skilled team, which can only be found in major cancer centers or pediatric oncology departments of large children's hospitals.

Eyelids and Conjunctiva: Like skin cancers, these are removed surgically with a section of normal tissue surrounding the tumors. A biopsy is done on the completely removed tumor. Plastic surgery may be necessary if removal has severely damaged the eyelid. Radiation is difficult with these tumors; chemotherapy is generally not used.

Tumors of the Orbit: These tumors are removed surgically, but the placement of the incision varies enormously, depending on the location of the tumor. Radiation is used only on a limited basis—for lympho-sarcoma of the orbit, or tumors that have metastasized to the orbit. Chemotherapy is not used for these tumors.

Experimental Treatments

For retinoblastoma, see CHOP, SJCRH (appendix H).

Doctors Who May Be Involved in Treatment

Ophthalmologist; therapeutic radiologist; medical oncologist.

Fatty Tissue

See "Bone."

Gallbladder

The gallbladder (*Vesica fellea*) is a pear-shaped sac on the underside of the liver, located in a hollow between the lobes of the liver. It serves as a reservoir for bile.

Cancer of the gallbladder is rare, and occurs primarily in older women. It is also associated with obesity and chronic problems with gallstones. Younger women who have had several children or those who have taken oral contraceptives also have some degree of risk.

Symptoms

Loss of appetite, nausea, weight loss, abdominal pain, temporary jaundice, recurrent and increasingly severe symptoms of gallstones. All symptoms are similar to those of benign gallbladder disease. It is usual not to discover cancer until the patient has gone in for surgery to treat noncancer disease.

Diagnosis and Staging

After a **medical history** is taken and a complete **physical examination** done, **X-rays** and a **gallbladder series** will be done. Stones may be seen, but it is hard to really look at the gallbladder with these tests. Laboratory tests include the alkaline phosphatase test and liver chemistries to see if there is liver involvement. There is no formal staging for cancers of the gallbladder.

Types of Cancers

Adenocarcinoma is the most frequent type of cancer found in the gallbladder; *epidermoid carcinoma* may also occur. Because of the location of the gallbladder, these cancers often invade the liver. Distant metastases may be found in the bones, lungs, and abdomen.

Treatment

These cancers do not respond to radiation or chemotherapy, so **surgery** is the treatment of choice. The operation is called a *cholecystectomy*, which is the complete removal of the gallbladder. Since the liver is usually involved at the time of diagnosis, the part involved

223

will be removed at the same time (this is called a *partial hepatectomy*). This operation is major surgery requiring a general anesthetic. The operation takes about an hour to an hour and a half, and the patient will remain in the hospital for six to eight days. After the operation, diet will be restricted because fats will be indigestible.

Since cancer of the gallbladder is almost never found in its early stages, prognosis is not good.

Gums

See "Head and Neck."

Head and Neck

Five to ten percent of all cancers involve sites in the head and neck. The term "head and neck cancers" refers to all those which effect the human body above the collarbone, excluding the brain and central nervous system. The head-and-neck region is the second most complex part of the body in terms of the numbers of structures, their proximity to one another, and the highly complex functions they perform. For ease of understanding, we have treated cancers affecting the eye, ear, thyroid, and esophagus in their own individual site sections even though they are located in this region.

In this section we will be discussing cancers that grow in the top portions of the respiratory and digestive system—specifically the structures in the nose, consisting of the *nasal cavity, nasal sinuses, nasopharynx, larynx* (voice box); and the structures of the mouth and throat—*lips, tongue, cheeks (buccal mucosa), gums, tonsils, hard palate, soft palate, floor of the mouth, oropharynx* (throat), *hypopharynx,* and *salivary glands.* (There are three large salivary glands: the *parotid,* on the side of the face near the ear; the *sublingual,* which is under the floor of the mouth; and the *submaxillary,* located in the upper part of the neck under the jawbone.)

In addition to these structures, cancer may also affect the *jawbone* (maxilla) and the *lymph glands* located on the sides of the neck (the "swollen glands" we refer to when we get an infection). Please refer to the diagram of the head and neck in Appendix A to locate all these structures.

Patients who risk developing head and neck cancers fall into various categories depending on the location of the cancer. Cancer of the *larynx* is five times higher for smokers than nonsmokers, and almost never appears in people who neither smoke nor drink. People in urban areas, those who use their voices in their work (actors, singers), and men 50–65 (90% of the patients are men) are at risk. Workers exposed to wood and metal dusts, and chemicals, and asbestos workers—particularly if they smoke—are at high risk.

Cancer of the *lips* has been linked to overexposure to the sun, pipe smoking, and syphilis. It is rare in blacks and seems to occur more often in men over forty. Farmers and sailors are in the high-risk occupational group.

Cancers of the *mouth* have been linked to smoking and alcohol (particularly when used together over a prolonged period of time), chewing tobacco, poor dental hygiene, badly fitting dentures, leukoplakia, vitamin-A deficiency, and to people who have a strong family history of cancer. They appear most often in people aged fifty to seventy.

Cancers of the *nasopharynx* are fairly uncommon, but appear more in urban areas and among populations who eat large quantities of salted fish (Eskimos). Leather workers are at high risk. Possible genetic and viral factors are being explored.

Salivary-gland tumors are usually benign. There may be a relationship between vitamin-A deficiency and these cancers and breast cancer and these cancers. They appear equally in men and women, most often around age 50. Hemangiomas have been known to appear in young children and infants: Although these tumors are benign, they tend to be malignant when they recur. They are quite common among Eskimos.

For cancers of the *throat*, smoking and drinking (particularly when done together) as well as chewing tobacco, leukoplakia, and a history of syphilis are causal factors. They are most common in men between the ages of 65 and 75.

Cancers of the *tongue* have similar origins to those of the mouth. There is also a condition called syphilitic glossitis which is precancerous, occurs most often in men between 50 and 70, and may recur in the cheek, floor of the mouth, or tip of the nose. Textile workers are in the high-risk group for tongue cancers, as are men over 40.

Common Characteristics of Head and Neck Cancers

As you can see from the preceding discussion, there are a score of specific sites in this region, and doctors divide these up into even smaller locations. We will discuss each of the sites listed above separately, but since they share many characteristics, they are categorized as a group.

All the sites in the head and neck are very close to each other. Thus if a cancer has spread at all, it may involve more than one site and you should read that section as well as the section on the primary site of your cancer.

Cancers of the head and neck generally do not metastasize widely in the body; rather, they spread by local invasion. The danger comes because, in this very confined space, even a locally invasive tumor may affect several vital systems: the respiratory system, the digestive system, the brain, and the central nervous system. Because we cannot survive without the effective functioning of these systems, locally invasive tumors can easily become life-threatening.

Cancers in this region frequently also spread to the lymph nodes in the neck. The enlarged nodes may provide the first symptom of cancers that in fact have begun at another site, and treatment often involves surgical removal of these lymph glands (this operation is called a *radical neck dissection*). Again because of the close quarters of the region, first symptoms may often include pain or pressure in the ears, or hearing loss, even when the ear is not involved.

Most cancers of the head and neck can be diagnosed at an early stage because they are accessible to examination by a doctor, dentist, or the patient. If caught in the early stages, they are highly curable.

Standard treatment for head and neck cancers is **surgery** and/or **radiation.** Chemotherapy is not used as a primary treatment, although it may be employed along with radiation for large tumors that have metastasized, both before and after surgery.

Diagnostic procedures for head and neck cancers include examination of all the structures of the head and neck, since, if the cancer has spread, it is most apt to do so locally.

If the cancer is not small, and affects more than just the outer layer of tissue, it is likely that a very sophisticated team approach will be needed in order to treat the cancer and rehabilitate the patient successfully. For this reason, patients with head and neck cancers should be treated at a major cancer center or major hospital that specializes in treating these cancers. Many head and neck cancers have a tendency to recur, and 15–20% of patients will develop second primaries.

Symptoms

The symptoms vary according to the site. Often the patient will feel no symptoms in the early stages. In many cases the development of cancer is preceded by a precancerous condition, particularly in the mouth, which has been noted by the patient, doctor, or dentist. This includes conditions like leukoplakia, which is seen as white patches or inflamed red areas. These should be watched closely and treated, and patients should immediately stop all tobacco use.

By site, the most common symptoms are:

226

CHEEK (buccal mucosa): Lump inside the cheek that persists and may become sore.

GUMS: Painful sore, sometimes under a denture; pain that doesn't go away following a tooth extraction; bleeding; difficulty chewing and/or swallowing.

HYPOPHARYNX: Shortness of breath; voice changes; coughing; foul breath; sore throat; difficult and painful swallowing.

LARYNX: Hoarseness; voice changes; weight loss; frequent throat clearing; coughing; noisy breathing; increasing pain as disease progresses.

LIP: Painless sore or ulcer on lip that may look like a cold sore but does not go away.

MOUTH: Numbness; swelling of lips and gums; difficulty chewing and/or swallowing; red or inflamed areas or white patches inside the mouth; a lump or thickening, discomfort when wearing dentures; bleeding.

NASOPHARYNX: Nasal obstruction and bleeding; altered hearing or slight loss of hearing; enlarged lymph nodes in the neck; stuffiness in the ears; swelling of cheek; bleeding mass in nose.

OROPHARYNX (throat): Sores in the mouth; earaches; painful swallowing; sometimes swollen glands in the neck; difficulty breathing.

PARANASAL SINUSES: May behave like sinusitis, with pressure, pain, bulging of cheek.

SALIVARY GLANDS: Painless, stony-hard lump below the ear in the cheek; dull pain; facial-nerve paralysis in some cases.

TONGUE: Sore on any part of the tongue—surface, edge, or the underside—that does not heal; painful chewing; deep red patches on the tongue, or white painless sores; swelling or thickening of the tongue; sore throat; a "wooden" or fixed tongue. Limited tongue movement, pain, odor, and excess saliva usually mean advanced disease in several types of mouth cancer, including the tongue.

TONSIL: Sore throat, excess salivation, and, in advanced cases, severe pain.

Diagnostic Procedures

A complete **medical history** will be taken and a **physical examination** done, including the lymph nodes in the neck. Dentists as well as doctors are trained in inspecting the mouth, gums, tongue, and throat for possible signs of head and neck cancers (cancers do not appear in the teeth). The physician (otolaryngologist—ear, nose, and throat specialist) will also examine the tonsils and the skin of the face for changes in warts and moles, or any abnormal masses and swellings.

A series of **X-rays** will be done, which may include chest X-rays to check for metastases to the chest, and X-rays of the skull, jaw, and bones of the sinuses. (Cancers of the gums and nasopharynx are likely to spread to nearby bones.) An X-ray of the larynx (laryngogram) may be done. An **upper GI** may be done.

Various types of **endoscopies** may be done, depending on the site of the tumor: a **laryngoscopy** will be used to examine the back of the throat, down to the esophagus; a *nasopharyngoscopy* is a similar procedure examining the nasal cavities and nasopharynx. In both procedures the doctor will examine the area visually and also take samples of tissues and cells for examination under a microscope.

If a salivary-gland tumor is suspected, a *sialogram* will be done. This is a **contrast-film X-ray** of the parotid gland.

Biopsies are usually done prior to treatment surgery, but in individual cases may not be done until the actual operation.

Types of Cancers

Squamous-cell carcinomas are the most common, they account for 90% of the cancers found in the oral cavity and may be found in the other sites as well. They are usually slow-growing, although tumors of the tongue and tonsil may be more aggressive. Squamous-cell carcinomas tend to recur within the first three years after treatment. Checkups are usually scheduled monthly for the first year, and then at progressively longer intervals through the first five years after treatment.

Adenocarcinomas (including *adenoid cystic carcinomas, mucoepidermoid carcinomas,* and *mixed tumors*) are found most often in the minor salivary glands that are dotted throughout the lining of the mouth, and may also be found in the major salivary glands. They may remain localized for long periods of time, but they may invade nearby structures (such as bone) and are very apt to recur. If located in the palate (most of these are), they are likely to involve not only the underlying bone but the maxillary sinus as well.

Malignant lymphomas are very rare (see also "Lymphomas" for discussion regarding treatment). *Malignant melanomas* are also rare (see also "Skin"). *Plasmacytomas* are most commonly found in the tonsil, but they are rare, localized, and curable with treatment. *Fibrosarcomas* may be found in the nasal cavity and paranasal sinuses. *Hypernephroma* is the most common tumor of the paranasal sinuses.

Treatment: An Overview

The most common forms of treatment for head and neck cancers are **surgery** and **radiation** (internal and external). The decision to use surgery, radiation, or both depends on the size and location of the tumor. Surgery involves removal of the tumor and a portion of the healthy tissue. Since these tumors frequently spread to the cervical lymph nodes in the neck, a radical neck dissection is frequently performed. For advanced tumors, surgery can be disfiguring and reconstruction is often required, involving **plastic surgery.** Plastic surgeons are very skillful in reconstructing bone, muscle, and skin so that a face can literally be "rebuilt" using healthy tissues from the patient (bone and skin grafts) or artificial materials and devices to replace missing bone and skin. One such device is an abdurator, which is a plug that fits into holes made in your own bone. Plastic surgery has been developed to a truly miraculous level, so that even a patient with major disfigurement may be able to look normal and function quite normally after reconstruction and rehabilitation.

Since surgical procedures for head and neck tumors may interfere with vital functions such as eating and breathing, they are often done in two or three stages. Some of the side effects of such surgery may not be pleasant, but they are temporary: The patient may not be able to fully open his jaw after some operations and will therefore have problems with chewing and swallowing; the patient may have difficulty speaking if a portion of the tongue must be removed.

If a radical neck dissection is done, a nerve will be cut which is connected to the muscles in your neck and upper back and controls arm motion. You will be put in an exercise program to regain control of the arm and to reacquire normal posture. Side effects of other surgical treatments are discussed below under "Treatments for Specific Sites."

Radiation is used both alone and in combination with surgery for primary curative treatment, for palliation of symptoms, and to treat local recurrences. When early tumors are found with no lymph-node involvement, radiation and surgery are often used together. When the tumor is larger, radiation may be used alone. When the tumor is advanced and has invaded bone, preoperative radiation or radiation plus **chemotherapy** may be used along with surgery.

Techniques are constantly being examined to improve the effectiveness of radiation treatments: For example, some types of cancers of the larynx have been successfully treated with radiation alone. If this is possible, then the voice box may be left intact, which is not always possible with surgery. If you have an early cancer where there may be a choice between surgery and radiation, you may wish to get opinions from both a head and neck surgeon and a therapeutic radiologist before deciding on a treatment plan.

Chemotherapy, immunotherapy, and **hormone therapy** techniques are being used in advanced cases of head and neck cancer (at times with radiation, at times alone) prior to surgery. (See also "Experimental Treatments" below.)

Treatments for Specific Sites

CHEEK (Buccal Mucosa): If the tumor is small and localized, **radiation** is used alone. If, however, the tumor is large and invasive, surgery is employed; a large area of the cheek will be removed and facial reconstruction will be required.

GUMS (Gingiva): With small tumors, **radiation** and **surgery** are used, preserving the jaw whenever possible. With large tumors, where bone invasion has taken place, more extensive surgery will be required: removing part of the jawbone and necessitating reconstructive surgery. Radiation will be used postoperatively.

HYPOPHARYNX: Preoperative **radiation** combined with **surgery** is the treatment of choice. Since metastasis to the lymph nodes in the neck has occurred in over 50% of the cases, neck dissection is usually necessary. Depending on the case, removal of part of the tongue may also be necessary. Reconstructive plastic surgery may be required, as well as physical and speech therapy. Postoperative radiation is used to prevent recurrence.

LARYNX: Most tumors of the larynx are benign. But if it is not, and the tumor is small, **radiation** alone may be used to preserve the patient's voice. If **surgery** must be done, it will be in the form of either a *partial* or *total laryngectomy*. A partial laryngectomy may be done if the tumor is confined to one vocal cord and the cord itself is mobile. This procedure removes the tumor and part or all of the single affected vocal cord. Afterward, the patient will be hoarse, but still able to speak. If, however, the tumor is large and extends beyond the vocal cords, a total laryngectomy will be performed, which means removing the entire voice box; the lymph nodes in the neck will be treated with radiation, surgery or both.

After both types of laryngectomies, the patient will have a *tracheostomy:* A slit is made in the front of the neck and trachea, and a tube is inserted so that the patient breathes through the tube, rather than through his nose. With a partial laryngectomy, the tube is removed after a few days and the patient breathes normally. After a total laryngectomy, the patient breathes through a permanent hole in the neck, which is called a stoma.

After a total laryngectomy, patients must learn to speak again—either with a technique called esophageal speech or with an artificial larynx. With esophageal speech, the patient learns to swallow air and then expel and articulate that air. It is similar to talking through a belch, but intelligible speech can be achieved through practice. An artificial larynx is either a mechanical or an electrical device that is held next to the throat to produce the vibrations no longer produced by the missing voice box. Patients begin the process of learning to speak through either of these means even before leaving the hospital.

There are associations all over the country for people who have lost their voice boxes. They can be contacted through your local chapter of the American Cancer Society and include the International Association of Laryngectomees, the Lost Cord Club, New Voice Clubs, and Anamilo Clubs. In all these organizations, laryngectomees and professionals work together to provide rehabilitation and emotional support for people who have a difficult adjustment to make.

LIP: Small localized tumors may be treated by simply removing them surgically. For premalignant lesions, like leukoplakia, a "lip shave" may be done: just scraping off the abnormal cells. If the tumor is large, or if it has spread to the bone or tongue, more radical surgery may be performed: removing the affected structures and lymph nodes, which necessitates reconstructive plastic surgery and rehabilitation. **Radiation** may also be used. The vast majority of cases never require this extensive treatment, because lip cancers are easy to diagnose in the early stages.

MOUTH: For some localized tumors of the mouth, *electrocoagulation* may be used (see "Eye" for details). For larger tumors, **surgery,** external **radiation,** and **radium implants** may be used, either alone or as a combined treatment with adjuvant **chemotherapy** (which is done for the purpose of "cleaning up" any stray cancer cells and/or relief of symptoms). If mouth tumors have reached into the jawbone, part of the jaw will have to be removed and reconstructive surgery done later.

NASOPHARYNX: Tumors of this area are very rare and are usually treated by **radiation:** External radiation is usually preferred, although **radium implants** are also used. The lymph nodes in the neck will receive external radiation as well. The dosage will vary depending on the size of the tumor and the cell type. For advanced tumors, a combination of external radiation, **surgery,** and radium implants is used.

OROPHARYNX: These tumors may be treated by external **radiation** and **surgery,** either alone or in combination. **Chemotherapy** may be used to clean up any stray cells. Surgery and radiation treatment in this location usually require reconstructive surgery and/or rehabilitation.

PARANASAL SINUSES: These tumors are very rare. External **radiation** is given prior to **surgery** to reduce the size of the tumor. The surgical procedure is called a *radical antrectomy* and involves removing the walls of the antrum (the bony cavern in which the sinuses are located) and, at times, reaching into the bones that form the orbit of the eye (the eye socket). Reconstruction by a plastic surgeon may be necessary in a later operation. Sometimes a radium mold is put into the defect created by surgery to remove any residue of the tumor.

SALIVARY GLANDS: Most salivary tumors are located in the parotid gland, and the usual treatment is surgical. In some tumors a *superficial parotidectomy* will be performed, which involves making an incision from the ear down the neck and removing the tumor and part of the facial nerve. In more serious cases, a *total parotidectomy* will be performed, which requires removing the entire parotid gland plus neck dissection. **Radiation, chemotherapy,** and estrogen treatments may also be employed. After surgery there will be the side effects described in our discussion of neck dissection (p. 230) as well as the possibility of partial facial paralysis. Reconstructive surgery may be necessary.

TONGUE: Specific treatments will vary depending on the location of the tumor and its size. Preoperative **radiation** may be used before **surgery,** particularly with small tumors. Surgical procedures may include a *hemiglossectomy* (removal of half the tongue), *radical neck dissection* (on one or both sides), *hemimandibulectomy* (removal of half the jaw), *glossectomy* (removal of the whole tongue). If the tumor is large or has spread and these radical procedures must be done, reconstructive surgery will be scheduled to repair the defects, as well as an extensive rehabilitation program.

TONSIL: The treatment is generally **radiation** therapy, particularly for lymphomas, which tend to occur. Some squamous-cell carcinomas are treated with preoperative radiation, surgical removal of the tumor and remaining tonsil (*tonsilectomy*), and *radical neck dissection.*

Experimental Treatments

Experimental treatments are being conducted in the areas of **surgery, radiation** [external—neuron, photon, and conventional—and internal], **chemotherapy, immunotherapy,** and **hormone therapy** in various combinations. Contact: CLB, COG, EST, NCOG, RTOG, SEG, SWOG, HNCP, MAYO, MDA, MSKCC, SFCC, VASAG, WSU, CCSF (see appendix H).

Doctors Who May Be Involved in Treatment

Head and neck cancers involve highly specialized treatment, usually by a team of specialists (both doctors and other therapists). For this reason it is strongly urged that patients with these cancers be treated at major cancer centers or large medical centers that work on head and neck cancers regularly. The primary treatment is surgery, done by an otolaryngologist (ear, nose, and throat specialist) or a general surgeon with advanced training or experience. Of the surgical subspecialties that deal with head and neck cancers—head and neck surgery, maxillofacial surgery, dental surgery, plastic surgery, and, possibly, neurosurgery or thoracic surgery—only the last three have special board certification. You should consult the American Medical Association's *American Medical Directory* to check out a surgeon's training and experience, and to see whether he/she is a member of the American Society for Head and Neck Surgery and the Society of Head and Neck Surgeons. Membership in either one means serious interest and experience in this field. One of the membership requirements for the American Society for Head and Neck Surgeons is that the surgeon must have performed thirty-five such operations in the previous year.

In addition to these surgeons, a therapeutic radiologist and medical oncologist will be on the team, as well as speech therapists and physical therapists.

Further Reading and Resources

Programs for laryngectomees are sponsored by the American Cancer Society. The National Cancer Institute also has specific programs to deal with the effects of treatment for these cancers.

For reconstruction of facial defects, contact:

Dr. Salvatore Esposito, Principal Investigator
Case Western Reserve University School of Medicine
2040 Adelbert Road
Cleveland, Ohio 44106

For maxillofacial prosthetic rehabilitation:

Dr. Douglas A. Atwood, Principal Investigator
Department of Prosthetic Dentistry
Harvard School of Dental Medicine
188 Longwood Avenue
Boston, Massachusetts 02115

For oropharyngeal rehabilitation:

Dr. Jerilyn A. Longemann, Principal Investigator
Northwestern University Medical School
303 East Chicago Avenue
Chicago, Illinois 60611

For laryngectomy:

International Association of Laryngectomees
219 East 42nd Street
New York, New York 10017
Phone: (212) 867-3700

For advanced prosthetics/orthodontics:

Dr. Hans R. Lehmeis, Principal Investigator
New York University
New York, New York 10016

For electronic laryngeal prosthesis:

Dr. Byron Bailey, Principal Investigator
Department of Otolaryngology
University of Texas Medical Branch
Galveston, Texas 77550

For comprehensive laryngectomy rehabilitation:

Dr. George A. Gates, Principal Investigator
University of Texas Health Science Center at San Antonio
7730 Floyd Curl Drive
San Antonio, Texas 78284

For voice changes after radiotherapy:

Dr. Raymond H. Colton, Principal Investigator
SUNY, Upstate Medical Center
Weiskotten Hall, Room 89
750 East Adams Street
Syracuse, New York

Hepatopancreatica

See "Ampulla of Vater."

Hodgkin's Disease

See "Lymphomas."

Hypopharynx

See "Head and Neck."

Ileum

See "Small Intestine."

Jaw

See "Head and Neck."

Jejunum

See "Small Intestine."

Kidney

The kidneys are situated at the back of the abdominal cavity, one on each side of the spinal column above the waist. Part of the urinary system, they excrete urine and help regulate the water, electrolyte, and acid base content of the blood. A person can live a normal life with one kidney.

Cancers of the kidney are found both in children and in adults. Children are subject to Wilms's tumor (also called nephroblastoma), which can develop in utero or appear up to age 8, the peak age being 2. With combination therapies using **surgery, chemotherapy,** and/or **radiation,** the cure rate for all stages is 50–90%, depending on the extent of disease at diagnosis. Children with Wilms's tumor should be treated at a major cancer center or large children's hospital with a pediatric oncology department experienced in treating this type of cancer.

In adults, kidney cancers are more common in men than in women, and women tend to respond better to treatment.

Cancers of the kidney may produce no symptoms in the early stages, so a large part of the kidney may be destroyed before the condition is diagnosed, and one-third of all patients have metastases at the time of diagnosis. The major form of treatment is **surgery,** with experimental programs being conducted using **radiation, chemotherapy,** and **immunotherapy.**

Persons at risk of developing kidney cancer include: men aged fifty to sixty; people with a family history of kidney cancer, a history of polycystic kidney disease, or kidney stones; tobacco users (cigarettes, pipes, cigars, and chewing tobacco); people who have used a drug called phenacetin for extended periods; and certain occupational groups: chemists; those who work with chloroform as an industrial solvent and in the manufacture of plastics; those who work with cadmium, which is used in the manufacture of electroplates, in welding, and in making storage batteries.

Symptoms

Fatigue; weight loss; fever of unexplained origin; anemia; loss of appetite; nausea; constipation; blood in the urine (this may come and

235

go). Some tumors may be so large that they can be felt. If there is a mass in the abdomen, pain in the flanks with accompanying muscle spasm, rapid pulse rate, and excessive sweating, the disease is usually advanced. Some patients may have hypertension. And in some patients the first symptoms actually come from metastases that have spread through the bloodstream to the bones, brain, and lungs (see those site sections for symptoms).

Diagnosis and Staging

In the doctor's office a complete **medical history** will be taken and a **physical examination** done, with careful palpation of the abdomen. Samples of urine and blood will be taken for laboratory tests, including **urinalysis** to detect blood or malignant cells in the urine and **CBC** and **SMA-12** analyses.

To detect metastases, **X-rays** will be taken of the chest and skeleton; a **bone scan** and a **liver scan** will be done; an **intravenous pyelogram** (IVP) will detect and locate masses in the kidney; **ultrasound** examination of the abdomen may discriminate between malignant and benign masses or cysts; a renal **angiogram** will be done, which is 90% accurate in diagnosing a tumor and extent of its growth; a **venacavogram** will be done; and a **tomogram** of the kidney, called an enphrotomogram, which can sometimes distinguish between a cyst and a tumor. **CAT scans** may be done of the pelvis and upper abdomen; the latter is particularly useful in detecting metastases to the liver. If ultrasound and the nephrotomogram have not been successful, a percutaneous **needle aspiration biopsy** may be performed on an inpatient basis. This is a controversial procedure, not widely used since it is felt that there is a potential risk of spreading the cancer along the path made by the needle. If it is considered necessary, it should be done in conjunction with a urologist, who should be prepared to operate should complications arise.

Types of Cancers

Adults are affected by two types of tumors. The first type, tumors of the renal parenchyma (the functional part of the kidney), are generally *adenocarcinomas*, which may be referred to as hypernephromas, renal-cell cancer (Garwitz tumors), or alveolar carcinoma. The second type, tumors of the renal pelvis, are generally *transitional-cell carcinoma*. These make up 7% of all renal cancers and are related closely to bladder cancer: During the course of the disease, the cancer often involves both the renal pelvis and the bladder.

Children are affected by *Wilms's tumor* or *nephroblastoma*.

Treatment

Surgery. Two different surgical procedures are employed. If cancer is confined to the kidney, the kidney is removed along with the nearby lymph nodes and the adrenal glands. This is called a *radical nephrectomy.* The surgery is done under general anesthesia and requires a two-to-three-week hospital stay. Drainage tubes will be left in after surgery to promote healing, and urine will be measured daily, since a side effect of the surgery may be suppression of urine.

If the tumor is a renal pelvis carcinoma, a *nephroureterectomy* will be performed, in which the ureter is removed as well as the kidney and lymph nodes, because these tumors may spread along the ureter and affect the bladder.

In the unlikely event that both kidneys are involved, the usual procedure is to try to save at least one kidney and then institute kidney *dialysis,* which consists of being connected to a dialysis machine through tubes permanently embedded in each arm. The machine takes over the function of kidneys that are not functioning, removing the liquid and chemicals in the blood, cleansing the blood of impurities, and sending it back into the body. Dialysis takes three to four hours, is completely painless, and must usually be done two to three times a week for life, unless a kidney transplant is successful.

Radiation. This may be used to shrink a large tumor before surgery, or to destroy cancer cells in the lymph nodes after surgery. It is not used instead of surgery as a primary treatment unless the disease is advanced when diagnosed. It is also used to treat bone and lung metastases and to alleviate bone pain. It may be used along with **surgery** and **chemotherapy** as a combined treatment plan for Wilms's tumor.

Chemotherapy. As mentioned above, chemotherapy is used along with **surgery** for Wilms's tumor. It is being used experimentally in adult kidney cancers.

Experimental Treatments

Experimental treatments are being conducted using **surgery, radiation, chemotherapy,** and **immunotherapy.** Adults may contact: EST, SEG, SWOG, MDA, OSU. Wilms's tumor is being studied by NWTS, CHOC, and SJCRH (see appendix H).

Doctors Who May Be Involved in Treatment

Internist, nephrologist (kidney specialist), urologist, medical oncologist, therapeutic radiologist.

Large Intestine (Colon, Rectum, Anus)

The large intestine begins at the small intestine (the meeting place is called the cecum), winds upward (ascending or right colon), across the abdomen (transverse colon), down (descending colon), makes an S-curve (sigmoid colon), and straightens out for the last twelve inches (rectum) to end in the anus, where solid wastes exit the body. The whole tube is about fifty-nine inches long. Of the cancers that affect the large intestine, 50% are in the rectum, 20% in the sigmoid colon, 15% in the right colon, 6–8% in the transverse colon, 6–7% in the descending colon, and only 1% in the anus.

There is a high rate of this type of cancer in the United States, mainly due to our diet, which is high in red meat and low in roughage (fiber). Individuals who are in the high-risk category for this type of cancer include: those over forty years old those who have a history of colon polyps; those who have had one cancer in this area, even if successfully treated; those who have a family history of colon cancer or other types of cancer; those who have a history of ulcerative colitis and familial polyposis (multiple polyps), as well as such conditions as Gardner's syndrome, Peutz-Jeghers syndrome (see "Small Intestine") and Crohn's disease (inflammation of the intestines).

Symptoms

Change in bowel habits (constipation, diarrhea, or alternation of the two); blood in the stool (either red or black); mucous discharge in bowel movement; iron-deficiency anemia without cause; weight loss; tenesmus (contraction of the anal sphincter muscle in spasms with pain and a persistent desire to defecate); crampy abdominal pain due to obstruction, which may also cause hemorrhaging and perforation of the bowel, which in turn may lead to symptoms of weakness, fatigue, loss of appetite. Complete obstruction of the intestine can occur rapidly and is marked by abdominal pain; this requires immediate emergency treatment (surgery).

Diagnosis

A thorough **medical history** is taken and a **physical examination** is done as well as a **manual rectal examination,** in which the doctor (after putting on rubber gloves) explores the rectum with his fingers while pressing on the outside of the abdomen. In women, he may put one hand in the vagina and one in the rectum to get a more accurate "feel" to detect polyps or tumors. While still in the doctor's office the patient will undergo a **proctosigmoidoscopy.** Laboratory tests will be done on blood, urine, and stool samples: These will include CBC,

SMA-12, CEA assay, and stool cytology (studying the components of the feces under a microscope). The patient will then undergo tests in the hospital, which may be done as an outpatient. These may include a **colonoscopy, lower GI,** chest and bone X-rays, **cystoscopy, intravenous pyelogram** (IVP), and **lymphangiogram.**

Types of Cancer and Staging

Cancers affecting this area include *adenocarcinoma, carcinoma,* and *epidermoid (squamous-cell) carcinoma.* Adenocarcinoma is the most common type in all but the anus, where epidermoid carcinoma is most prevalent. These cancers usually spread by local invasion to nearby organs. They metastasize via the lymph channels and bloodstream. The most common sites for metastases are the liver, lung, bone, and, in women, the ovary. These tumors have a tendency to recur.

The cancers are usually staged on five levels:

Stage 0   (TIS, NO, MO)—*in situ*
Stage I   (TO-2, NO-X, MO)—contained within bowel wall
Stage II   (T3-5, NO-X, MO)—extended beyond bowel wall but no spread to regional or distant organs
Stage III (any T, N₁, MO)—spread beyond bowel wall with regional involvement
Stage IV   (any T, any N, M₁)—spread beyond bowel wall with distant metastases.

Treatment

Surgery is the first—and, at times, only—step in treatment of these cancers. The procedures vary from minor operations (the removal of polyps and small obstructions while doing the diagnostic proctosigmoidoscopy) that can take place in a doctor's office, to major surgery removing large portions of the large intestine or other abdominal organs and requiring an ostomy for the elimination of wastes from the body. The type of operation depends entirely on the location, size, and stage of the tumor, and the sex, age, and general health of the patient. Major surgical procedures include:

Colectomy   removal of part or all of the colon. The surgeon will remove the tumor and a portion of healthy tissue on either side. If enough of the colon is left, he will sew the two ends together and you will be able to function normally. If not, he will do a
Colostomy   in which an opening (called a stoma) is created in the abdominal wall, and feces diverted via a tube to a disposable, plastic bag on the outside of the body. Colostomies may be temporary (to allow time for the colon to heal) or permanent. If the colectomy involved removing a portion of the colon that would leave less than three to four inches of the lower part of the rectum, a permanent colostomy is necessary.

239

There are numerous specific names for the above operations, based on the precise part of the large intestine that is being resected (removed); your surgeon will explain these to you. In addition, if other organs in the abdominal cavity (such as the bladder or the uterus) have been affected by the cancer, they too will be removed at the same time. In certain cases, when normal major surgery is not advisable, *cryosurgery* may be done (see chapter 8). If the tumor has metastasized to other organs, and the spread is limited to those organs, they may be removed: A pulmonary resection may be done for the **lung,** an oophorectomy for an affected **ovary.** (See those sites for details of the procedures.)

All major surgical procedures require hospitalization of three to four weeks. You will be required to check into the hospital several days before the actual operation for preoperative tests and to clear out your intestinal tract as much as possible: Antibiotic drugs will be given to kill bacteria that might cause infection, and you will be put on a liquid diet to make the large intestine as "clean" as possible before surgery (these procedures have greatly reduced the number of postoperative complications). If you are anemic, blood transfusions may be given, and you will have an IV in your arm for several days feeding you vitamins and minerals. All of this is aimed at making you as healthy and strong as possible prior to surgery. At times surgical procedures must be done in several stages (like the Babcock and Bacon operations, which are "pull through" procedures—the colon is pulled through the anus for removal), in which case hospitalization will be longer.

Surgery is often part of a treatment plan using **radiation** and **chemotherapy** (see "Combined Therapies" below).

Colostomies involve a major period of adjustment for the patient. See chapter eight for a full explanation of ostomies. Support services are listed at the end of this chapter.

Radiation. Adenocarcinomas of the rectum are usually radiosensitive, but radiation as a primary treatment is used only for patients who have inoperable cancers. External radiation is given for palliative relief of symptoms, or to relieve obstruction and stop hemorrhages. An experimental program is under way at the Highland Hospital in Rochester, New York, using implants of radium needles every few weeks as a possible alternative to surgery for some localized nonadenocarcinoma tumors.

Chemotherapy. Most chemotherapy treatments are still experimental. Single drugs are still being tested; combination chemotherapy as a primary treatment has not been tested yet. Chemotherapy is being used after surgery to prevent recurrences in patients with lymph-node involvement.

240

Combined Therapies and Experimental Treatments

Because cancers of the large intestine affect so many Americans (they are the second leading cause of cancer deaths in males over 35, third in females 35–54, second in females 55–74 and the leading cause of cancer deaths in women over 75), major efforts are under way to find the most effective treatments for these cancers. Rectal cancer appears to be responding extremely well under an experimental "triple treatment": **surgery**, followed by four to six weeks of **radiation** treatments, followed by eighteen months of **chemotherapy.** Rectal cancer has a nasty habit of coming back, but this triple treatment has cut the recurrence rate in half: from 52% in patients treated with surgery alone, to 21% in patients getting the triple treatment. There are still no statistics available on long-term survival rates. Dr. Philip Schein of Georgetown University, who is the chairman of the Gastrointestinal Tumor Study Group, has said: ". . . we stopped doing surgery alone in our study last February. . . . And if one were going to select a therapy today, I think one would go with the triple treatment."

Experimental Programs: CLB, EST, GTSG, NSABP, RTOG, SEG, SWOG, MAYO, MDA, MSKCC, MTS, SFCC, VASAG, WSU, MICRC, NCCTG, SJCRH, WCCC, WFU (see appendix H).

Doctors Who May Be Involved in Treatment

Proctologist, therapeutic radiologist, medical oncologist.

Resources

Patients who have had ostomies often have a difficult adjustment to make (see chapter 8 on surgery). There is a nationwide network of support groups. Contact:

United Ostomy Association
1111 Wilshire Boulevard
Los Angeles, California 90016
Phone: (213) 481-2811
(Contact your local American Cancer Society for the nearest local chapter.)

Larynx

See "Head and Neck."

Leukemias

Leukemias are cancers of the blood or circulatory system. They usually start in the bone marrow, which is the factory that produces the various types of blood cells. White blood cells are produced in the spleen and lymph nodes as well as in the bone marrow. Leukemias do not usually show up in the form of tumors, but rather are characterized by the production of enormous numbers of white blood cells, which never reach maturity and cannot do the regular work of healthy cells. The result is that the blood cannot carry enough oxygen (this is the effect on the erythrocytes or red blood cells); the body bleeds and bruises easily (the effect on the platelets or thrombocytes, which control the clotting mechanism); and the body becomes extremely susceptible to infection (the effect on the white blood cells called granulocytes, lymphocytes, and leukocytes).

The exact causes of leukemias are unknown. There seems to be a genetic predisposition to developing some forms of leukemias, and it is known that exposure to radiation or treatment with certain anticancer drugs can lead to leukemia. People who work with benzene are also considered at high risk. Theories linking leukemias to viruses are being explored, and a major research effort is under way in the field of immunology.

Leukemias are generally divided into two broad groups: *acute* and *chronic*. Acute leukemias are characterized by poorly differentiated, immature white blood cells. They are generally severe, more commonly found in children (average age: four) and, if untreated, rapidly fatal. The white blood cells accumulate rapidly and invade such organs as the liver and spleen as well as the lymph nodes. Normal bone marrow is replaced by abnormal cells. Acute leukemias can progress very rapidly to a fatal stage as patients suffer from severe anemia, central-nervous-system involvement, and a marked tendency to hemorrhage. The usual goal of treatment of acute leukemia is cure or complete remission.

For patients with chronic leukemias, the treatment goal is palliation and control of the disease rather than cure. Chronic leukemias are characterized by well-differentiated mature white blood cells. Excessive numbers of these white blood cells are found in the bone marrow, spleen, and liver. Chronic leukemias progress slowly and respond to treatment.

Acute and chronic leukemias may be further subdivided into the following types:

ACUTE: Lymphocytic
                  Lymphocytic or lymphoblastic (ALL)

242

               undifferentiated
               prolymphoblastic
          Monocytic
               acute monocytic or monoblastic (AMonoL)
          Myelogenous
               granulocytic (AGL)
               myelocytic (AML)
               myelomonocytic (AMML)
               erythroleukemia (EL)
               promyelocytic (AProL)
               oligoblastic
CHRONIC:
          Chronic myelocytic or granulocytic (CML)
          Chronic lymphocytic (CLL)

These various forms of leukemias affect different age groups, produce different symptoms, progress in different patterns, and are treated differently. Therefore, we will discuss the four major types of leukemias (AML, ALL, CLL, and CML) separately. However, there are certain aspects of diagnosis and treatment that are shared, and we will discuss these before getting into the specific types of leukemias.

Diagnosis

Leukemias may be the easiest form of cancer to diagnose, particularly from a patient's point of view. In addition to the usual **medical history** and complete **physical examination,** all definitive tests are done on blood samples and bone-marrow samples. Blood samples are easily taken in the doctor's office. **A bone-marrow aspiration** and **bone-marrow biopsy** will be done in the hospital. Should the leukemia prove difficult to classify, patients should have their slides read by a specialist in this type of diagnosis—a hematopathologist—at a major cancer center. This is particularly important since the exact type of leukemia makes a difference in the kind of treatment that will be effective. (See the explanation of CBC in chapter 5 for an explanation of the various blood tests.) Other diagnostic procedures may be scheduled, depending on the particulars of each case and the type of treatment program the patient wishes to enter. They may include chest **X-ray, lymphangiogram,** kidney-function tests, **liver-spleen scan, CAT scan** of the head, **lumbar puncture, bone scan.**

Treatment Techniques: An Overview

Chemotherapy is the mainstay of treatment for all leukemias. Occasionally a patient may develop enlarged organs or lymph nodes, which may be treated with external **radiation** or **surgery.** Should the leukemia affect the central nervous system, a combination of chemotherapy (administered directly into the fluid surrounding the spine via a lumbar puncture) and external radiation of the brain will be used. Total body irradiation (external) and internal radiation using radioactive phosphorus administered through an IV may be used in treating some chronic leukemias. **Immunotherapy** is experimental at present.

Both the leukemia and the treatments themselves must be monitored extremely closely because of the many severe consequences and complications that may arise: anemia, hemorrhaging, and life-threatening infections. Treatment of these problems may require transfusions of whole blood, platelets, or white blood cells, and intravenous instillations of fluids and/or antibiotics. If bone-marrow function is severely depressed, the patient may become a candidate for an experimental procedure called *bone-marrow transplant,* in which a compatible donor (preferably a brother or sister, who theoretically has a compatible immune system) gives some of his/her bone marrow to replace the diseased marrow in the patient. The procedure has shown some encouraging results with patients in their first remission, although it is usually not attempted unless other measures have failed.

ALL

Characteristics

ALL is primarily a childhood leukemia, occurring most commonly under the age of 10. It is the most common form of childhood cancer. Patients usually have symptoms for only a few months before the disease is diagnosed, and secondary infections are usually present. There may also be bone destruction with pain resembling that of rheumatoid arthritis. With ALL there is a marked reduction in the numbers of white blood cells that fight infection (granulocytes), and infection is the usual cause of death. Remission occurs in 80–90% of cases treated with combination chemotherapy, and survival rates are improving all the time. However, at the moment about half the patients can be expected to have relapses.

Symptoms

Bruise easily; tire easily; frequent nosebleeds; bleeding gums; frequent infections; bone pain; persistent fever; symptoms of urinary inflammation; in boys the testes may be involved. Fifty percent of all patients have pancytopenia, which is a reduction in the numbers of all types of blood cells. Patients usually have enlarged spleen and lymph nodes.

Treatment

Treatment is carried out in two phases. The first is called the induction phase, and utilizes high-dose combination **chemotherapy** plus treatment of the central nervous system. Many patients already have CNS leukemia (meningeal leukemia) at the time of diagnosis, and because it develops so frequently even if it not present, prophylactic treatment is given. The goal in this phase is to obtain a complete remission. The patient will have to repeat the bone-marrow exams approximately every two weeks as a monitoring procedure. If the patient has not obtained a complete remission after six weeks of intensive therapy, he/she should be referred to a cancer center that can offer more advanced, experimental forms of treatment.

Complete remissions are achieved in 85–95% of the patients. Once this has been achieved, the second phase of treatment (maintenance phase) begins. This usually involves three to five years of low-dose combination chemotherapy. The goal of this phase is to prolong the remission and possibly produce a cure. Frequent bone-marrow and spinal-fluid examinations will be done to catch any relapses at the earliest possible point. For male patients there is a risk of involvement of the testes, and **biopsy** of these organs at the end of treatment is recommended.

Patients who have relapsed can be re-treated with combination chemotherapy: Complete remissions can be obtained but are usually of short duration. At this point some patients would be considered for bone-marrow transplantation.

AML

Characteristics

This is the most common leukemia in adults over 40, although it can occur at any age. It is characterized by a marked decrease of platelet production, which puts the patient in danger of massive internal hemorrhaging. White cells are also decreased, with the result that infections are common and often do not respond to antibiotics given in normal doses. Without treatment, patients usually survive only a few months. Treatment produces remission in 40–60% of patients, but the recurrence rate is high. Death is often caused by infection.

Symptoms

The onset of symptoms may be quite sudden, with fever and chills brought on by an acute systemic infection. Patients may also

245

experience anemia, which produces fatigue and pallor, and bleeding— usually from the gums or gastrointestinal tract. The bleeding is caused by severe platelet reduction, and may be light or very heavy. Enlargement of the lymph nodes is common. In some cases there may be an enlarged spleen. Other symptoms may include bone pain, obstruction of the ureters, and, if the central nervous system is involved, headaches and double vision.

Treatment

There are three phases to treatment for AML. The first is the induction phase, where high-dose combination **chemotherapy** is given to produce remission. Because bleeding and infections are such a serious problem for this type of leukemia, and even the insertion of a needle to give chemotherapy drugs presents a danger, the patient is hospitalized and is under constant care and supervision for the three to six weeks necessary for this phase of treatment. Supportive therapies are often given in the form of various kinds of transfusions (white cell, red cell, platelets); and antibiotics, antimetabolites, and immunotherapy drugs may be used until the bone marrow starts to function normally again.

Several weeks after this phase is completed, the patient will be rehospitalized for the consolidation phase, in which lower doses of combination chemotherapy are given. The patient is then placed on long-term maintenance therapy at still lower doses, which can be given on an outpatient basis. If there is central-nervous-system involvement, it will be treated in the same way described above for ALL.

AML is less responsive to treatment than ALL. Approximately 50% of the patients achieve a complete remission. Children respond better than adults, and adults over 60 respond the least frequently. If relapse occurs, a second remission can be obtained with chemotherapy, but it is usually of short duration.

CML

Characteristics

CML accounts for 20% of all leukemias in the United States and usually affects adults 20–50 years old. Most patients with CML have a chromosomal abnormality called the Ph or Philadelphia chromosome (only 10% do not). It is the only known chromosomal abnormality associated with leukemia. The disease usually stays chronic for three or four years, controllable by chemotherapy, but then a bone-marrow failure or "blast crisis" occurs. This makes it an acute disease and there is increasing anemia, which does not respond to treatment. From this point on, the disease is usually considered fatal, although patients have responded to treatment and returned to a chronic form of the disease.

Symptoms

The symptoms of CML develop slowly. There may be recurrent infections, easy bruising and bleeding, fatigue, and abdominal discomfort due to an enlarged abdomen. Patients may perspire heavily, lose weight, and be unable to tolerate heat. As the disease progresses they may experience bone pain and persistent fevers.

Treatment

Treatment for CML is aimed at controlling the disease through maintenance therapy—correcting abnormal blood counts and relieving symptoms. **Chemotherapy,** external **radiation,** or internal radiation (with radiophosphorus) may be used. When the blast crisis occurs, treatment is changed, and in younger patients bone-marrow transplants are sometimes used. If there is central-nervous-system involvement, cranial radiation is given. Treatment is given on an outpatient basis; when the blast crisis occurs, treatment must be done on an inpatient basis.

CLL

Characteristics

CLL is usually a disease of later life (60–70) with slight male predominance. It is the most common type of chronic leukemia, and encompasses several subgroups of leukemias, such as T-cell CLL, hairy-cell leukemia, and lymphosarcoma-cell leukemia. Patients are very apt to develop secondary infections since immunity is impaired, and there is a high frequency of second malignancies. There is usually spleen involvement, with accompanying enlargement of the spleen.

Symptoms

CLL often has no symptoms and is spotted during a routine physical examination. When symptoms do occur, they may include weight loss, fatigue, low-grade fevers, and night sweats. Occasionally, enlarged lymph nodes, an enlarged spleen, enlarged liver, or new skin lesions that may itch are the first signs.

247

Treatment

Often no treatment is necessary at first, since in many cases this is a very slow-growing form of leukemia. When necessary, the disease can be kept under control and symptoms relieved with external radiation (to alleviate weight loss, bleeding problems, and bone marrow failure) and internal radiation (radioactive phosphorus given by IV to correct irregularities in blood-cell composition). Prednisone has been used with some success in decreasing the tendency to bleed and in reducing lymph-node and spleen enlargement. Most patients respond satisfactorily to treatment given on an outpatient basis for a minimum of six months.

Experimental Treatments

Major research is being conducted in treating leukemias, and these programs do present the cutting edge of treatment development, so they should be explored. Treatments include **chemotherapy, radiation, immunotherapy,** and **bone-marrow transplants.** Experimental programs are being conducted for all types of leukemias at the National Cancer Institute in Bethesda, Maryland, as well as through the cooperative groups listed below (see appendix H):

ALL (including acute undifferentiated leukemia [AUL] and stem-cell leukemia): CCG, CLB, SEG, SWOG, MDA, MSKCC, SFCC, MIDWEST, SJCRH.
AML (all types): CCB, CLB, EST, NCOG, SEG, SWOG, MDA, MSKCC, SJCRH, UCLA, YALE.
Chronic Leukemias: CLB, EST, SEG, SWOG, SCG, SLT, MDA, MSKCC.
Other Leukemias: CCG, PVSG, SEG, SWOG, MDA, MSKCC, YALE.

Doctors Who May Be Involved in Treatment

Hematologist, medical oncologist, therapeutic radiologist.

Resources

For children with leukemia, see chapter 13, "Children with Cancer." It is recommended that children with leukemia be treated at a major cancer center or children's hospital with a large pediatric oncology department.

Liver

The liver is the largest (weighing several pounds) and one of the most complex organs in the body. It is located on the upper right side of the abdomen, under the rib cage, and is composed of two lobes and the bile ducts that run into the duodenum. Technically a part of the digestive system, it performs many functions—converting worn-out red blood cells into bile; regulating hormone levels; producing proteins necessary for blood clotting; storing sugar and vitamins A, D, E, and K; regulating the amount of sugar circulating in the blood; and controlling cholesterol levels. Clearly a person cannot survive without a liver, although the liver has tremendous recuperative powers and can function with 80% of it removed. Even though liver cancers do spread, death from this type of cancer is usually due not to the metastases but to liver failure.

Primary cancers of the liver are very rare—about 2% of all cancers. It is, however, a common site of metastases for other forms of cancer, particularly lung, breast, and gastrointestinal cancers. It is important to remember that metastatic tumors in the liver are not "liver cancer": Treatment and prognosis for these cancers are based on the primary sites from which they spread.

In the United States, people at high risk of liver cancer include those who work with arsenic and vinyl chloride (used in making plastics), and people who have taken testosterone, a synthetic male hormone used by athletes to improve muscle development and also used in sex-change procedures.

Patients with inoperable primary liver cancer should consider experimental treatments, since presently the prognosis is very poor, with only 1% surviving five years and most dying within six months of diagnosis.

Symptoms

Jaundice; a general feeling of malaise and fatigue; weight loss; a feeling of abdominal fullness or bloating due to ascites (the accumulation of fluid in the abdominal cavity); a dull pain in the upper abdomen, which may become more acute with deep breathing; pain in the shoulder that radiates to the back and becomes more severe over time.

Diagnosis and Staging

A complete **medical history** will be taken and **physical examination** done with careful examination of the abdomen, since many liver tumors can be felt as hard, enlarged masses. Blood samples will be analyzed in the laboratory: **CBC, alkaline phosphatase** test, and the **BSP** (bromsulphalein) test. If cancer is present, the levels of the latter two will be elevated.

In the hospital, the patient will have **X-rays, tomograms, CAT scan, liver scan, angiogram,** and possibly a new procedure called a *radiologic catheter invasion,* in which a dye is injected through a catheter and pictures are taken of the highlighted blood vessels; since the liver has so many blood vessels, this test not only gives an accurate picture of

249

the vessels but also shows up irregularities in the structure of the liver itself.

Definitive diagnosis will be made using a **needle biopsy**, which is usually done on an inpatient basis. An exploratory **laparotomy** may be done for staging purposes. The diagnostic and staging procedures are very thorough since a tumor in the liver is most commonly a sign of some other form of cancer, not liver cancer. A treatment plan will not be worked out until doctors are absolutely sure whether the tumor is a primary liver cancer or one that has spread to the liver from another site. There is no formal staging system in use at this time.

Types of Cancers

Hepatomas (hepatocellular carcinomas) and *cholangiocarcinomas* account for half of all liver tumors. Hepatomas usually involve both lobes of the liver, and they metastasize to the adrenal glands, lungs, and bones. Cholangiocarcinomas begin in the small bile ducts and spread by invading the liver itself.

Hemangiosarcomas seem to be increasing in incidence and are linked to industrial exposure to vinyl chloride. They are mixed tumors consisting of sarcoma cells and hemangiomas, which are benign tumors of dilated blood vessels. *Mixed sarcomas* are very rare, but when they appear they spread to other parts of the liver as well as to distant lymph nodes in the regions of the lung and brain. *Hepatoblastomas* are a very rare liver cancer found in children, and are granular tumors. *Adenocarcinomas* are found in the bile ducts.

Treatment

For primary liver cancers that involve a single tumor confined to one lobe, a surgical procedure called a *total hepatic lobectomy* is performed: This involves removal of the tumor and part, or all, of the healthy tissue in that lobe. The operation is a major one, done under general anesthesia, and requires about two weeks of hospitalization. At the time of diagnosis, however, most liver cancers are inoperable.

For inoperable cancers, **chemotherapy** is being tried using a technique called *hepatic artery infusion,* which is a form of regional chemotherapy: A catheter is placed directly into the blood vessels going to the liver so that the drugs are concentrated in the liver. Experiments are also being done with liver transplants, and also with various combinations of drugs and combining drugs with **radiation.**

See: EST, NCOG, RTOG, SEG, SWOG, SFCC (appendix H).

Doctors Who May Be Involved in Treatment

Gastroenterologist, abdominal surgeon, medical oncologist, therapeutic radiologist.

Lung

The lungs occupy most of the space in the chest cavity. They wrap around the heart, the blood vessels going to and from the heart, and the esophagus. Air gets into the lungs through the windpipe (trachea), which branches into the lungs and further subdivides into small passages called "bronchial tubes" or "bronchi." Each lung is divided into lobes: The right lung has three lobes, the left lung has two.

Lung cancers are adult diseases. This is partly because, with the exception of oat-cell carcinoma, lung cancers are slow-growing—it takes twenty years for them to go from a single abnormal cell to a symptom-producing, detectable cancer. They also tend to be symptom-free until they become advanced, making early detection uncommon and effective treatment difficult. The lungs themselves are vital organs, and lung cancers tend to spread (through the blood and lymph systems as well as invasion) to other vital parts of the body: the brain, liver, bones, and heart.

The causes of lung cancers only begin to play a role in people's lives in their mid-teens and early twenties. Smoking is the primary cause of lung cancer: Epidemiologists consider that 90% of the deaths due to lung cancer could be prevented if no one smoked. Exposure to air pollution in and near factories and mines also causes cancer, and generally does not become a factor until people enter the labor market. Workers with particular susceptibility to lung cancers include ship-yard workers, miners, construction workers, chemical workers, asbestos workers, and copper-smelting workers, to name a few. All of the people employed in these occupations double their chance of developing lung cancer if they also smoke, and lung cancer among asbestos workers occurs almost exclusively among smokers. Other people in the high-risk group include patients with a history of tuberculosis, chronic bronchitis, and emphysema.

Symptoms

The first symptoms may be related either to the primary tumor or to the metastases. The primary tumor may cause: a persistent cough lasting more than three weeks; chronic chest pain; difficulty in breathing, or wheezing when breathing; coughing up blood; difficulty swallowing; or hoarseness caused by the tumor pressing on the esophagus. In later stages, pneumonia may develop or there may be an accumulation of fluid in the chest cavity. In many cases the primary tumor itself may produce no symptoms, but the metastases do. This is why people suspected of having brain tumors or bone tumors have chest X-rays as part of the initial diagnostic procedure: Often these tumors have metastasized to these sites from the lungs.

251

Diagnosis

After taking a thorough **medical history** and doing a **physical examination,** the following procedures may be employed: chest **X-ray;** chest **tomogram; fluoroscopy** (to watch the lungs in motion); **gallium scan; bone scan;** and **liver scan.** A variety of procedures are used to determine the exact location of the tumor and to obtain cell and tissue samples for examination under a microscope. These include a **bronchoscopy, bone-marrow biopsy, scalene-node biopsy,** and **thoracentesis,** as well as the following:

Thorascopy: Done in the operating room under general anesthesia. An incision is made between the ribs and the lung is deflated, like a balloon. The entire lung and surrounding structures are examined and a biopsy is obtained. After the procedure, the lung is reinflated.

Mediastinoscopy: Using a local anesthetic, a small incision is made in the neck near the breastbone (mediastinum) and lymph nodes are removed. The test is used to determine whether the cancer is operable, whether it has spread behind the mediastinum, and for obtaining tissue samples. It can be done on an outpatient basis.

Percutaneous needle biopsy: Using a local anesthetic, a hollow needle is inserted through the chest to remove tissue from the lung. The procedure can be done on an outpatient basis and takes only a matter of minutes.

Sputum examination: The patient coughs up a sample of mucus for examination under the microscope to see if cancer cells are present. This procedure can often detect cancers too small to be seen in an X-ray, and will be done several times in the course of the diagnostic process to make sure that the changes that have taken place in the mucus are constant.

Before any surgical procedure is done, the patient will have a *pulmonary-function test.* This is a procedure that determines how well the lungs are working in terms of the volume of air that can be inhaled and exhaled, and also the flow rate of air in and out of the lungs (measured in liters per minute). Depending on the condition of the patient and the information that is needed, the procedure can take anywhere from a few minutes to two hours.

Most of the procedure can be done using a machine called a "spirometer." This is a small box that contains a bellows or a small drum inverted over water. A tube leading from the side of the box is placed in the patient's mouth (nose clips are usually employed to prevent air leaks and to make sure the patient breathes only through the mouth). The patient breathes into and out of the tube, expanding the bellows or moving the drum up and down. The movement (which shows the volume and flow) is recorded on a moving chart on the top of the box by a pen attached to the bellows or drum. The nurse, technician or doctor who is doing the test will ask the patient to breathe in different ways. The patient may be asked to breathe air that has been mixed with specific amounts of helium or nitrogen.

The procedure can be done with the patient at rest (sitting) or while doing exercise. There is no pain involved, but the patient may feel fatigued when the test is over. Some patients, especially those who have difficulty breathing normally, may experience a feeling of suffocation when the nose clips are put on. The test can be done at bedside, in a doctor's office, or in a special room called a "pulmonary function laboratory."

There is also a diagnostic procedure called a *thoracotomy*, but because it is also a surgical treatment procedure, it is described below under "Surgery."

Types of Cancers

There are over a dozen types of cancers that begin in the lungs, but four of them make up 90% of all cases: *oat-cell (small-cell) carcinoma, epidermoid (squamous-cell) carcinoma, adenocarcinoma,* and *large-cell carcinoma.* Although knowledge of the precise cell type of cancer is important in designing treatments for all lung cancers, two distinctions made by oncologists are very important from the patient's point of view.

First of all, they divide lung cancers into oat-cell and non–oat-cell types. This is done because oat-cell carcinoma behaves very differently from all other lung cancers: It is fast-growing, it is sensitive to radiation and chemotherapy, and surgery is not used in the treatment plan. It is important that patients diagnosed with oat-cell carcinoma be treated at a major cancer center that has experience with newly developed treatment techniques. This used to be the most lethal form of lung cancer, but the newer treatments have made the picture brighter. All other lung cancers are slow-growing, and surgery is the primary curative treatment. Squamous-cell carcinomas are centrally located, spread by local invasion, and are more associated with smoking than are the other types of lung cancer. If found early, there is a high cure rate. Adenocarcinoma of the lung metastasizes widely (brain, bones, adrenal glands, liver—almost any organ in the body) and is usually confined to one lobe of the lung. Women and nonsmokers commonly have this type of lung cancer. Large-cell carcinoma behaves similarly to adenocarcinoma.

The other distinction oncologists make is whether the non–oat-cell lung cancers are operable. Since surgery is the primary treatment for these cancers, this is very important. Over 50% of all lung cancers are inoperable, either because of their location or because at the time of diagnosis they have spread too far for surgery to be effective.

253

Treatment

Surgery. Before any surgery is done, there must be a thorough knowledge of not only the type of cancer involved but how advanced it is (i.e., it must be carefully staged). Surgery will only be an effective cure if the tumor is localized, and small enough to be completely removed. In some cases surgery may be performed to relieve symptoms even if the tumor cannot be removed entirely. This is usually followed by **radiation** treatment.

All surgical procedures for lung cancer are major surgery, and are done under general anesthesia. The operations take from two to three hours and require two to three weeks of hospitalization. After surgery you may experience a great deal of pain, which does go away, and shortness of breath. There will be a tube running out of your chest (temporarily sewn to your skin to keep it in place) to drain excess fluid. The fluid will be bloody at first, but after a few days it will get lighter and there will not be as much of it. This is normal. You will also be asked to cough to keep your lungs clear, and to do simple arm and leg exercises and breathe deeply. All of these things hurt at first but are necessary. The nursing staff will monitor you closely so that blood clots, irregular heart rhythms or, in rare cases, respiratory failure, can be dealt with immediately and successfully.

There are three surgical procedures used in treating lung cancer. The *thoracotomy* is technically an exploratory operation in which the chest cavity is opened for the purpose of diagnosis. If lung cancer is found and is operable, one of two procedures will be done: a *lobectomy*, which is the removal of a lobe of one lung; or a *pneumonectomy*, which is the removal of an entire lung.

Radiation. External radiation may be the primary treatment for some Stage I cancers, but it is usually used by itself to treat inoperable cases, or cases where lung cancer has recurred after having been successfully treated by surgery. It is also used as palliative treatment for brain and bone metastases and to relieve symptoms like coughing and shortness of breath by shrinking inoperable tumors in the lung. Radiation is used experimentally to control metastases and increase survival time, and preliminary results are encouraging. It is also used in combined primary treatment with **chemotherapy** for oat-cell carcinoma.

Chemotherapy. Chemotherapy is used as a primary treatment only for oat-cell carcinoma. It may be used as palliative therapy for all lung cancers. Most chemotherapy treatment plans for all forms of lung cancers are experimental (see below).

Experimental Treatments

Experimental treatments are being carried out using **surgery, radiation, chemotherapy,** and **immunotherapy** (see appendix H).

254

Oat-cell carcinoma: CLB, EST, NCOG, SEG, SWOG, MAYO, MDA, MSKCC, WPL, CA-LUN, CCSF, NCCTG, NUTR, RPMI, WFU, National Cancer Institute/VA Hospital.

Non–oat-cell cancers: CLB, COG, EST, NCOG, RTOG, SEG, SWOG, WDP, BCRC, LCSG, MAYO, MDA, MSKCC, MTS, VALG, VASAG, VASOG, WPL, WSU, CCSF, NC-LUN, RPMI, UARIZ, UCLA, WFU, CAN-NCIC, CAN-OCI.

Doctors Who May Be Involved in Treatment

Thoracic surgeon, therapeutic radiologist, medical oncologist.

Further Reading

"Progress Against Cancer of the Lung" and "What You Need to Know About Lung Cancers," both available free from the Office of Cancer Communications, NCI, Building 31, Room 10A18, Bethesda, Maryland 20205.

Barbara G. Cox, *Living with Lung Cancer* (Rochester, Minnesota: Mayo Foundation, 1977), $2.55. Order from: Schmidt Printing, Inc., 1416 Valley High Drive, NW, Rochester, Minnesota 55601.

Lymphomas

Lymphomas are cancers of the lymphatic system. The abnormal lymph cells usually appear as congregations, which enlarge the lymph nodes, form solid tumors in a variety of locations in the body, or, rarely, like leukemia, circulate in the blood. They are usually fast-growing.

The classification system of lymphoma is complex, and not all physicians agree on one scheme. Lymphomas are usually divided into two large groups: Hodgkin's disease and non-Hodgkin's lymphomas. In addition, we will also discuss one type of non-Hodgkin's lymphoma, mycosis fungoides (MF), separately at the end of this chapter. MF is a non-Hodgkin's lymphoma that invariably involves the skin, and is therefore classified separately.

Under a microscope, lymphoma tissue often resembles normal lymph tissue. Pathologists often disagree about the cancerous potential of a given sample, or about the exact type of lymphoma being observed. If there is any doubt as to the diagnosis, patients should ask that their tissue samples (slides) be reviewed by several experienced pathologists.

Hodgkin's Disease

Hodgkin's disease is a form of lymphoma that now has a 90% complete remission rate in early-stage disease. Both combination **chemotherapy** and **radiation** therapy are used as standard treatments. Hodgkin's disease can occur at any age, but has two peak periods: between the ages of 15 and 34, and after 50. Males and females are equally susceptible.

Symptoms

The symptoms of Hodgkin's disease vary from patient to patient and may include enlarged lymph nodes in the neck, groin, or armpit; fatigue; pain after drinking alcohol; itching; nausea and vomiting; weight loss; fever or night sweats.

Diagnosis and Staging

A **medical history** will be taken and a complete **physical examination** done, with attention paid to lymph nodes, spleen, liver, and pain in bones. Laboratory tests of the blood and urine will be done. If one of the easily accessible lymph nodes (neck, groin, armpit) is involved, initial diagnosis may be made by removing these through minor surgery for microscopic examination. If these nodes are not involved, conclusive diagnosis must wait for complete staging, which requires a **bone-marrow biopsy, lymphangiogram, intravenous pyelogram (IVP), abdominal** and/or **chest CAT scan, liver scan, spleen scan,** and **bone scan;** all can be done on either an inpatient or outpatient basis. Surgical diagnostic/therapeutic procedures for the procurement of tissue samples for microscopic examination may include a **laparotomy** with a **wedge biopsy** of the liver, and a **splenectomy** (removal of the spleen— the patient can live without it).

In planning treatments, very careful diagnostic and staging procedures will identify the exact cell type and the pattern of cancer spread. Clinical staging (CS) should follow what is called the Ann Arbor Classification:

Stage I   Involves a single lymph node region.
Stage II   Involvement of two or more lymph node regions on the same side of the diaphragm.
Stage III   Involvement of lymph-node regions on both sides of the diaphragm.
Stage IV   Spread of the disease outside the lymph system.

Each stage is then divided into A and B categories: "A" patients have no generalized symptoms; while "B" patients have had either unexplained weight loss of more than 10% in the six months before diagnosis, or unexplained fever with temperatures above 38° C (100.4° F).

The diagnostic and staging process is not complete without examination of commonly affected tissues and cells under a microscope. This is called "pathological staging" (PS), and the same system is used as in clinical staging. An example of how this information would look on a patient's chart would be: CSIIA, PS III$_s$A. This means that the patient is in clinical stage II with no general symptoms, but after the laparotomy it was found that he is actually in Stage III, with disease in the abdominal lymph nodes and spleen. This example represents a common occurrence: The patient has been "up-staged" based on careful diagnostic efforts. The up-staging will result in the use of different and more effective treatment.

Types of Cancers

Hodgkin's disease has been classified by several systems. The old system divided it into three groups: paragranuloma, granuloma, and sarcoma. The current system, the Ryle Classification, divides it into lymphocyte predominance, nodular sclerosis, mixed cellularity, and lymphocyte depletion.

Treatment

Depending on the stage, type, and specific location of the disease and condition of the patient, **radiation, chemotherapy,** or a combination of both may be used for the purposes of cure.

Radiation. Stages I (A&B), II (A&B), and IIIA are usually treated by megavoltage external radiation, given in one or two four-week periods.

Chemotherapy. The standard chemotherapy combination for Hodgkin's disease is called MOPP (nitrogen mustard, Oncovin (vincristine), procarbazine, and prednisone). It is given in twenty-eight-day cycles over a period of months; the exact length of treatment varies from case to case. It is usually used in advanced cases (Stages IIIB and IVA&B). Chemotherapy may also be given in combination with radiation in advanced cases and in cases where there are large tumors.

NOTE: With careful staging and treatment, the high remission rate for Hodgkin's disease often means a "cure" for many patients. Both radiation therapy and chemotherapy are technically difficult to administer correctly; the details and duration of treatment need to be carefully planned and executed. Patients are advised to seek out physicians who are experienced in treating Hodgkin's disease.

Experimental Treatments

Despite the high complete remission rate in some stages, experiments continue for those types of Hodgkin's disease that still do not respond well to current treatments, and also for the purpose of refining treatment techniques. Contact: CCG, CLB, EST, RHDG, SEG, SWOG, MDA, MSKCC, SFCC, CHOP, YALE, CAN-NCIC (see appendix H).

Non-Hodgkin's Lymphomas

The most confusing aspect of explaining non-Hodgkin's lymphomas is the terminology. The old names for this group of lymphomas were lymphosarcoma, reticulum-cell sarcoma, and giant follicular lymphoma. But these were not useful classifications in describing how the diseases progressed and how they responded to treatment. The most widely accepted of the newer classification systems is called the Rappaport Classification. It is based on various combinations of the following characteristics: whether the pattern is *nodular* (the cells are clumped in the lymph node) or *diffuse* (spread out); whether the types of cells affected are *histiocytes* or *lymphocytes* or *mixed;* and how well *differentiated* the cells are. This has led to the identification of eight types of non-Hodgkin's lymphomas:

NLWD	Nodular lymphocytic well-differentiated lymphoma
NLPD	Nodular lymphocytic poorly differentiated lymphoma
NHL	Nodular histiocytic lymphoma
NML	Nodular mixed histiocytic-lymphocytic lymphoma
DLWD	Diffuse lymphocytic well-differentiated lymphoma
DLPD	Diffuse lymphocytic poorly differentiated lymphoma
DHL	Diffuse histiocytic lymphoma
DUL	Diffuse undifferentiated (non-Burkitt) lymphoma

The rule of thumb in prognosis is that, without effective treatment, nodular is better than diffuse, lymphocytic is better than histiocytic, and well differentiated is better than poorly differentiated. However, experimental combination drug chemotherapy has produced excellent results with DHL. Non-Hodgkin's lymphomas also include mycosis fungoides and Burkitt's lymphoma.

Symptoms, Diagnosis, and Staging

The symptoms, diagnostic process, and staging of non-Hodgkin's lymphomas are similar to those of Hodgkin's disease, with the following exceptions:

· Non-Hodgkin's lymphomas may show up almost anywhere in the body, often with primary sites outside the lymph nodes: For example, the gastrointestinal tract is a common site for non-Hodgkin's lymphoma to arise. In many of these cases there has been confusion with less serious diseases or other forms of cancer before lymphoma was finally diagnosed. Since lymphoma responds to very different forms of treatment than other cancers that affect this region, it is very important to have an accurate diagnosis.

· Because the gastrointestinal tract is often involved, an **upper** and **lower GI series** and other tests for this system (including **endoscopy**) may be performed. Although the abdominal region is explored in staging both types of lymphomas, for non-Hodgkin's lymphomas **laparoscopy** may be substituted for a laparotomy, and splenectomies are not routinely performed.

· The diffuse lymphomas can involve the coverings of the brain (the meninges) and the fluid that bathes the brain (the cerebrospinal fluid). Some of this fluid is usually examined by a **spinal tap** (**lumbar puncture**).

· It does not spread in a regular pattern like Hodgkin's disease does. Hodgkin's disease usually spreads to adjacent lymph nodes, and is therefore predictable. Non-Hodgkin's lymphomas do not.

Treatment

Treatments vary depending upon the specific cell type of lymphoma, the patient's condition, and the stage of the disease. Early-stage nodular lymphomas may not require any immediate treatment, but should be monitored closely. Pathologically staged I and II diffuse lymphomas are usually treated with **radiation.** In cases where radiation fails to provide a complete remission, **chemotherapy** provides effective retreatment.

For Stage II and IV nodular and diffuse lymphomas, the primary treatment is high-dose combination chemotherapy. Radiation may be used to reduce the size of tumors before chemotherapy starts, or as consolidation treatment after remission has been achieved with chemotherapy.

Non-Hodgkin's lymphomas are diseases in which the details of treatment are technically demanding. Recent advances in knowledge about lymphoma treatment have been rapid, and the cures have emerged only in the last five to ten years. Patients should be treated in major medical or cancer centers by physicians experienced in designing and administering curative forms of treatment.

Experimental Treatments

Involvement in a Phase III experimental program should be considered the cutting edge of standard treatment for non-Hodgkin's lymphomas because the interim results of ongoing protocols are promising. Patients should contact the National Cancer Institute or the following cooperative groups: CCB, CLB, EST, SEG, SWOG, MDA, SMKCC, SFCC, CHOC, SJCRH, WFU, YALE, CAN-UICC (see appendix H).

Mycosis Fungoides

Mycosis fungoides is a very rare type of lymphoma that is usually discussed separately because it behaves so differently from other lymphomas: It is slow-growing, affects the skin, and remains on the skin for years before spreading to other parts of the body. It is very difficult to diagnose because the symptoms are similar to those of other, less serious skin diseases; only in advanced cases are there enough lymphoma cells concentrated on the skin to make a confirmed diagnosis by a pathologist possible. For this reason, even though the symptoms may have been noted for years and the patient may even have been under the care of a skin specialist (dermatologist), it is usually not diagnosed in people under 40.

Symptoms

A chronic, intermittent, itchy rash that can appear anywhere on the surface of the body. In the early stages it appears as patches of thick, scaly skin (called plaques) that look like eczema or psoriasis.

Diagnosis

Diagnosis can only be made on the basis of **biopsy**—examination under a microscope of affected skin cells removed by minor surgery in the doctor's office after a **medical history** and complete **physical examination** have been done. To determine the extent of the disease, the patient may be asked to undergo the following procedures: **chest tomograms**, pulmonary-function tests (see "Lung"), **liver-spleen scan, gallium scan,** and **lymphangiogram.** Immunological laboratory tests may be done on blood and urine samples given by the patient.

Treatment

Treatment depends on the stage of the disease. Stage I, the premycotic stage, produces the symptoms described above. In this stage it is almost impossible to get a confirmed diagnosis, and treatment focuses on relieving the itching—with soothing baths, antihistamines, and creams containing steroid hormones. In Stage II, the infiltrative stage, the abnormal cells (reticuloendothelial cells) spread into the lower levels of the skin, producing very thick patches that can be studied under a microscope. In Stage III the disease spreads through the lymph channels to various parts of the body.

Treatment involves **radiation** (electron-beam therapy) and/or **chemotherapy.** Chemotherapy may be topical (the application of nitrogen mustard), or systemic (IV and pills), or combinations of drugs.

Experimental Treatments

Experimental programs to determine the best forms of treatment are being conducted at the National Cancer Institute/VA Hospital and SWOG (see appendix H).

Doctors Who May Be Involved in Treatment

Dermatologist, therapeutic radiologist, medical oncologist. Because of the difficulties involved in diagnosis, the rarity of the disease, and the team effort necessary for its effective management, it is advisable for patients to contact one of the centers that have the most expertise in dealing with mycosis fungoides.

Melanoma

See "Skin."

Mouth

See "Head and Neck."

Myeloma

See "Bone."

Nasopharynx

See "Head and Neck."

Nasal Cavities

See "Head and Neck."

Nerves

See "Brain and CNS."

Nose

See "Head and Neck."

Oropharynx

See "Head and Neck."

Ovary

Ovarian cancers are unfortunately subject to the "Catch-22 syndrome" of all cancers that grow deep within the body: They are easy to cure if found early, but they are almost never found early because they are hidden deep within the abdomen and produce no symptoms in the early stages. Once you have been diagnosed as having ovarian cancer, you must get treatment immediately: Untreated ovarian cancer is fatal in a very short time—the average is ten months. Even if your first set of treatments does not cure you, this type of cancer is being worked on with new, more effective treatments being developed all the time. If you can buy time now, it is likely that you will be able to live a long time.

Symptoms

There are no symptoms in the early stages. As the tumor grows the woman may feel pelvic pressure, and/or fullness in the abdomen; she may notice unusual bleeding or absence of menstruation. In very advanced stages she may feel pain and there may be an abnormal accumulation of fluid (ascites) in the abdominal cavity. These symptoms are commonly ignored by women when they first appear; younger women may dismiss them as normal fluctuations in the body during the menstrual cycle, or attribute them simply to overeating. Since ovarian cancer most commonly affects women between 40 and 60, the symptoms may be dismissed as being part of menopause. Even your gynecologist may not be able to spot the cancer when it is small. Mildly enlarged cystic ovaries (a cyst is an abnormal sac containing gas, fluid, or semisolid material; cystic ovaries have cysts on them) are fairly common in younger women and are usually ignored. Ovarian cancer is not detectable on a Pap smear (that test is used only to diagnose cervical cancer).

Diagnosis

Your gynecologist will discuss your **medical history,** give you a thorough **physical examination** and **pelvic examination,** do a Pap smear, and may do a **paracentesis** or cul-de-sac **aspiration;** a needle is placed through the vaginal wall into the space between the vagina and the rectum to draw out any fluid for microscopic examination. She will also palpate your breasts for lumps. If there are any, she may do a **needle biopsy** to see if they are benign or malignant. All of this takes about an hour.

The next part of the diagnostic work-up must take place in the hospital, although these procedures can be done on an outpatient basis: **mammogram, upper** and **lower GI series, intravenous pyelogram (IVP).** The final diagnostic procedure is a **laparotomy:** This is major surgery and is usually done as part of a "cancer operation"—an operation that includes both diagnostic and treatment procedures. This will be discussed under "Treatment" below.

Types of Ovarian Tumors

Epithelial-cell tumors make up 90% of ovarian tumors. Most are adenocarcinomas. The epithelium is the covering of all surfaces in the body, both inside and outside—your skin, the surfaces of organs like the ovary or stomach, and the inside surfaces, like the lining of your blood vessels. The other 10% are made up of various other tumor types.

Celioblastomas act differently depending on how large they are. When these tumors are small, they act like fibromas (a benign tumor, made up of the fibrous tissue that forms the structure of the ovary). When they are large they act more like cystadenomas. They can grow to an enormous size.

Dysgerminomas are rare germ-cell cancers, often mixed in with other tumors, like teratomas. They are very sensitive to radiation. After successful treatment, if it is going to recur at all, 80% of the cases will recur within the first year after diagnosis; patients who remain free of the disease for two years have a good future.

Endometrioid tumors are named for their similarity to adenocarcinoma in the endometrium (uterus). They are not very malignant, but they tend to recur; the patient must have regular checkups.

Hormonal or *feminizing* tumors are the *granulosa-cell tumor* and the *theca-cell tumor* (*thecoma*). These tumors are generally not found during a woman's reproductive years, and they may or may not be cancerous. Granulosa-cell tumors usually occur in childhood, and symptoms include "precocious puberty"—early onset of menstruation, early breast development, and early development of pubic hair. Theca-cell tumors usually appear during or after menopause.

Krukenberg tumors are usually found on both ovaries and are very malignant. They may start in the ovary, or may start in the stomach and spread to the ovary. Under a microscope they are noted for having signet-ringlike cells.

Squamous carcinoma has cells that look flat and scaly under a microscope. If the tumor is found in only one ovary and is removed completely, the survival rate is good.

Sarcomas are very malignant tumors—they spread easily and quickly. The cells are packed very closely together, and they generally affect the connective tissue that makes up most of our body (muscles, skin, bones, etc.).

Teratomas are tumors made up of many different types of tissue, many of them coming from the part of the body where the tumor grows. They are broken down into three types: *solid* teratomas, which are very rare, usually grow in children or very young women, and are considered malignant unless proven otherwise; *embryonal (immature)* teratomas, which are germ-cell tumors and may combine with other types of germ-cell tumors (like choriocarcinomas, which are found in the uterus), and are usually found in only one ovary; and *adult (mature)* teratomas, germ-cell tumors that are only cancerous in 2% of the cases—the other 98% are fairly common benign tumors in older women—and also are usually found only in one ovary.

There are two kinds of tumors that are *usually not cancerous* but can become cancerous on occasion (doctors describe them as having "low malignancy potential"). *Cystadenomas* make up 50% of all cancerous and noncancerous ovarian tumors. On the rare occasion that they become cancerous, the survival rate is 35%. *Dermoid cysts* are the other kind of generally noncancerous tumor. They are probably congenital, and they account for nearly half of all ovarian cysts that occur in childhood.

You may also hear the term "unclassified carcinoma." The classification systems that are used for the different cancers are very detailed but not complete. Some cancers simply do not fit into any convenient slot, so they are considered "unclassified."

Grading and Staging

Several different systems are used for grading ovarian tumors; the following is the one used by the American College of Obstetricians and Gynecologists:

Stage I: Tumor growth is limited to the ovaries.
Stage IA: Tumor growth is limited to one ovary with no ascites.
Stage IB: Tumor growth is limited to both ovaries with no ascites.
Stage IC: Tumor growth in one or both ovaries with ascites present which have malignant cells in the fluid.
Stage II: Tumor growth is in one or both ovaries *and* there is tumor growth in other parts of the pelvic region.
Stage IIA: Tumor growth and/or spread is confined to the uterus and/or fallopian tubes.
Stage IIB: There is tumor growth in other pelvic tissues.
Stage III: There is tumor growth in one or both ovaries and it has spread to the abdomen.
Stage IV: There is tumor growth in one or both ovaries and it has spread outside the abdominal (peritoneal) cavity.

Treatment

Treatment for ovarian cancers always begins with **surgery,** and then may continue with **radiation** and/or **chemotherapy.**

Surgery. One operation will often involve several procedures, named for what is done and what is removed. For ovarian cancers, the surgeon will want to look at and feel the entire abdominal cavity and get tissue samples from any suspicious area. This exploratory procedure, involving a long incision up the front of the patient's abdomen, is called a **laparotomy.**

The surgeon will then look at, and appropriately deal with, the areas that have been or are likely to be affected by the cancer, including the ovaries, fallopian tubes, and uterus. Women generally refer to removal of any of these organs as a "hysterectomy." In fact, a *hysterectomy* is the removal of the uterus. A *salpingo-oophorectomy* is the removal of the ovary and its fallopian tube. Removal of both ovaries and fallopian tubes is called a *bilateral salpingo-oophorectomy.* There are two kinds of hysterectomies: vaginal and abdominal. In both cases, the uterus is removed. With a vaginal hysterectomy, the uterus is removed by going through the vagina. With an abdominal hysterectomy, the surgeon goes in through the abdominal wall. The usual surgery is a total abdominal hysterectomy (TAH) and a bilateral salpingo-

265

oophorectomy (BSO). You will be walking the day after surgery and released from the hospital in about a week.

This operation means that you can no longer bear children, and you will no longer have menstrual periods. It does not mean you will immediately gain fifty pounds, suffer unbearable depressions, have crying jags, or no longer enjoy an active sex life.

It is possible that the laparotomy will be done as a separate procedure. In this case there will be five to seven days between the laparotomy and the TAH & BSO. This may happen because the surgeon wants to consult with the pathologist and the oncologist to map out the specific treatment plan. If there is no spread at all, they may opt for a vaginal hysterectomy, which is a less serious operation than an abdominal hysterectomy. There may be "suspicious" places in the abdominal cavity which might or might not be handled surgically, and this decision would be made not by the surgeon alone but in consultation with the oncologist (who is not present at the laparotomy), based on possible treatment options.

In addition to these procedures, while you are on the operating table an *omentectomy* may be performed. The omentum is a fold of membrane going from the stomach to neighboring organs in the abdominal cavity. An omentectomy is the removal of that membrane if it seems to be involved with the spread of cancer. It may be performed as a preventive measure; but it is a controversial procedure and is usually not done unless there are signs that the cancer has spread. After the bulk of the cancer is removed by surgery, **radiation** and/or **chemotherapy** may be used. If the cancer is very widespread, it is possible that no surgical treatment will be done.

A second laparotomy may be done at the end of your total treatment to make sure that the radiation and/or chemotherapy has done its job and that no more such treatment is needed.

Radiation. Radiation therapy may be given in the form of **internal radiation** implants or **external** radiation, which is given to the whole abdomen in the form of rays, usually from a material called "cobalt 60." Treatment will begin no sooner than one week, but no later than four weeks, after surgery. NOTE: Radiation has not been successful in treating recurrences of ovarian cancer. Should that happen, the doctor will usually recommend a **chemotherapy** program, not more radiation.

Chemotherapy. Chemotherapy treatments are given both in high doses for curative purposes and in low doses for maintenance. Some treatments involve only one drug, others use a combination.

Experimental Treatments

CCG, EST, GOG, NCOB, SEG, SWOG, MAYO, MDA, MSKCC, MTS, OCSG, SFCC, WSU, YALE, CAN-NCIC (see appendix H).

Doctors Who May Be Involved in Treatment

Gynecologist, abdominal surgeon, medical oncologist, therapeutic radiologist, gynecological oncologist.

Palate

See "Head and Neck."

Pancreas

The pancreas is a gland that functions as part of the digestive and endocrine systems. It is about five inches long and divided into three sections: The head is nestled into the duodenum (small intestine); the tail runs into the spleen; the body runs between the two ends. The common bile duct comes out of the gallbladder and liver, joins the pancreatic duct, and feeds into the small intestine through the head of the pancreas. The pancreas manufactures digestive juices and insulin. The latter is manufactured by special cells called "beta cells" or "islets of Langerhans." Alpha cells secrete glucagon, a hormone that also affects sugar levels in the blood.

Cancers of the pancreas tend to be slow-growing, but because they cannot be felt in regular physical examinations and often exhibit no symptoms for a long time, diagnosis is usually not made until the cancers are far advanced. If untreated, death occurs most frequently from obstructive liver failure.

Cancers of the pancreas account for 2–3% of all cancers; however, a rise in the number of cases in the past several years make it now more common than cancer of the stomach. People who are at risk of developing pancreatic cancers include those over 30, males, smokers, drinkers, coffee drinkers, chemists, chemical engineers, coke workers in steel plants, workers in rubber and paint plants, and dye manufacturers.

Symptoms

Pancreatic cancers often produce no symptoms until they are well advanced. Then they may appear as one or more of the following: jaundice; back pain; weight loss; weakness; loss of appetite; fever and chills; bile-colored or dark urine; clay-colored stools; very itchy skin; abdominal pain; diabetes; depression and anxiety.

267

Diagnosis

A complete **medical history** and **physical examination** will be done, including a **rectal examination** (see "Large Intestine"). Laboratory studies on blood and urine samples will include **CBC**, **cytological studies, serum alkaline phosphatase test,** and fasting blood sugar test. Liver function studies (see **liver scan**), **upper** and **lower GI series, CAT scan, ultrasound** examination of the abdomen, and an *ERCP* (endoscopic retrograde cholangiopancreatography) will be done. The ECRP is a form of **endoscopy** in which a special scope is swallowed and threaded into the duodenum. A small catheter, located within the endoscope, is then inserted into the pancreatic duct. Cell samples may be taken and a dye injected into the pancreas, after which **X-rays** are taken.

Definitive diagnosis must be made on the basis of tissue samples (although both ultrasound and ERCP are highly accurate in diagnosing these tumors). This is usually done using a surgical procedure called a **laparotomy,** which may be done at the same time as, or prior to, treatment surgery, when a biopsy is made.

Types of Cancers

Ninety percent of all cancers of the pancreas are *adenocarcinomas.* Two-thirds of these occur in the head of the pancreas with accompanying conditions of pancreatitis (inflammation of the pancreas) and duct obstructions. *Islet cell tumors* are not common.

Tumors are divided into two types: *functioning* and *nonfunctioning* (extremely rare). Functioning islet-cell tumors spread to the liver, as do adenocarcinomas, but the prognosis is better. *Cystadenocarcinomas* are very slow-growing tumors, also rare, and also with a better prognosis than adenocarcinomas.

Treatment

The primary form of treatment for pancreatic cancers is **surgery.** As mentioned above, an exploratory laparotomy and biopsy will be performed, which includes examination of the liver and surrounding lymph nodes. Since most cancers of the pancreas have already spread by the time they are diagnosed, further surgery may not be indicated.

Two types of procedures are employed for tumors that are resectable. In a *partial pancreatectomy,* or *Whipple procedure,* part of the pancreas and the surrounding lymph nodes are removed, as well as the duodenum, part of the stomach, and the common bile duct. In a *total pancreatectomy,* the entire pancreas is removed; if all or part of the pancreas is removed together with the duodenum, the procedure is called a *pancreatoduodenectomy*. The operation can take anywhere from one to six hours depending on what has to be removed and how many of the gastrointestinal structures have to be relinked with bypass procedures (see "Large Intestine," "Small Intestine"). The patient will be hospitalized for several weeks, and may require transfusions, IV feedings, and other special care during the first few days. Total convalescence takes up to six months. Since the removal of the pancreas means that no insulin will be produced by the body, the patient will have to remain on a permanent low-fat, low-sugar diet.

For unresectable tumors, palliative surgery may be performed to alleviate symptoms. This may come in the form of bypass operations to relieve obstructions, or neurosurgical procedures like **nerve blocks** to relieve severe pain.

Radiation combined with **chemotherapy** may be given postoperatively to relieve symptoms and provide short-term remission.

Experimental Treatments

Because pancreatic cancers are not discovered until they are advanced, and are not treated successfully by standard radiological and chemotherapy techniques, they have one of the worst prognoses of any form of cancer: The five-year cure rate is less than 2%, and usually the time between onset of symptoms and death is only a matter of months.

For this reason, all patients with pancreatic cancers may want to seriously consider becoming involved with experimental programs using chemotherapy and radiation techniques, either alone or in combination, being conducted by CLB, EST, NCOG, SWOG, GTSG, MSKCC (see appendix H). The National Cancer Institute is conducting experiments using high-dose radiation during surgery.

Doctors Who May Be Involved in Treatment

Gastroenterologist, gastrointestinal surgeon, therapeutic radiologist, medical oncologist. Because of the seriousness of the surgical procedures and the expertise needed for accurate diagnosis, patients should seek out a highly experienced treatment facility for this type of cancer, in either a major medical center or comprehensive cancer center.

Papilla of Vater

See "Ampulla of Vater."

Penis

The penis is the male organ of copulation and the passage for urine. Primary cancers of the penis are extremely rare, but those at highest risk are uncircumcised males aged 50–70 with poor hygiene. (Contrary to superstition, intercourse with a female who has cervical cancer does not cause penile cancer.) Cancers of the penis when found and treated in the early stages have a five-year survival rate of 85–90%. If the cancer has spread to the lymph nodes in the groin, the five-year rate shrinks to 30–40%. Since lesions on the penis usually result from venereal disease or cancer, a doctor should be consulted immediately when a lesion appears.

Cancers of the bladder, testicle, prostate, and kidney (the rest of the genitourinary system) can spread to the penis. Treatment for these metastatic cancers will be the same as that described for their primary sites, not necessarily the treatment described below.

Symptoms

The usual symptoms are a sore or ulcer on the tip of the penis that does not heal, although it is rarely painful; a lump in the groin; discharge from the penis, which is caused by an infection and may irritate and itch; bleeding upon erection; or erection without sexual desire.

Diagnosis

After the doctor takes a **medical history** and does a complete **physical examination**, a **biopsy** is done under local anesthetic. Circumcision (removal of the foreskin) may be necessary in order to expose the lesion for biopsy.

Treatment

Chemotherapy and radiation are not effective with primary cancers of the penis, so **surgery** is the treatment of choice. If diagnosed in an early stage, an operation called a *partial penectomy* will be done, removing the lesion or tumor and part of the penis and leaving a stump for sexual activity and urination. Later stages will require a *total penectomy*—amputation of the entire penis. The lymph nodes in the groin may also be removed in a procedure called an *inguinal lymphadenectomy* (see "Testes" for description).

If the cancer has metastasized to the penis from another site, the tumor will be removed surgically and **radiation** treatments given to relieve the pain that these metastases often cause.

Doctors Who May Be Involved in Treatment

Urologist, therapeutic radiologist.

Prostate

The prostate is a gland found only in men; it produces the milky fluid that is mixed with semen during ejaculation. It is located under the bladder and surrounds the urethra, the tube that carries urine from the bladder to the outside of the body. It is comprised of three lobes: the median lobe and two lateral lobes.

The prostate is quite susceptible to a variety of conditions, including benign tumors; in fact, the majority of tumors of the prostate are benign. It is common for the prostate to become enlarged after age 40. Although cancer of the prostate is uncommon in younger men, it is the second most common form of cancer in men over 60. Those at increased risk of prostate cancer are those over 55 years of age, black men, and married men.

Cancer of the prostate is very slow-growing, and is generally considered a chronic disease. If the cancer is detected in the early stages, while still localized in the prostate, it is quite curable; for this reason, regular rectal examinations in men over 40 are important. Since these cancers grow slowly, are often without symptoms, and generally affect older men, the usual cause of death is from other age-related diseases (heart and lung conditions) rather than from prostate cancer.

Symptoms

The disease usually does not produce symptoms until it is advanced. The most common symptom is a hard lump that may be found in a routine physical examination. Some symptoms may be caused by enlargement of the prostate, such as bleeding from the penis; difficulty in starting or stopping urination; painful urination; dribbling; and, if the tumor obstructs the flow of urine, frequent urination and/or bedwetting. (NOTE: These symptoms are *not* specific to cancer; rather, they indicate a problem with the prostate which should be checked with a doctor immediately.) Often the first symptoms come from metastases, rather than the tumor itself: for example, backache or sciaticalike pain, and swelling of the legs.

Diagnosis

In the urologist's office, a complete **medical history** will be taken and you will have a complete **physical examination** including a rectal examination: After putting on rubber gloves, the doctor will put his finger into the rectum and actually feel the prostate gland. Ninety percent of tumors can be felt.

Laboratory tests will be done on samples of blood and urine. They include serum factor analysis, **acid phosphatase test,** and blood urea nitrogen (BUN) tests. In larger medical centers, enzyme and hormone

271

assays may be done. Experimental tests are being developed by the Prostate Cancer Project of the National Cancer Institute to detect prostate cancer before it metastasizes, but these are not usually available.

A definitive diagnosis cannot be made until a **biopsy** is done and tissues examined under a microscope. A **needle (aspiration) biopsy** is usually done, but if the patient is having severe problems due to prostate enlargement and surgery is being done in order to alleviate those problems, a biopsy may be taken at the same time.

The extent of metastases will be checked with skeletal and chest **X-rays,** an **intravenous pyelogram (IVP),** and **bone scans,** since cancer of the prostate most frequently spreads to the bones, lungs, and lymphatic system.

Staging

Tumors are staged in four groups: T_1 tumors are encapsulated within the prostate and are surrounded by normal tissue; T_2 tumors are also completely within the prostate but make a bulge in the usual contour of the gland and are beginning to break out of the capsule; T_3 tumors go beyond the capsule; T_4 tumors are immovable or involve structures next to the prostate. Staging classifications will include whether only one or many tumors are involved, whether the nearby lymph nodes are involved, and the exact location of metastases, if any.

Types of Cancers

Most cancers of the prostate are *adenocarcinomas*. Prostate cancers are radiosensitive and estrogen-dependent, making hormone therapy a treatment option (see "Cervix" for a detailed explanation).

Treatment

Standard treatments for cancer of the prostate include **surgery, radiation,** and **hormone therapy.** Chemotherapy is not used as a primary treatment, although it may be employed if relapse occurs.

Surgery. The type of operation that may be done depends on the size of the tumor and the extent of involvement.

For small tumors, a procedure called *transurethral resection* (TUR) of the prostate may be performed. This involves no incision and uses **cryosurgery** as a technique. After the patient has been anesthetized, using a spinal or general anesthesia, a tubelike instrument called a "resectoscope" is inserted through the penis. Layer after layer of the tumor cells are destroyed by touching them with an electric wire loop. After each layer is killed, the dead cells are removed by a washing process until the tumor is gone. If any bleeding occurs, the sources are also sealed off using the electric current. A catheter will remain in place for several days to help with urination. The patient is usually discharged from the hospital in ten days and is able to urinate normally.

For larger tumors a *total prostatectomy* is necessary. There are several types of prostatectomies, all of which include the removal of the prostate gland and seminal vesicles. In a *suprapubic* prostectomy, an incision is made below the navel, the bladder is opened, and the prostate tissue is removed by the surgeon's fingers through the urethra. In a *retropubic* prostatectomy, the incision is made in the same place, but no incision is made into the bladder. In a *perineal* prostatectomy, the incision is made between the legs, in front of the rectum, close to the gland. The bladder is not cut into.

With all prostatectomies, a catheter is left in place for seven to ten days to help with urination, and the patient may go home after about ten days. Pain is only moderate and is controllable with medication. About a month's convalescence is required. After the operation the patient is sterile; and if nerves have been damaged during surgery, the patient may no longer be able to have an erection. If so, he should ask his urologist about devices that can be permanently implanted in the penis so that intercourse is again possible. A few patients will find that their ability to control their urine has been impeded by the operation. This can usually be corrected through exercise.

Radiation. Radiation treatments may be **internal,** in the form of seeds implanted in the prostate, or **external** megavoltage radiation. Radiation treatments are used for very early, small tumors, for tumors that cannot be treated surgically, and to treat metastases. The results have been good. Radiation may also be used to treat bone pain caused by metastases. Radiation therapy may temporarily cause diarrhea and bleeding in the urine.

Hormone Therapy. Since prostate tumors are estrogen-dependent, the manipulation of hormone levels in the body can relieve symptoms and retard tumor growth. Using various techniques, the levels of male hormones are decreased. This may be done by removal of the glands that produce male hormones (the testes, in a procedure called an *orchiectomy*), or by the patient taking oral estrogens in the form of diethylstilbestrol (DES) or cortisone. If the disease recurs or the patient does not respond to hormonal management, the adrenal glands, which also produce male hormones, may be removed. This is called a *surgical adrenalectomy.* The hormones produced by the adrenal glands can be counteracted by administering cortisone followed by a maintenance dosage of prednisone; this is called a *medical adrenalectomy.* Male-hormone release may be reduced further by the removal of the pituitary gland (hypophysectomy). Adrenalectomies usually do not prolong life, but they relieve symptoms and pain; hypophysectomy

273

may retard the disease process as well as reducing pain. Hormone therapy may result in certain cardiovascular conditions, impotence, and enlarged breasts.

Experimental Treatments

Experimental treatments are being given in **chemotherapy, hormone therapy,** combinations of chemo- and hormone therapy, **radiation,** radiation and hormone therapy. See: EST, NCOG, NPCP, RTOG, SEG, SWOG, UORG, MDA, WSU, WFU, YALE (appendix H).

Doctors Who May Be Involved in Treatment

Urologist, medical oncologist, endocrinologist, therapeutic radiologist, urological surgeon.

Rhabdomyosarcoma

See "Bone."

Salivary Glands

See "Head and Neck."

Sinuses

See "Head and Neck."

Skin

Cancers of the skin are the most common types of cancer in the United States: Over 400,000 new cases appear each year. With the exception of malignant melanoma, the victims of skin cancer are not counted in most cancer statistics because these cancers are fairly easy to detect and cure by surgery, and thus generally do not pose the life-threatening hazard presented by other forms of cancer. Skin pigmentation is nature's way of protecting against skin cancers, so these cancers tend to be Caucasian diseases, with the highest incidence showing up in fair-skinned people, among the elderly, and in people whose work exposes them to factors that can lead to skin cancers: outdoor workers (sunlight is carcinogenic), people exposed to abnormal amounts of radiation (radiologists, technicians, patients receiving radiation treatment), and people who work around certain chemicals (coal tar, aromatic hydrocarbons, arsenic, etc.).

Skin cancers are generally divided into two large groups: malignant melanoma, and nonmelanoma skin cancers. These will be discussed separately in this section.

Nonmelanoma Skin Cancers

Types and Symptoms

There are two major types of nonmelanoma skin cancers. *Basal-cell carcinoma (basal-cell epithelioma)* is the most common type, comprising 80% of these cancers. They are usually found around the nose, eyelids, cheeks, and backs of the hands—all areas that have had long-term exposure to sunlight. It is a fairly slow-growing cancer and can appear in three forms:

1. The nodule-ulcerative form, which is the most common. It is raised off the surface of the skin, its center is ulcerated, and the outer edge looks beaded and rolled-in toward the center. In early stages the skin covering the tumor looks pearly; after it ulcerates it looks crusty.
2. The superficial, sharply marginated plaque. The border is a raised, shiny thread; the center may be covered with scales or superficial ulcers.
3. The pigmented nodular or superficial form.

Basal-cell carcinomas, although slow-growing, spread by direct invasion and, if left untreated, can invade bone and cartilage. They have been called "rodent ulcers" because of this tendency to invade. They do not metastasize.

Squamous-cell carcinomas may appear in a wide range of forms: They may be scaly or ulcerated, an elevated node, a punched-out infiltrating ulcer, an ulcer with turned-out edges, or a large spongy tumor. It does infiltrate, and affected tissues become hard. Lymph nodes may or may not be involved, but in very late cases widespread metastases may occur. These cancers can be caused by constant local irritation, or by heat, or exposure to radiation. They may appear on top of old scars. They are commonly found on the ear, face, hands, lower lip (trumpet players are susceptible), and neck, and in people over 60.

275

Several skin conditions should be watched carefully, as they are considered premalignant. *Xeroderma pigmentosum* is an inherited condition and involves areas of the skin that are exposed to the sun. *Keratosis* occurs most frequently in older people who have had long exposure to the sun and is a thickening of the skin in a small area, often scaly. *Hyperkeratosis* is similar to keratosis but generally involves a small area of skin, usually found on the hands and face. *Bowen's disease (intraepidermal squamous-cell carcinoma)* usually appears on areas of the skin not exposed to the sun and wind, and is usually a reddish-brown scaly patch.

In addition to the two basic types, there are a series of very rare cancers that affect the skin: malignant *epithelial-cell tumors,* which develop from the sweat and sebaceous glands; and *dermatofibrosarcoma protuberans,* which looks like clusters of nodules. Malignant *lymphoma* and *mycosis fungoides* are discussed in the section on lymphoma. *Kaposi's sarcoma* and *leiomyosarcoma* are discussed under "Bone."

Diagnosis and Staging

The patient will have a complete **physical examination** and a **medical history** will be taken, with particular attention paid to any familial history of skin cancers. Diagnosis is made on the basis of a **biopsy:** Small tumors may have an **excisional biopsy,** which may also be curative surgery. Larger tumors may be examined using an **incisional** or **punch biopsy.**

Staging classifications are usually as follows:

Tis   Carcinoma *in situ*
T_1 Tumor of 2 cm or less, completely superficial
T_2 Tumor of 2–5 cm, or with minimal infiltration
T_3 Tumor of more than 5 cm, or with deep infiltration of the dermis
T_4 Tumor extends to other structures, like cartilage, muscle, or bone

Treatment

Surgery and **radiation** are the primary methods of treatment. In early stages, (Tis–T_2) the patient may have a choice, depending on the location of the tumor.

Surgery. Small early cancers may be removed in the doctor's office using a local anesthetic. It is most often indicated for T_3 and T_4 tumors; for residual or recurrent tumors after radiation treatment, or in cases where there is bone involvement; and when tumors develop on top of scars. Depending on the location of the cancer and how deep it is, reconstructive plastic surgery may be necessary to repair any defects. In general, surgery involves removing the tumor and a margin of healthy tissue around it.

There are several types of surgical techniques used. *Electrosurgery* uses an electric needle and a curette (a small, rakelike tool). The curette scoops out some of the cancer, and the electric needle is applied to burn off the remaining abnormal cells. This can be done in the doctor's office with a local anesthetic, and is only used with small tumors (1 cm or less). *Excision surgery* is the standard type of surgery, done with a scalpel. The tumor and a margin of healthy tissue are removed. *Chemosurgery* uses chemicals, usually zinc chloride, to remove the cancer cells. The chemical is applied, and given several hours to work. The site of the tumor is examined under a microscope to see if any abnormal tissue remains, and, if so, another application is made. *Cryosurgery*, freezing the cells with liquid nitrogen, is used only on tiny cancers and precancerous lesions.

Radiation (external). This may be used instead of surgery which would disfigure the patient—such as on the face and ears. It is also employed with high-risk or elderly patients considered unsuitable for surgery.

Chemotherapy. This is used mainly in the form of topical 5-FU cream for superficial and precancerous lesions. For recurrent cancer that cannot be controlled with surgery or radiation, patients have been helped by systemic chemotherapy.

Immunotherapy. DNCB cream has been used in skin metastases and multiple superficial lesions. Injections of immunotherapy drugs may also be used in advanced cases.

Experimental Treatments

There are no formal experimental treatment programs for non-melanoma skin cancers because they are already so curable. Basal-cell carcinoma is considered 100% curable. If there is no lymph-node involvement and the patient receives adequate treatment, the cure rate for squamous-cell carcinoma is 95%. If the lymph nodes are involved, the rate is about 70%.

Doctors Who May Be Involved in Treatment

Treatment should be given by a qualified dermatologist, with the addition of a therapeutic radiologist if radiation treatment is to be used, a plastic surgeon if reconstructive surgery is necessary, and an ophthalmologist if the cancer is on the eyelid.

Malignant Melanoma

Malignant melanoma is a rare cancer (1–2% of all cancers), but has had an increasing incidence in the last twenty years; in many countries the mortality rates have doubled. Unlike other skin cancers, it grows very rapidly and spreads to distant sites very quickly. It is extremely important that this type of cancer be detected in its earliest stages: If caught before it spreads, it is considered 100% curable by simple surgery; after it has spread, the cure rate drops dramatically to 10–20%.

Melanomas most commonly start in pigmented cells (nevi) in the skin, although they can also be found in the eye, intestines, vagina, and vulva. It may start in an existing mole or in a new area. Melanomas are highly invasive and spread throughout the bloodstream and lymphatic system. The most common sites for metastases are the lungs, brain, and liver, although they can spread anywhere in the body. It is common for a person who has developed one melanoma to develop more, so patients who have been successfully treated must be monitored carefully.

Melanomas are most common in light-skinned people with freckles. In white women, melanomas occur most often on the lower limbs; in white men, on the trunk. Black patients most often develop melanomas on the soles of the feet. Certain families seem prone to developing melanomas. Sun exposure can be a factor.

Symptoms

The following list of eight melanoma danger signs has been put out by the National Cancer Institute:

1. Change in size of a mole: Sudden increase in size is of special concern; slow change is much more common.
2. Change in color of a mole: Of special concern is the mixing of shades of red, white, and blue, or a sudden darkening of brown or black shades.
3. Change in mole surface: Watch for scaliness, flaking, oozing, erosion (as when a scab comes off), ulceration, bleeding; appearance of a nodule or bulging, mushrooming mass.
4. Change in how a mole feels to the touch: Getting hard, getting lumps.
5. Change in shape or outline of a mole: Finding an irregular, notched border where it used to be regular and smooth; sudden elevation of a surface that used to be flat.
6. Change in skin around a mole: Spread of pigment from the edge of the mole into skin that used to be normal-looking; finding redness or swelling (inflammation); development of satellite pigmentation (that is, nodules of pigmentation next to, but not a direct part of, a mole).
7. Onset of new feelings or symptoms in a mole: Feeling itchy, tender, or painful.
8. Sudden appearance of a new pigmented lesion in an area of skin that used to be normal.

Diagnosis and Staging

A complete **medical history** will be taken, with focus on skin problems, exposure to high-risk situations, and family history of skin cancer or other types of cancers. The doctor will then give the patient a complete **physical examination,** with careful examination of the skin all over the body, including the hard-to-see areas on the back, back of the neck, buttocks, genital area, and scalp. Diagnosis will be made on the basis of an **excisional biopsy,** which can be done in the doctor's office under a local anesthetic. If the lesion is quite large, an **incisional biopsy** may be done. At times melanoma may be difficult to diagnose under a microscope, so the patient should have the diagnosis confirmed by a pathologist experienced in this type of cancer (dermatopathologist).

Staging procedures may include palpation of the lymph nodes and a **lymphangiogram.** Laboratory tests include **urinalysis, CBC,** and an examination of stool samples. The patient may also be scheduled for chest **X-rays** or **tomograms, brain scan, liver scan,** and/or **cardiac catheterization.**

Melanoma may be staged as follows:

Stage I   Localized
Stage II   Spread to regional lymph nodes
Stage III   Distant spread to lymph nodes; multiple tumors on skin; and/or has spread beneath skin to other sites.

Another system classifies the tumors as: T_1, flat tumors; T_2, nodular tumors; T_3, tumors with satellite nodules.

Types of Malignant Melanomas

There are three types: *Superficial spreading melanoma* (SSM) and *nodular melanoma* (NM) start from already existing moles; *lentigo maligna melanoma* (LMM), also called Hutchinson's freckle, is quite rare and is associated with sun exposure in fair-skinned people. Superficial spreading melanoma accounts for two-thirds of all melanomas.

All types grow and spread very quickly. There have been cases of spontaneous regression with melanomas. Some regressions are partial—the original tumor goes away, but the metastases continue to grow—but occasionally a complete regression occurs. These spontaneous regressions are very rare.

Treatment

Standard treatment is **surgery,** and may be done at the same time as the biopsy, or the curative surgery may be done later. The pro-

279

cedure involves the removal of the tumor and a *wide* (2–3″) margin of healthy tissue around it. Some type of plastic surgery and skin grafting is usually required to repair the defect. If the melanoma arises on the hands or feet, amputation of the digit may be necessary. If the lymph nodes are involved, they will be removed if appropriate; melanomas on the middle of the back may spread either up or down, and so many lymph nodes may become involved that removing them all is not advisable.

Since people who have developed one malignant melanoma are at high risk for developing others, the patient will be monitored closely and expected to take precautionary measures after the cancer has been successfully removed. The patient should stay out of the sun and use sunscreens with a high sun protection factor (SPF). *Consumer Reports* of June 1980 evaluated sunscreens and gave the highest rating (SPF 15+) to the following products: Black Out Cream Lotion, Coppertone Super Shade Sunblocking Lotion, Total Eclipse Sunscreen Lotion, Elizabeth Arden Suncare Sun Blocking Cream, Bain de Soleil Ultra Sun Block Creme, Clinique 19 SPF Sun Block, and Estee Lauder Sun-Cover Creme. The patient should also have regular monthly self-examinations, and twice-a-year examinations by a dermatologist. Patients with a familial history of malignant melanomas and "B–K moles" should be checked every three months during periods of mole growth.

Experimental Treatments

Chemotherapy and **immunotherapy** are being intensively studied, particularly in regard to advanced, disseminated melanomas or regionally confined metastases. Patients with advanced disease should contact: EST, NCOG, SEG, SWOG, MAYO, MDA, MSKCC, WSU, CA-MEL, NC-MEL, OK-MEL, PA-MEL, WFU, CAN-NCIC (see appendix H).

Resources

A booklet called "Early Detection of Primary Cutaneous Malignant Melanoma" is available from your local chapter of the American Cancer Society. It has good pictures that can help in identifying suspicious moles.

Doctors Who May Be Involved in Treatment

Dermatologist (for diagnosis); general surgeon with experience in dealing with cancers, particularly melanomas; plastic surgeon; medical oncologist. Since malignant melanomas are rare cancers, initial diagnosis and treatment should be carried out in major cancer centers or hospitals with experience in this type of cancer.

Small Intestine

The small intestine is a twenty-foot loop consisting of three parts: the duodenum, which receives food from the stomach, bile from the liver and gallbladder, and pancreatic juices; the jejunum; and the ileum, which joins up with the large intestine.

Tumors of the small intestine are rare, and only about half of those are cancerous. The many types of benign tumors that affect the small intestine may go undetected throughout a patient's life. It is thought that cancers of this site are related to a high consumption of fat and protein. Patients with certain preexisting conditions are at risk: Gardner's syndrome is a condition in which the patient develops multiple polyps in the duodenum before age 20. It is an inherited condition, and there is a high risk of developing a malignancy. Patient's with Peutz-Jeghers syndrome also develop multiple polyps at an early age, again due to a genetic pattern. Although only 5% of patients with this syndrome actually develop malignant tumors, they require close supervision and regular checkups.

Symptoms

Obstruction within the small intestine produces severe abdominal cramps and pain. There may also be rapid weight loss, vomiting, anemia, bleeding, and the patient may experience what is called the "malabsorption syndrome"—an inability of the body to absorb nutrients from food being digested.

Diagnosis

The doctor will take a **medical history** and do a complete **physical examination,** including examination of the skin and mucous membranes for symptoms associated with Peutz-Jeghers syndrome. In the hospital, the patient may be scheduled for an **upper** and **lower GI series,** abdominal and chest **X-rays, duodenoscopy,** bone-marrow **biopsy, liver scan,** and laboratory analyses of blood, urine, and stool samples. An exploratory **laparotomy** may be performed.

For staging classifications, see "Large Intestine."

Types of Cancers

Primary cancers of the small intestine include *carcinomas,* the most common form; *carcinoid tumors; lymphomas* (see "Lymphomas" for diagnostic and treatment procedures for this type of cancer); and occasionally *adenocarcinomas.* Carcinoid tumors, also called *argentaffinomas,* can be either benign or very slow-growing malignant tumors. On the rare occasions when they do spread, they go to the liver, lungs, bones, and large intestine.

281

The small intestine is a common metastatic site for tumors whose primary sites are the pancreas or the stomach. See those site discussions for diagnosis and treatment of those cancers.

Treatment

Surgery is usually the first—and possibly the only—method of treatment. Depending on the size of the tumor, its exact location, and whether it has spread, surgery may both remove and cure the cancer, or—if the tumor cannot be completely removed—surgery may alleviate blockages and pain.

Before any surgical procedure, the patient is usually put on a low-residue diet with protein supplements. If the tumor has created a serious health problem, the patient may be placed on a special high-calorie/high-nutrient IV called a TPN (total parenteral nutrition—see the chapter on surgery) to build up his strength.

The actual surgical procedure used depends on the size, location, and spread of the tumor. Descriptions of the most common procedures follow.

Intestinal resection—the tumor and part of the healthy intestine around it are removed and the remaining sections of the intestine are sewn together.

Wedge resection—similar to the intestinal resection, but a part of the mesentery is also removed. The mesentery is a fan-shaped fold of the peritoneum (the lining of the abdominal cavity) which encircles the jejunum and ileum. Hospitalization for both these procedures is about two weeks.

When the tumor affects the duodenum, a *pancreatoduodenectomy* may be performed (see "Pancreas").

If the tumor is growing in the lowest section of the small intestine, the terminal ileum, two procedures may be performed: an *ileotransversostomy* and a *colectomy*. The first is a colostomy done at the point where the ileum joins the transverse colon; the second is the removal of part or all of the colon. See "Large Intestine" for details.

Radiation and **chemotherapy** are not used as primary treatments (except for lymphomas), but as adjuncts to surgery to clean up what is left, or as treatment if the tumor or the condition of the patient make surgery impossible.

Experimental Treatments

The prognosis is good for patients with localized carcinoid tumors and some lymphomas, but quite poor for those with adenocarcinomas or unresectable tumors. Those patients may want to inquire into the experimental programs in **chemotherapy** and **immunotherapy** being

282

conducted by SEG, SWOG, GTSG, MDA, MSKCC, SFCC, VAMC, and UCLA (see appendix H).

Doctors Who May Be Involved in Treatment

Gastroenterologist, abdominal surgeon, endocrinologist, medical oncologist, therapeutic radiologist.

Soft-Tissue Sarcomas

See "Bone."

Spinal Cord

See "Brain and CNS."

Stomach

The stomach is part of the gastrointestinal system, located between the esophagus and the small intestine.

Stomach cancer—usually referred to as gastric cancer—used to be the most common cancer among men in this country, but the rise in smoking has now given lung cancer that distinction. There has also been a decrease in the incidence of gastric cancer, which has been attributed to the increased use of refrigerators and the decreased use of food preservatives such as nitrates.

People at risk of developing stomach cancer include: those who are poor; those whose diet has included large amounts of smoked foods, pickled vegetables, cabbage, or foods grown in soil that contains a lot of peat; those with a family history of gastrointestinal cancers; people with stomach ulcers (these occasionally become malignant); and those with a history of gastritis, gastric polyps, pernicious anemia, acanthosis nigricans (a rare chronic inflammatory skin disease), or anachlorhydria (the absence of free hydrochloric acid in the stomach). Stomach cancer is most prevalent in patients in their sixties. Men contract this type of cancer twice as often as women.

Gastric cancer usually begins in the lining of the stomach. When it infiltrates, it penetrates the stomach wall and may cause obstruction

283

and the vomiting of blood. Regional metastases to nearby lymph nodes, liver, pancreas, and ovary may be found. Krukenberg tumor arises in the stomach and generally spreads to both ovaries. Stomach cancer may also spread to distant sites using the lymphatic system, most commonly finding its way to the lungs, bone, and occasionally the skin.

Stomach cancers are usually not diagnosed until they are quite advanced. The prognosis depends on the degree of penetration into the stomach wall, the involvement of the lymph nodes, and the extent of metastases. Because it is usually diagnosed in the later stages, the cure rate is only 10%.

Symptoms

There may be no symptoms at all until the disease is advanced, and even then the symptoms may be quite similar to those of less serious stomach disorders. Symptoms may include bloody stools, chest pain, indigestion, belching, loss of appetite, weight loss, weakness, and pain. As the disease progresses, the patient may vomit.

Diagnosis and Staging

A complete **medical history** will be taken and a **physical examination,** including a rectal examination (see "Large Intestine") will be done. Samples of blood, urine, and stool will be analyzed in the laboratory. An **upper GI** and **lower GI** will be done, as well as a **gastroscopy,** during which a **biopsy** will be taken. Exfoliative cytology will be done, in which the lining of the stomach is brushed and washed in order to get cell samples. To determine the extent of metastases, if any, **X-rays** of the chest and skeleton will be taken and a **liver scan** done. All of this can be done on an outpatient basis.

There are several systems of staging gastric cancers. It is most easily thought of in four stages:

Stage I Tumor is confined to the lining and connective tissue of the stomach.

Stage II Tumor has involved the stomach wall, but there is no penetration.

Stage III Tumor has penetrated stomach wall; there may be regional metastases but no distant metastases.

Stage IV Tumor has penetrated stomach wall, and both regional and distant metastases are identified.

Types of Cancers

Ninety percent of all stomach cancers are *adenocarcinomas.* One to three percent are non-Hodgkin's *lymphomas* (see "Lymphomas"). Treatment and prognosis for lymphomas are very different than for other stomach cancers. In fact, it is more accurate to say that a person with lymphoma in the stomach does not have stomach cancer but has lymphoma which happened to show up in the stomach. *Epidermoid cancers*, which usually affect the upper part of the stomach, are thought to have spread from the esophagus. Tumors in the stomach may look like polyps, or be ulcerating or infiltrating.

Treatment

Surgery. Surgery is the primary method of treatment. The operation is called a *gastrectomy*. A *subtotal* or *partial* gastrectomy involves removing a part of the stomach. A *total* gastrectomy is the removal of the entire stomach. When a total gastrectomy is done, the regional lymph nodes, the spleen, and some of the intestine are usually removed. A person can live a normal life-span without a stomach. The major adjustment involves eating smaller quantities of food and more meals per day (six or eight) so that you do not overload the remaining intestinal tract. Digestion is made easier by sticking to a high-protein diet.

As part of the surgery, reconstruction of the intestinal tract must be done; this process is called *anastomosis*. In a partial gastrectomy, the remaining upper part of the stomach is joined to the jejunum, a loop of the small intestine. The procedure is called a *gastrojejunostomy* and is done when a tumor involves the lower part of the stomach. If the tumor involves the upper part of the stomach, the entire stomach must be removed. This procedure requires even more extensive reconstruction, as the jejunum is connected to the esophagus, which entails opening the chest wall and the abdomen.

The patient will be admitted to the hospital up to five days before the scheduled operation. During this time he will be put on a liquid diet and his stomach will be "washed out" with a gastric tube several times. He may also get supportive treatment (transfusions, nutritional IV's, pain medication) to prepare him for the surgery. The operation is a major one requiring several hours and is done under general anesthesia.

After surgery the patient is fed by a nasogastric tube that goes through the nose and down past the esophagus. This tube also removes gas and air that may accumulate and cause pain. Gradually the patient will be given food by mouth, starting with liquids and graduating to solid bland food. Vitamin deficiency and anemia are common side effects and can be controlled by consumption of additional nutrients. Many patients suffer from the "dumping syndrome" after gastric surgery. This refers to weakness, nausea, and vomiting caused by the stomach ridding itself of food too quickly. As the stomach and intestinal tract adjust to the reconstruction and the patient adheres to the proper diet, the syndrome passes.

About two weeks of hospitalization is required after this surgery and another month of recuperation at home. Depending on the case, **chemotherapy** or **radiation** may follow the surgery.

Many cancers of the stomach are inoperable, either because the disease is too widespread at diagnosis or because of technical problems with the surgery. In some cases surgery will be performed for palliation of symptoms, or for removal of only part of the tumor to allow other forms of treatment to be more effective.

Radiation may be used as primary treatment if the tumor affects the junction of the esophagus and stomach. Generally it is used as adjuvant therapy after surgery, either to cure lymphomas (usually used with chemotherapy) or to reduce the severity of symptoms. Radiation has limitations in this area of the body because the doses needed to kill cancer would also kill the healthy tissue of the many vital organs in the region.

Chemotherapy is used mainly to relieve symptoms and in experimental programs (see below).

Experimental Treatments

Experimental treatments are being conducted using **chemotherapy, immunotherapy,** and **radiation.** There are protocols both for adjuvant treatment after surgery and for primary treatment of tumors that cannot be treated surgically. Contact: GTSG, CLB, EST, NCOG, SWOG, GUMO, MAYO, MDA, MSKCC, VASAG, SEG, SFCC, NC-VAMC, NCCTG, RPMI, UCLA, CAN-UICC (see appendix H).

NOTE: Preliminary evidence on experimental treatments for advanced gastric cancer has shown an improved response rate, but as yet no improvement in cure rate.

Doctors Who May Be Involved in Treatment

Gastroenterologist, abdominal surgeon, medical oncologist, therapeutic radiologist.

Testes

The testes are the male genital glands (gonads) that produce the male reproductive cells, or spermatozoa, and the male hormone testosterone. Testicular cancers grow from cells in the gonads that actually create the sperm. The right side is involved more often than the left side, and bilateral testicular tumors are rare. Although testicular cancers themselves are quite rare, they are very malignant and are the leading cause of death by cancer in men 29–35 years old. Death is usually caused by the cancer having spread to the lungs, but there is a good chance of complete cure if testicular cancer is found in the early stages. All lumps in this area should be checked immediately, since very few benign tumors are found here.

Patients at high risk of developing testicular cancers are those with undescended testicles. Rarely, there may be a family predisposition to testicular cancers. It is less common in the black population than among whites, and the usual age range is from 20 to 35 years old, but it has been found in newborns and men 50–60 years old.

Symptoms

Painless lump in the testes; an enlarged testicle; feeling of heaviness in the scrotum, sometimes with pain and swelling; hormonal imbalance that causes breast enlargement, loss of sexual potency, or loss of sex drive. Some patients notice the first symptoms after a blow to the testicle or lifting an unusually heavy object.

Diagnosis and Staging

A complete **medical history** will be taken and **physical examination** done which may detect the presence of the tumor. *Transillumination* (exposing the testicle to strong light) will be used to detect a tumor, and laboratory tests will be done on blood and urine samples, with particular attention to tests called *HCG (human chorionic gonadotropin)* and *AFP (alpha fetal protein)* which detect hormones that act as "tumor markers." By monitoring these hormones, the doctor not only can confirm the presence of cancer but can also tell whether or not the patient is responding to treatment.

To determine whether the tumor has spread outside the immediate area of the testicles, the following procedures may be done: chest **X-ray** and **tomograms** of the lungs; an **IVP** to detect urinary obstructions; **angiogram;** inferior **venacavogram, lymphangiogram: CAT scan** of the chest and/or abdomen; and **ultrasound** examination of the abdomen. A **biopsy** of the testicle is not done until the actual surgery for removal of the testicle, since the testis must be removed through the groin rather than through the scrotum. (The scrotum is actually a part of the abdominal wall; an incision in the scrotum might cause the cancer to spread into the abdominal tissues.)

Testicular tumors are staged on three levels:

Stage I_A Tumor confined to the testis
Stage I_B Microscopic involvement of retroperitoneal lymph nodes
Stage II   Macroscopic involvement of retroperitoneal lymph nodes
Stage III   Extension beyond retroperitoneal lymph nodes

Types of Cancers

The most common forms of testicular cancer are *seminomas,* which comprise 40% of testicular tumors. They spread through the lymph system to the liver, lung, adrenal glands, and bone, and can cause obstruction of the ureters. The rest are called *nonseminomas;* these are more malignant, spread through the bloodstream, and are less sensitive to radiation therapy than seminomas. In this group are several specific types of cancers including *teratomas, embryonal-cell tumors,* and *choriocarcinomas* (very rare, though extremely malignant). Some tumors are of mixed cell types, including several of those listed above.

Treatment

Surgery. Surgery is usually the first step in the treatment of all forms of testicular cancer. The basic operation is called a *radical orchiectomy,* in which one or both testicles are removed. The incision is made through the groin, and the testicles and all tubes are removed. If the cancer has not involved the scrotum (the outside skin sac), an artificial testicle may be inserted at this time or in a subsequent operation. If both testicles are removed, the patient will become sterile but not necessarily impotent.

With nonseminomas, a radical *lymphadenectomy* may also be performed to determine the extent of the disease. This is an extremely difficult and time-consuming operation that may require as much as eight hours. The operation consists of removing all of the lymph nodes on one side of the abdomen up to the kidneys. If necessary, it may be done on both sides.

A frequent complication of the lymphadenectomy is retrograde ejaculation: Although the patient with one testis continues to produce sperm, the sperm do not make their way out of the penis at the time of ejaculation—hence he may become functionally sterile.

If cancer is present in the lymph nodes, **radiation** and/or **chemotherapy** will be needed. If no cancer cells are present, further treatment is usually not required.

Ninety percent of recurrences happen in the first year after treatment, therefore monthly checkups will be scheduled, which will include a physical exam, chest X-ray, and blood tests. Recurrences detected early are very curable.

Radiation. Radiation therapy is the standard treatment after a radical orchiectomy for seminomas. It may be used on the abdominal lymph nodes as well as locally. If the seminoma is advanced, the patient may be treated with systemic **chemotherapy** prior to the radiation therapy.

If a nonseminoma is present, radiation is usually combined with

chemotherapy. After a lymphadenectomy, radiation may be given to patients with only a few malignant lymph nodes, and this may eradicate any stray cancer cells. Radiation is only used when the lymph nodes are small and there are no tumor masses; it is not used when there is an extensive abdominal tumor.

Chemotherapy. This is used either alone (for nonseminomas and for testicular cancers that have spread) or after the orchiectomy and/or lymphadenectomy has been performed. Many experimental programs are being conducted (see below).

Experimental Treatments

Experimental protocols are being conducted using **chemotherapy, radiation,** and **surgery** in various combinations. Contact: EST, NCOG, SEG, SWOG, TCIS, MDA, MSKCC, SFCC, WFU, National Cancer Institute (see appendix H).

Doctors Who May Be Involved in Treatment

Urologist; therapeutic radiologist; medical oncologist. This is a rare cancer and should be treated at a major hospital or cancer center that has experience with this type of cancer and has appropriate working teams of specialists and support services. Care must be taken to ensure very close follow-up after treatment, particularly for the first two years.

NOTE: If both testicles are removed, or as a *possible* side effect of treatment, the patient may become sterile. Should he want to have children after treatment, he should investigate the possibility of putting sperm in a sperm-bank prior to treatment, realizing that this is usually expensive, only 50% effective, and that sperm only remain viable for two years. All questions regarding sterility, use of a sperm bank, or possible sexual dysfunction should be discussed with your doctors prior to treatment.

Tongue

See "Head and Neck."

Tonsils

See "Head and Neck."

289

Thyroid

The thyroid gland is located in the neck, under the Adam's apple. It consists of three sections: two lobes on either side of the windpipe, and the section connecting the lobes, called the "isthmus." One of the ductless glands of the endocrine system, it produces hormones that regulate metabolism.

An enlargement of the thyroid gland is called goiter. Goiter, a condition linked to excesses and deficiencies of iodine in the diet, is a benign condition. There is, however, a higher risk of developing thyroid cancer among patients with goiter or a family history of goiter.

Cancer of the thyroid is extremely rare, and is the most chronic of all cancers: generally slow-growing, with patients having a near-normal life expectancy. Thyroid cancers affect women more frequently than men, concentrate in the 30–60 age range (although they can appear at any age), and affect whites more than blacks. Thyroid cancer is linked to radiation exposure: High levels of thyroid cancer developed among the surviving populations of Hiroshima and Nagasaki; and several years ago, when radiation treatment was given quite freely for acne, ear infections, tonsil infections, thymus-gland enlargement, it was discovered that this group was at high risk for developing thyroid cancer.

Symptoms

The first symptom of thyroid cancer is an enlarged thyroid gland. Later symptoms may include difficult breathing and swallowing, hoarseness, or a hard lump. Vocal-cord paralysis may indicate invasive thyroid cancer.

Diagnosis

A **medical history** will be taken and complete **physical examination** done. Most thyroid cancers are found in routine physical examinations or by patients who notice collars getting too tight. The thyroid is examined by a **thyroid scan. Ultrasound** examination may also be performed. To check on the extent of the tumor and possible metastases, an **upper GI**, chest **X-rays** or **tomograms,** and X-rays of the neck and skeleton will be done. A **laryngoscopy** will be done to view the vocal cords. If a thyroid cancer does metastasize, it usually does so to the lungs, bone, and lymph glands in the neck.

Types of Cancers

Papillary carcinoma is the most common form. It may occur in one or both lobes of the thyroid and may remain localized for years. It spreads to the lymph nodes early, and much later may develop distant metastases via the bloodstream.

Follicular thyroid carcinoma is usually confined to one lobe of the thyroid and is less apt to spread to the lymph nodes. It may recur and is considered fast-growing.

Anaplastic carcinoma of the thyroid is very malignant, extremely rare, and is noted for fast growth and early spread to distant parts of the body.

Generally, thyroid cancers are slow-growing and metastasize late. Patients should note that involvement of the lymph nodes does not indicate quickly spreading cancer, as it does in most other forms of cancer.

Treatment

Standard treatment may include **surgery** and **hormone therapy,** alone or in combination.

If the thyroid scan is abnormal but no lump or nodule is present, the patient is treated with hormones by mouth and checked closely to make sure that a lump does not develop. If it does, surgery is indicated.

When surgery is indicated, a *thyroidectomy* is performed. This can be a *partial* thyroidectomy, also called a *lobectomy,* in which only part or all of one lobe is removed; or a *total thyroidectomy,* in which the whole thyroid plus the lymph nodes in the neck may be removed. When possible, part of the thyroid is left intact because it performs a vital function. The operation takes two to four hours under general anesthesia and about a week of hospitalization. If surgery severely impairs thyroid function, the patient is given oral doses of the thyroid hormone for the rest of his or her life. **Hormone therapy** may also be given for a short time after surgery to allow the gland to heal and to control any remaining malignant cells.

Anaplastic cancers of the thyroid are generally considered to be inoperable.

Radiation. Radioactive iodine (**internal radiation**) is used with metastatic thyroid cancers. A large dose of radioactive iodine is given every three to four weeks until the tumor no longer absorbs it. The radioactive iodine gives a high dose of radiation to the tumor without affecting the normal tissue. **External radiation** may be given for lymph nodes in the neck, rather than surgical treatment, and for palliation of symptoms.

Chemotherapy has not yet proven effective with these cancers (see "Experimental Treatments" below).

Experimental Treatments

Phase I and II chemotherapy experiments are being done on advanced and metastatic thyroid cancers by SEG and MDA (see appendix H).

Doctors Who May Be Involved in Treatment

Endocrinologist, endocrine surgeon, nuclear-medicine specialist, therapeutic radiologist.

Ureter

See "Bladder."

Urethra

See "Bladder."

Uterus

The uterus is part of the female reproductive system: the womb in which a baby grows. It lies between the fallopian tubes, which carry the eggs from the ovaries, and the cervix, which is actually the lower part of the uterus that connects with the vagina. The lining of the uterus is called the "endometrium." The term "uterine cancer" often includes invasive cervical carcinomas.

Cancers of the uterus comprise 4% of all cancers, but are the leading form of cancer affecting the female reproductive system (excluding carcinoma *in situ* of the cervix). Because it presents symptoms early, it is often diagnosed early and, therefore, treated successfully. These cancers appear most often in postmenopausal women of the 50–60 age group. It affects white women more than black women, and higher income groups more often than lower income groups. Women at increased risk are those who are obese (with associated conditions of hypertension and diabetes) and those who have never had children, have a history of irregular periods, or who have received prolonged estrogen therapy.

292

Symptoms

The most common symptom is unusual vaginal discharge and/or bleeding. Any bleeding after menopause is abnormal. During menopause the normal pattern is one of gradually decreasing flow, with periods coming farther and farther apart. Any bleeding between periods, with intercourse, and/or the advent of heavy, frequent flows at any age should be investigated. Other symptoms include low abdominal pain and back pain. Precancerous conditions that should be watched carefully are atypical hyperplasia, which is an overgrowth of the cells in the lining of the uterus, and polyps, which frequently grow in the uterus.

Diagnosis and Staging

A **medical history** will be taken and a complete **physical** and **pelvic examination** will be done. The patient's entire menstrual and menopausal history should be given in detail, along with mention of any estrogens, oral contraceptives, and medications prescribed. Procedures designed specifically to diagnose the cancer may include an *aspiration curettage* (a tube called an "endometrial aspirator" is put into the vagina, threaded through the cervix into the uterus, and removes tissue from the uterus for examination under a microscope) and a *Gravelee test* (a tube is inserted through the cervix into the uterus, a stream of fluid is injected, and the resulting fluid-mixed-with-cells is collected for examination).

The most reliable method of collecting tissue samples for biopsies is a *D&C (dilatation and curettage)*—a common surgical procedure. The patient will be hospitalized for twenty-four hours because a general anesthetic is used. Going in through the vagina, the doctor uses a curette to scrape the inside wall of the uterus. All material collected this way is sent to the laboratory for analysis. Pelvic exam under anesthesia is often done at the same time as the D&C. A Pap smear is *not* reliable for diagnosing endometrial cancer, since the abnormal cells tend to stay inside the uterus, but one will be done as part of the initial evaluation.

Other procedures will be done to determine if the cancer has spread. Blood samples will be taken for a CBC and serum electrolyte assay. **Urinalysis** will be done on urine samples. An **EKG** will be given. Additional procedures may include a chest **X-ray; IVP; sigmoidoscopy** and **cystoscopy** to check for spread to the bladder or rectum; **bone scan** and **liver scan.** In advanced cases a **lymphangiogram** may be done to check for lymph-node involvement. If this is positive, a fine-needle **aspiration** will be done as well as a **CAT scan** of the pelvis.

Cancer of the uterus is staged as follows:

Tis   (Stage o)   Carcinoma *in situ.*
T_1 (Stage I)   Cancer confined to the body (corpus) of the uterus.
T_2 (Stage II)   Cancer involving the cervix, but still confined to the uterus as a whole.
T_3 (Stage III)   Cancer extending outside the uterus, including spread to the vagina, but remaining inside the pelvis.
T_4 (Stage IV)   Cancer has spread to the bladder or rectum or extends beyond the true pelvis.

Types of Cancers

Generally, uterine cancers are *adenocarcinomas:* These include *adenoacanthoma* and *adenosquamous*. On rare occasions *squamous carcinoma* and *sarcomas* may be found. Unlike other cancers affecting the uterus, sarcomas are fast-growing and can spread quickly to the lymph nodes, pelvic structures, and distant sites via the bloodstream. The subtypes of sarcomas that may be found in the uterus include *leiomyosarcoma, endometrial stromal sarcoma, mixed mesodermal sarcoma,* and *carcinosarcoma.* Because of the early onset of symptoms and the thick muscle coat of the uterus (myometrium) which checks the usual tendency of adenocarcinomas to invade and spread, uterine cancers can be found in the early stages. If found in stages Tis or T_1, the cure rate is 75–90%, depending on the cell type and grade of cancer.

Choriocarcinoma is a rare, highly malignant tumor of the placenta, usually affecting women under 35. It may start during pregnancy, causing a spontaneous abortion, or it may start after delivery. This tumor grows very rapidly and spreads to the lungs. There is a high incidence of these tumors in China, and it is thought to be caused by protein deficiency, malnutrition, and multiple pregnancies.

Treatment

For early-stage adenocarcinomas, **surgery** plus **radiation** is the treatment of choice. Sarcomas are treated with surgery plus radiation and **chemotherapy.**

Surgery. For Tis and T_1 cancers, curative surgery is used in the form of a *total abdominal hysterectomy* and *bilateral salpingo-oophorectomy* (see "Ovary" for a complete description), in which the uterus, ovaries, and fallopian tubes are removed. At times the lymph nodes in the pelvis may also be surgically removed. **Radiation** and **chemotherapy** may be used postoperatively. Choriocarcinoma is particularly responsive to chemotherapy. Women who have carcinoma *in situ* and want to have children should discuss **hormone therapy** with their doctors.

Radiation. Radiation may be used alone, preoperatively and/or postoperatively. It is used alone for very advanced cases, or when a patient's general health rules out surgery, or the cancer is inoperable, or in very early stages.

When radiation is given prior to surgery, the treatment course is usually completed four to six weeks before the operation. Preoperative radiation may be internal, in the form of intracavity implants of radium; or external cobalt radiation. Both forms of radiation may also be given after surgery.

Hormone and Chemotherapy. With uterine cancers, chemotherapy and hormone therapy are usually combined, and given after surgery and/or radiation. It has been found that large doses of progesterone can offer relief from symptoms and prolong life in advanced cases. This hormone has also proven effective in treating metastases that appear later in the course of the disease. About 30% of advanced uterine cancers will show some response to progesterone. Methotrexate has been very effective in treating choriocarcinoma. Standard chemotherapy usually consists of the administration of alkalyzing and progestational agents. At this point, most chemotherapy is experimental, but shows promising results (see below).

Experimental Treatments

Experimental treatments are being conducted using **chemotherapy** and **hormone therapy,** usually after surgery and radiation treatments have been completed. Contact: EST, GOG, NCOG, CAN-NCIC, SWOG, MDA (see appendix H).

Doctors Who May Be Involved in Treatment

Gynecologist, gynecological oncologist, therapeutic radiologist, medical oncologist, endocrinologist, immunologist.

Vagina

The vagina is the birth canal, extending from the vulva to the cervix. Cancers of the vagina are extremely rare and occur mainly in women over 50. High-risk women include those who have dysplasia, leukoplakia, and vaginal adenosis. Also at risk are women who were exposed *in utero* to DES and other nonsteroid estrogens. These estrogens were given to women who were otherwise unable to carry a child to term. A small percentage (0.4/1000) of daughters exposed to DES in the womb have developed clear-cell cancers.

295

Symptoms

Vaginal discharge; spotting or bleeding between periods; bladder discomfort and/or irritation; a lesion or lump.

Diagnosis and Staging

The gynecologist will take a complete **medical history** and do a **physical examination** that includes a **pelvic examination.** In his office, he may perform a **colposcopy** which includes a **Schiller test,** and a **biopsy.** Laboratory tests will be done on blood and urine samples: **CBC, urinalysis, BUN,** and **liver-function tests. X-rays** will be taken of the chest, and an **intravenous pyelogram** will be done. A **cystoscopy** and/or **sigmoidoscopy** may be performed to rule out bladder or rectal involvement. After these tests are completed, the cancer will be staged as follows:

Stage I	Tumor confined to the wall of the vagina.
Stage II	Has penetrated the wall of the vagina but has not reached the pelvic wall.
Stage III	Tumor has reached the pelvic wall.
Stage IV	Cancer goes beyond pelvis or has invaded nearby organs (rectum, bladder).
Stage IVA	Tumor has spread to nearby organs.
Stage IVB	Tumor has spread to distant organs.

Types of Cancers

Most cancers of the vagina are *epidermoid carcinomas. Alenocarcinomas, malignant melanomas,* and *sarcomas* may also be found. Clear-cell adenocarcinomas have a high rate of recurrence, as do invasive cancers. The vaginal wall is also a common site of metastases from cancers of the cervix, vulva, ovary, and uterus.

Treatment

Treatment will depend on the type and location of the tumor and also on the patient's age, whether she wants to have children, maintain sexual activity, etc. **Radiation** and **surgery** are both used as primary treatments.

In early lesions, especially with clear-cell cancers in young women, treatment may involve surgical removal of the tumor plus internal radiation. This approach is limited because these cancers tend to spread quickly to the pelvic lymph nodes. For carcinoma *in situ,* a *vaginectomy* (removal of the vagina) may be performed. A new vagina can often be reconstructed with plastic surgery.

All invasive lesions require radical radiation therapy or radical surgery. In Stages I and II, a radical hysterectomy (see "Ovary") and vaginectomy may be performed. Surgery is indicated only if the upper posterior portion of the vagina is involved. Radiation treatment is an alternative to surgery and usually includes both **internal** radiation and **external** pelvic irradiation.

If other portions of the vagina have been affected, more extensive surgery *(exenteration)* involving the removal of some or all of the nearby organs (bladder, urethra, rectum) and/or the pelvic lymph nodes may be necessary. Along with these procedures, an ostomy may be performed (see "Large Intestine" and "Bladder").

Experimental Treatments

Chemotherapy, radiation, and **immunotherapy** experiments are being conducted on advanced and metastatic cases by GOG and SWOG (see appendix H).

Doctors Who May Be Involved in Treatment

Gynecologist, gynecological oncologist, therapeutic radiologist, medical oncologist, plastic surgeon.

Vulva

The vulva is the outermost part of the female reproductive system. It includes the opening of the vagina, the lips (labia majora and minora), and the clitoris. Cancers of the vulva are extremely rare, usually affecting women in the 50–65 age group. *In situ* vulvar cancer seems to be increasing in the 30–40 age group.

Symptoms

In the early stages there are often no symptoms. When they do occur, they are similar to those of noncancerous conditions: burning, itching, bleeding, pain, discharge, feeling a lump. The presence of leukoplakia (white patches) may or may not be significant; it must be biopsied to determine whether it is a sign of dysplasia, carcinoma *in situ*, invasive cancer, or simply a thickened layer of vulvar skin (hyperkeratotic area).

Women should not use steroid creams to treat itching until they have been examined by a gynecologist.

Diagnosis and Staging

Many cancers of the vulva are first seen and felt when the gynecologist does a routine **pelvic examination.** If there are suspicious lesions, a **colposcopy** may be performed as well as a **punch** or **excisional biopsy,** which is done with a local anesthetic. Laboratory tests will be done on samples of blood and urine, including a **CBC** and **urinalysis.** If the biopsy is positive, other tests done in the hospital will determine if the cancer has spread to the lymph nodes, other parts of the reproductive system, rectum, urinary tract, liver, and lungs. These may include **X-rays, intravenous pyelogram (IVP), lower GI, cystoscopy, proctoscopy,** liver-function tests, **lymphangiogram,** and **liver** and **bone scans.** Cancers of the vulva are often diagnosed in the very early stages when they are completely curable. They are staged as follows:

Stage I   A tumor of 2 cm or less which is confined to the vulva.
Stage II   Larger than 2 cm, confined to the vulva.
Stage III   Any size tumor that has spread to the vagina, anus, or urethra, with or without involvement of the lymph nodes in the groin which are movable.
Stage IV   Tumor has spread to the bladder, bone, rectum, or other distant site or lymph nodes in the groin which cannot be moved.

Types of Cancers

Eighty percent of vulvar cancers are *squamous-cell carcinomas* and are usually found in women over 50, but may affect younger women as well. Researchers are currently looking at a possible relationship of this cancer to a virus called "herpes simplex." *Malignant melanomas* comprise 5% of these cancers. This type of cancer often appears in younger women and can occur during pregnancy, posing a danger to the placenta and fetus. These can be seen on pelvic examination. Other vulvar cancers include *basal-cell carcinoma* (common in older women, and generally spread by invasion rather than metastasis), *adenocarcinomas, sarcomas, fibrosarcomas,* and *mixed tumors. Paget's disease* is a specific histological type of vulvar cancer that has a high rate of recurrence and is often associated with an underlying invasive cancer or breast or rectal adenocarcinoma.

Lesions often appear on both sides of the vulva (bilateral lesions) before vulvar cancer is diagnosed. Tumors of the vulva spread to the nearby lymph nodes fairly early, and commonly invade the vagina. Distant metastases are rare, although they are known to spread to the lung, liver, and bones. Death is usually due to infection and hemorrhaging caused by invasion of the cancer into the urinary and anal openings.

Treatment

Standard treatments include **surgery, radiation,** and **chemotherapy.** In very early stages, the cancer may be treated with a cream that contains 5-FU. If this does not cure it after two applications, a *vulvectomy* will be performed. A *simple vulvectomy* involves removal of the skin layer of the vulva. It is followed by a skin graft. A *total* or *radical* *vulvectomy* is performed if the cancer has already become invasive. The labia and clitoris will be removed, as will the nearby lymph nodes *(pelvic lymphadenectomy)*. In this operation, incisions are made on the inside of both sides of the groin. After radical vulvar surgery, reconstructive surgery may be done to repair the vulva using skin flaps from the legs. The patient can still become pregnant, although delivery will probably be by cesarean section.

The preferred method of treatment for *in situ* cancers is local excision or simple "skinning" vulvectomy with a skin graft. Standard treatment of invasive vulvar cancer is radical vulvectomy with groin-node dissection (removal). Other surgical procedures may be employed if the cancer has spread outside the vulva (see "Large Intestine," "Vagina," and "Bladder").

The main complication of surgery is pulmonary emboli (blood clots in the lungs). Often the legs swell and the wound may not heal well because of the amount of tissue removed and technical problems with closing the wounds securely in this region of the body. The operation can be done using a general or regional (epidural) anesthetic, and generally requires at least two weeks' hospitalization.

Radiation has a very limited role in the treatment of vulvar cancers and usually serves as palliative treatment. Newer techniques currently being developed may prove useful in the future.

Chemotherapy, at times in conjunction with **immunotherapy,** is being investigated with some vulvar cancers, particularly with malignant melanoma. Chemotherapy may be used to treat metastases. It has had limited results to date.

Experimental Treatments

Experimental treatments using **chemotherapy, radiation, immunotherapy,** and **surgery** are being conducted for Stage III and Stage IV cancers by: GOG, SWOG, and MDA (see appendix H). (Stage I and II cancers have an 80–95% cure rate using standard treatments.)

Doctors Who May Be Involved in Treatment

Gynecologist, gynecological oncologist, therapeutic radiologist, medical oncologist, plastic surgeon.

PART III

Appendices

Appendix A

ANATOMICAL DRAWINGS AND DIAGRAMS

LYMPHATIC SYSTEM

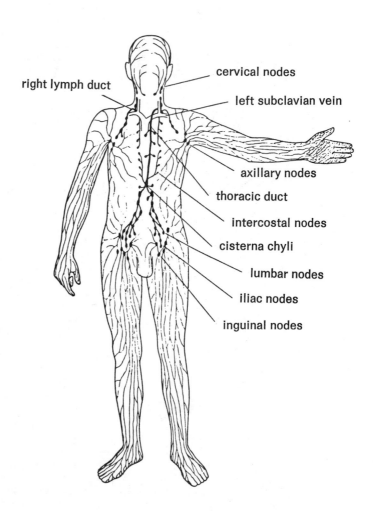

Source: H. S. Mayerson, "The Lymphatic System," *Scientific American*, 208 (6): 81 (June 1963).

RESPIRATORY SYSTEM

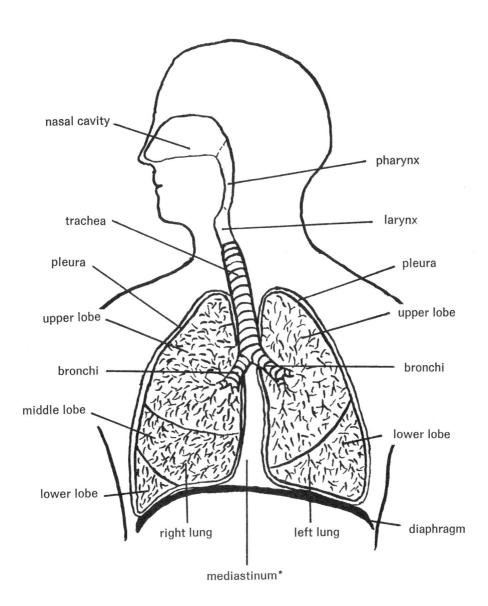

nasal cavity

pharynx

larynx

trachea

pleura

pleura

upper lobe

upper lobe

bronchi

bronchi

middle lobe

lower lobe

lower lobe

diaphragm

right lung

left lung

mediastinum*

* The mediastinum is the space between the lungs which contains major blood vessels and nerves; part of the trachea and esophagus; the heart; and the thymus gland.

DIGESTIVE SYSTEM

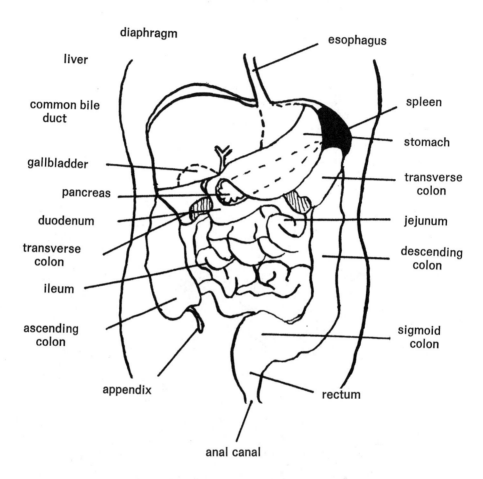

diaphragm

esophagus

liver

spleen

common bile duct

stomach

gallbladder

transverse colon

pancreas

jejunum

duodenum

transverse colon

descending colon

ileum

ascending colon

sigmoid colon

appendix

rectum

anal canal

LIVER-PANCREAS-SPLEEN-DUODENUM

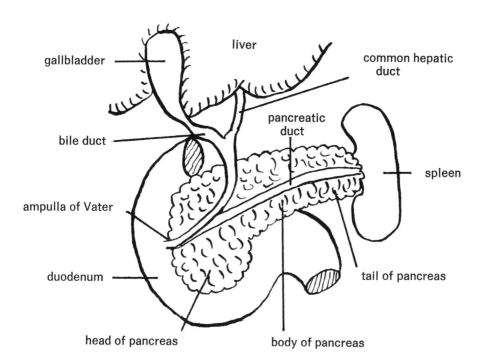

ENDOCRINE (HORMONE) SYSTEM

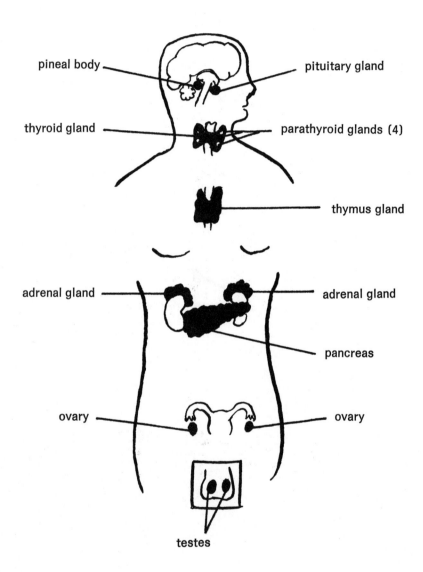

pineal body

pituitary gland

thyroid gland

parathyroid glands (4)

thymus gland

adrenal gland

adrenal gland

pancreas

ovary

ovary

testes

FEMALE GENITOURINARY SYSTEM

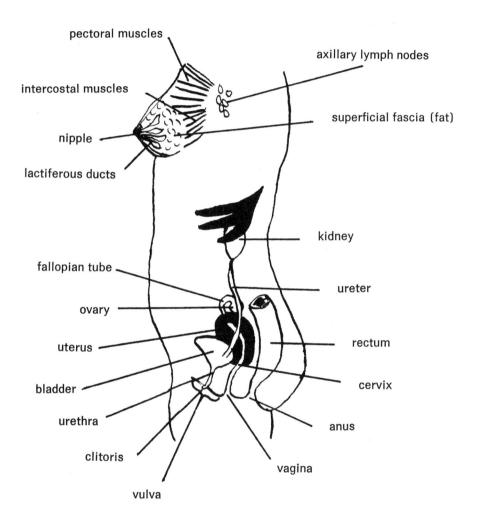

pectoral muscles

axillary lymph nodes

intercostal muscles

superficial fascia (fat)

nipple

lactiferous ducts

kidney

fallopian tube

ureter

ovary

uterus

rectum

bladder

cervix

urethra

anus

clitoris

vagina

vulva

MALE GENITOURINARY SYSTEM

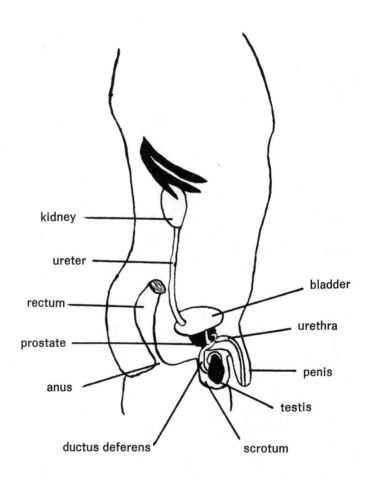

STRUCTURES OF THE BRAIN, HEAD, AND NECK

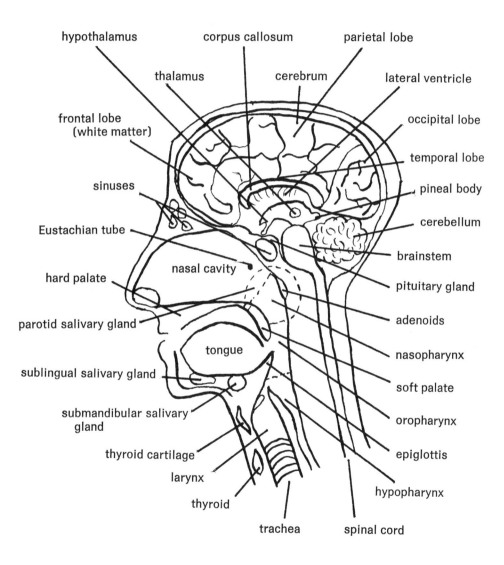

hypothalamus

corpus callosum

parietal lobe

thalamus

cerebrum

lateral ventricle

frontal lobe
(white matter)

occipital lobe

temporal lobe

sinuses

pineal body

Eustachian tube

cerebellum

hard palate

nasal cavity

brainstem

parotid salivary gland

pituitary gland

adenoids

tongue

nasopharynx

sublingual salivary gland

soft palate

submandibular salivary
gland

oropharynx

thyroid cartilage

epiglottis

larynx

hypopharynx

thyroid

trachea

spinal cord

Appendix B

BENIGN TUMORS— A PARTIAL LIST

Always Benign

Adenoma
Angioma (hemangioma)
Basophilic tumor
Chondroblastoma
Cystadenoma
Eosinophilic tumor (sweat gland)
Fibroma
Fibromyoma (leiomyoma)
Ganglioneuroma
Granular cell myoblastoma
Hemangioma (angioma)
Hemangiomatosis
Keloid
Leiomyoma (fibromyoma)

Lipoma
Lymphangioma
Multiple benign cystic epithelioma
Multiple hemorrhagic hemangioma
    of Kaposi
Myoma
Neurofibromatosis
Neuroma, not otherwise specified
Osteoma
Pigmented nevus (mole)
Pseudomucinous cystic tumor
Rhabdomyoma
Serous papillary cystic tumor
Squamous cell papilloma

Potentially Malignant

Chondroma
Fetal fat cell lipoma
Hemangioendothelioma
Hydatidiform mole
Lymphendothelioma (lymphangio-
  endothelioma)

Myxoma
Osteochondromatosis
Plexiform neuroma
Synovioma

Benign or Malignant

Adrenal cortical rest tumor (testis)
Argentaffinoma
Arrhenoblastoma
Branchioma
Chromophobe tumor
Cystosarcoma phyllodes
Feminizing tumor
Functionally hyperactive para-
  thyroid tumor
Functionally hyperactive thyroid
  tumor
Functioning islet cell tumor
Ganglioglioma
Giant cell tumor of bone
Glioblastoma multiforme
Glioma, not otherwise specified
Glomangioma
Granulosa cell tumor
Gynandroblastoma
Hamartoma

Hemangiopericytoma
Interstitial cell tumor
Meningioma
Mixed tumor, salivary gland type
Mixed tumor, not otherwise
  specified
Nonfunctioning islet cell tumor
Papillary or polypoid tumor, not
  otherwise specified
Paraganglioma
Pheochromocytoma
Rete cell tumor
Schwannoma
Sebaceous tumor
Sertoli cell tumor
Sweat gland tumor
Teratoma
Theca-cell tumor (thecoma)
Thymoma
Virilizing tumor

313

CANCER DEATHS—
PRESENT, PROJECTED,
AND PREVENTABLE

Leading Causes of Cancer Deaths by Age and Sex—1977*

	Under 15		15–34		35–54		55–74		75+	
	Male	Female	Male	Female	Male	Female	Male	Female	Male	Female
	Leukemia 54%	Leukemia 50%	Leukemia 34%	Leukemia 27%	Lung 62%	Breast 42%	Lung 57%	Breast 32%	Lung 33%	Colon & Rectum 38%
	Brain & Nervous System 34%	Brain & Nervous System 36%	Brain & Nervous System 20%	Breast 27%	Colon & Rectum 15%	Lung 22%	Colon & Rectum 17%	Colon & Rectum 23%	Prostate 29%	Breast 25%
	Bone 6%	Kidney 5%	Testis 19%	Brain & Nervous System 18%	Pancreas 8%	Colon & Rectum 12%	Prostate 12%	Lung 23%	Colon & Rectum 22%	Lung 13%
	Kidney 4%	Bone 5%	Hodgkin's Disease 16%	Uterus 16%	Brain & Nervous System 8%	Uterus 12%	Pancreas 8%	Ovary 11%	Stomach 8%	Pancreas 11%
	Connective Tissue 3%	Connective Tissue 4%	Melanoma 12%	Hodgkin's Disease 11%	Leukemia 7%	Ovary 12%	Stomach 6%	Uterus 11%	Bladder 8%	Uterus 10%

* From: Vital Statistics of the United States, 1977.

315

Estimated New Cancer Cases and Deaths by Sex and Site—1981*

Site	Estimated New Cases			Estimated Deaths		
	Total	Male	Female	Total	Male	Female
All Sites	815,000**	403,000**	412,000**	420,000	227,500	192,500
Buccal Cavity & Pharynx (Oral)	26,600	18,400	8,200	9,150	6,300	2,850
Lip	4,600	4,100	500	175	150	25
Tongue	4,800	3,200	1,600	2,000	1,400	600
Salivary Gland				700	450	250
Floor of Mouth	9,600	5,700	3,900	525	400	125
Other & Unspecified Mouth				1,550	1,000	550
Pharynx	7,600	5,400	2,200	4,200	2,900	1,300
Digestive Organs	194,500	99,700	94,800	110,500	57,600	52,900
Esophagus	8,800	6,200	2,600	8,100	5,800	2,300
Stomach	23,900	14,500	9,400	13,900	8,400	5,500
Small Intestine	2,100	1,100	1,100	700	350	350
Large Intestine	83,000	38,000	45,000	46,200	21,500	24,700
Rectum	37,000	20,000	17,000	8,700	4,700	4,000
Liver & Biliary Passages	13,000	6,000	7,000	9,400	4,600	4,800
Pancreas	24,200	12,700	11,500	22,000	11,500	10,500
Other & Unspecified	2,500	1,200	1,300	1,500	750	750
Respiratory System	135,800	99,000	36,800	110,100	81,000	29,100
Larynx	10,700	9,000	1,700	3,700	3,100	600
Lung	122,000	88,000	34,000	105,000	77,000	28,000
Other & Unspecified Respiratory	3,100	2,000	1,100	1,400	900	500
Bone, Tissue, Skin	20,900	10,700	10,200	10,050	5,800	4,250
Bone	1,900	1,100	800	1,750	1,000	750
Connective Tissue	4,700	2,600	2,100	1,600	800	800
Skin: Melanoma	14,300	7,000	7,300	6,700***	4,000	2,700

Breast	110,900	900	110,000	37,100	300	36,800
Genital Organs	151,600	75,200	76,400	46,400	23,700	22,700
Cervix, Invasive	16,000	—	16,000	7,200	—	7,200
Uterus	38,000	—	38,000	3,100	—	3,100
Ovary	18,000	—	18,000	11,400	—	11,400
Prostate	70,000	70,000	—	22,700	22,700	—
Testis, Other Genital, Male	5,200	5,200	—	1,000	1,000	—
Other & Unspecified Genital, Female	4,400	—	4,400	1,000	—	1,000
Urinary Organs	54,600	38,000	16,600	18,700	12,200	6,500
Bladder	37,000	27,000	10,000	10,600	7,300	3,300
Kidney & Other	17,600	11,000	6,600	8,100	4,900	3,200
Eye	1,800	900	900	400	200	200
Brain & Central Nervous System	12,100	6,700	5,400	10,200	5,600	4,600
Endocrine Glands	10,800	3,300	7,500	1,500	600	900
Thyroid	9,900	2,800	7,100	1,050	350	700
Other	900	500	400	450	250	200
Leukemias	23,400	13,000	10,400	15,900	8,900	7,000
Other Blood & Lymph	39,500	20,900	18,600	21,600	11,200	10,400
Hodgkin's Disease	7,100	4,100	3,000	1,700	1,000	700
Multiple Myeloma	9,400	4,800	4,600	6,700	3,400	3,300
Other Lymphomas	23,000	12,000	11,000	13,200	6,800	6,400
All Other & Unspecified Sites	32,500	16,300	16,200	28,400	14,100	14,300

* Incidence estimates are based on rates from the NCI SEER Program 1973–1977. These statistics were prepared by Edwin Silverberg, Project Statistician, Department of Epidemiology and Statistics, American Cancer Society, New York. *Ca–A Cancer Journal for Clinicians*, vol. 31, no. 1, January/February 1981, pp. 20–21.

** Carcinoma *in situ* and nonmelanoma skin cancers are not included in the totals for estimated new cases. Carcinoma *in situ* of the cervix accounts for 45,000 new cases annually. Nonmelanoma skin cancers account for 400,000 new cases annually.

*** Melanoma 5,000; other skin 1,700.

Estimated Preventable Deaths from Cancer[*]

	Type	Expected deaths	Preventable deaths
Cancer associated with cigarette smoking	Lung & some larynx	80,000	70,000
+ alcohol	Head & neck	7,500	5,000
	Esophagus	6,000	
+ industrial exposure	Bladder	9,000	5,000
	Liver	9,800	
Cancer associated with aspects of diet	Breast	30,000	5,000[a]
	Colon & rectum	30,000	10,000
Other factors	Uterine cervix	7,500	3,000[a]
	Melanoma & other skin	5,000	1,500

[a] Achievable mostly through earlier diagnosis by application of known techniques.
[*] From Marvin A. Schneiderman, "Sources, Resources, and Tsouris," in *Persons at High Risk of Cancer: An Approach to Cancer Etiology and Control*, ed. Joseph F. Fraumeni, Jr. (New York: Academic Press, 1975), p. 452.

Early Detection: Checkup Schedule for the General, Low-Risk Population

In March 1980 the American Cancer Society revised its guidelines for the scheduling and specific types of tests that should be used to detect cancer, in *low-risk, symptom-free* people. The schedule reflects increased risks due to age and sex.

These guidelines produced quite an uproar in the medical community when they were announced, and the disagreement in two areas should be known by the public. (1) The ACS eliminated chest X-rays and sputum-cytology tests completely. The National Cancer Institute is at odds with this recommendation for heavy smokers over 45, since these tests are the only way to detect lung cancer in the early stages. NCI recommends yearly chest X-rays for this group. (2) The ACS rescheduled the Pap tests for every three years, rather than every year. The American College of Obstetrics and Gynecology strongly recommends annual pelvic examinations and Pap smears for women over 20, or younger women who are sexually active.

A "cancer checkup" is a special physical that includes examination of the oral cavity, neck, thyroid gland, other glands and lymph nodes, breasts, and abdomen. It also includes a pelvic exam for women, examination of the testes in men, a rectal exam, laboratory examination of a stool sample, and a thorough look at every part of the skin, from the scalp to the soles of the feet.

318

Checkup Schedule for the General Population

Procedure	Sex	Age	Frequency
Cancer Checkup	M&F	over 20	every 3 years
	M&F	over 40	every year
Pelvic Exam	F	20–40	every 3 years
		over 40	every year
Pap Test	F	20–65[a]	every 3 years[b]
Breast Self-Examination	F	over 20	every month
Breast Physical Examination	F	20–40	every 3 years
Mammogram	F	35–40	one baseline exam
		under 50	consult physician
		over 50	every year
Endometrial Tissue Sample	F	menopause[c]	menopause
Manual Rectal Exam	M&F	over 40	every year
Sigmoidoscopy	M&F	over 50	every 3 years[d]
Stool Slide Test	M&F	over 50	every year
Chest X-ray	not recommended for any population		
Sputum Cytology	not recommended for any population		

[a] Should be done on women under 20 who are sexually active.

[b] After two initial Pap tests, done a year apart, are both negative; high-risk women should have them done more frequently.

[c] Particularly for women with a history of infertility, obesity, failure of ovulation, abnormal bleeding, or estrogen therapy.

[d] After two initial examinations, done a year apart.

319

Appendix D

PROGNOSIS
STATISTICS

These are all the latest statistics available on the five-year survival rates for cancers. We have divided the table into two sections: "Official Statistics" and "Update."

The "official statistics" are the latest statistics put out by the National Cancer Institute for the major types of cancer. ("Cancer Patient Survival," Report #5. DHEW Publication no. [NIH] 77-992. These figures were most recently quoted in "Cancer Statistics, 1981," *Ca—A Cancer Journal for Clinicians*, vol. 31, no. 1, January/February 1981.) Please note that although these statistics appeared in 1977, they are based on data gathered in 1965–69. Therefore they only tell how well patients did on treatments that were available at that time.

The "update" provides newer statistics or improved-outlook information based on accepted studies done with newer therapeutic techniques over the last fifteen years. There have been many advances with rare cancers that were not included in the official list—which is why there are no "official statistics" for those types of cancer. Also, some advances have been made in one type of cancer affecting a particular site, but not the others.

Prognosis Statistics

	Official Statistics							
	Male			Female			Percent diagnosed in local stage	Update
Site	All Stages	Local	Regional	All Stages	Local	Regional		
Bladder	62	71	23	62	76	16	82	Tis/T$_1$ 80%, T$_2$ 40–50%, T$_3$ & T$_4$ 20–30%
Bone								Osteogenic Sarcoma 50%+ Rhabdomyosarcoma 50%+ Ewing's Sarcoma 50%+
Brain	25	25	20	33	33	37	88	Varies tremendously depending on location; new breakthroughs in experimental chemotherapy; astrocytomas curable in children
Breast	—	—	—	65	85	56	48	T$_1$/T$_2$ 90% with radiation and surgical removal of tumor
Buccal Mucosa								70% with no node involvement 35% with node involvement
Cervix								*In situ*, 100%
Colon & Rectum	44	71	23	46	72	47	44	T$_1$ 70–85%, T$_2$ 40–60%, T$_3$ 30%, T$_4$ 10%
Esophagus	3	4	5	6	7	10	27	Much improved outlook for preventing recurrences using surgery + radiation + chemo
Eye								Retinoblastoma 50%+ Melanoma of the choroid 50%+
Gallbladder								3%
Gums								60% without node involvement 40% with node involvement
Hodgkin's Disease	53	—	—	57	—	—	—	90% using radiation or chemo

Official Statistics

Site	Male — All Stages	Male — Local	Male — Regional	Female — All Stages	Female — Local	Female — Regional	Percent diagnosed in local stage	Update
Kidney	41	70	39	43	66	40	45	Wilms's Tumor 90%
Larynx	63	80	38	59	75	34	62	T_1 80–90%; others 50%
Leukemias (total)	14	—	—	15	—	—	—	ALL 50%+; 90% remissions / AML 40–60% remissions
Lip	84	87	66	85	89	—	84	
Liver	6	15	1	9	29	5	26	
Lung	8	28	10	13	51	15	17	Chemotherapy for oat cell carcinoma produces regression lasting 1–2 years
Lymphoma (non-Hodgkin's)								
Lymphosarcoma	34	—	—	37	—	—	—	{Very much improved prognosis with newest
Reticulosarcoma	18	—	—	19	—	—	—	(experimental treatments (60%+)
Burkitt's Lymphoma								80%+
Mouth	45	64	38	56	78	40	44	With treatment, patients may live five years
Multiple Myeloma	17	—	—	16	—	—	—	Current experimental programs working on advanced stages
Ovary	—	—	—	34	78	40	44	
Pancreas	1	5	2	2	6	5	15	30–40%
Paranasal Sinuses								
Pharynx (all)	21	35	21	30	47	29	20	
Penis								Stage I 85–90%; Stage II 60%; with node involvement 20%

Site								Notes
Prostate	57	70	61	—	—	—	61	
Skin								
Melanoma	61	76	47	75	85	41	73	Considered 100% curable in earliest stages; with node involvement, 20%
Nonmelanoma								95% with no node involvement; 75% with node involvement; 50–70% after recurrence
Small Intestine								Carcinoid tumors 50%+ Adenocarcinomas 20–25%
Stomach	12	39	15	14	41	13	18	Increased response rates with some experimental programs
Testes								50–60%
Thyroid	80	100	83	87	97	87	54	70% without node involvement 25% with node involvement
Tongue	32	55	24	44	61	30	41	15% for tumors on posterior third
Tonsils								50–75% without node involvement 25% with node involvement
Salivary Glands								Adenoid cystic carcinomas 85% Squamous cell carcinomas 20%
								Overall: T_1 70–85%, T_2 40–60%, T_3 30%, T_4 10%
Uterus	—	—	—	66	83	46	63	Choriocarcinoma 80%+
Vagina								Stage I 55%; Stage II 31%
Vulva								Early stages 75% Metastases or large tumor 8–10%

Appendix E

PHYSICIAN SPECIALTIES

The *American Medical Directory,* published by the American Medical Association, lists doctors practicing medicine in more than eighty areas of specialization. Forty of these areas are under the jurisdiction of AMA specialty boards (see Appendex F). Some of these specialties are self-explanatory; for the others we offer very brief descriptions.

Adolescent Medicine—general practice focusing on teen-agers.
Aerospace Medicine—the study, diagnosis, and treatment of the human body as affected by or in a state of high-speed air or space travel or extraterrestrial environments.
Allergy—the study, diagnosis, and treatment of hypersensitivity of body cells to specific substances.
Allergy and Immunology.
Anesthesiology—deals with the pharmacological, physiological, and clinical basis of anesthesia, its use, and related fields: pain, resuscitation, and intensive respiratory care.
Bronchoesophagology—specializes in endoscopies of the trachea (windpipe), bronchial tree, and the esophagus.
Bloodbanking
Cardiovascular Diseases—the study and treatment of diseases of the heart and circulatory system.
Dermatology—study, diagnosis, and treatment of skin diseases.
Dermatopathology—study of the cell characteristics of skin lesions; a type of pathology.

Diabetes—the study, diagnosis, and treatment of diabetes.

Emergency Medicine—practice focused on the types of high-risk/fast-action medical situations found in hospital emergency rooms.

Endocrinology—the study, diagnosis, and treatment of malfunctions of internal secretions, hormones, and glands.

Family Practice—a general practitioner.

Gastroenterology—study, diagnosis, and treatment of the stomach and intestines.

General Preventive Medicine—specializes in preventing, rather than curing, disease.

Geriatrics—study, diagnosis, and treatment of diseases and malfunctions that occur in old age.

Gynecology—study, diagnosis, and treatment of the female reproductive system.

Hematology—study, diagnosis, and treatment of blood diseases.

Hypnosis—practice includes the use of hypnosis for therapeutic purposes.

Immunology—the study, diagnosis, and treatment of diseases and functioning of the immune (disease-fighting) system.

Infectious Diseases—study, diagnosis, and treatment of diseases transmitted by microorganisms.

Internal Medicine—focuses mainly on the diseases and functions of internal organs, from neck to hips; see Appendix F for subspecialties of internal medicine.

Laryngology—specializes in the study, diagnosis, and treatment of the larynx (voice box).

Legal Medicine—specializes in the legal aspects of medical practice, particularly for use in offering expert medical testimony in trials.

Maxillofacial Surgery—specializes in surgery on the jaw and face.

Neoplastic Diseases—specializes in the study, diagnosis, and treatment of benign and malignant tumors.

Nephrology—study, diagnosis, and treatment of the kidneys.

Neurology—study, diagnosis, and treatment of the nervous system.

Neonatal-Perinatal Medicine—specializes in the study, diagnosis, and treatment of newborn babies.

Neurology, Child—specializes in the neurology of children; also called "pediatric neurology."

Neuropathology—specializes in the study and diagnosis of the nervous system; a form of pathology.

Nuclear Medicine—a combined specialty of internal medicine, pathology, and radiology, using radioactive materials placed inside the patient for study, diagnosis, and treatment.

Nuclear Radiology—see "Nuclear Medicine."

Nutrition—practice focuses on the role of nutrition in maintaining health.

Obstetrics—specializes in the care of pregnant women, delivery, and aftercare.

Obstetrics and Gynecology

Occupational Medicine—specializes in job-related diseases.

Oncology—study, diagnosis, and treatment of cancer.

Ophthalmology—study, diagnosis, and treatment of the eyes.

Otology—study, diagnosis, and treatment of the ears.

Otorhinolaryngology—ear, nose, and throat specialist.

Pathology—study of the causes of diseases and the structural and functional changes in the body and its cells due to disease.

325

Pathology, Clinical—a subspecialty of pathology that relates directly to the diagnosis of disease and the care of patients as well as the prevention of disease.

Pathology, Forensic—a subspecialty of pathology that uses the results of pathological examinations in legal proceedings.

Pediatrics—general practice focusing on children.

Pediatrics, Allergy—subspecialty of pediatrics that focuses on allergies in children.

Pediatrics, Cardiology—specializes in study, diagnosis, and treatment of heart and circulatory problems in children.

Pediatric Endocrinology—study, diagnosis, and treatment of the functioning of the endocrine system (internal secretions, hormones, glands) in children.

Pediatric Hematology-Oncology—specializes in blood diseases and related cancers (leukemias, lymphomas, Hodgkin's disease) in children; may be called in to oversee chemotherapy treatments in adults for these and other kinds of cancers.

Pediatric Nephrology—specializes in children's kidney diseases and malfunctions.

Pharmacology, Clinical—specializes in the use of drugs in patient care.

Physical Medicine and Rehabilitation—specializes in helping patients to resume normal life after debilitation due to accident, disease, or treatment.

Psychiatry—study, diagnosis, and treatment of mental disorders.

Psychiatry, Child—study, diagnosis, and treatment of mental disorders in children.

Psychoanalysis—a specific method of psychiatric therapy originated by Sigmund Freud.

Psychosomatic Medicine—specializes in the relationship between mind and body in maintaining health, in the origin of diseases, and in the healing process.

Public Health—a very broad field of medicine with many subspecialty areas that focuses on the study of diseases and its causes (as well as methods of diagnosis, treatment, and, particularly, prevention) as they present themselves in the population as a whole.

Pulmonary Diseases—specializes in study, diagnosis, and treatment of diseases of the lungs.

Radioisotopic Pathology—a subspecialty of pathology that employs radioisotopes.

Radiology—the study, diagnosis, and treatment of disease using radiant energy.

Radiology, Diagnostic—specializes in the use of radiology for diagnosis only.

Radiology, Pediatric—specializes in the use of radiology for the study, diagnosis, and treatment of children.

Radiology, Therapeutic—specializes in the use of radiology for the treatment of patients.

Rheumatology—the study, diagnosis, and treatment of diseases of the musculoskeletal system.

Rhinology—study, diagnosis and treatment of the nose.

Surgery, Abdominal—a subspecialty of surgery that deals only with the abdominal cavity.

Surgery, Cardiovascular—a subspecialty of surgery that deals only with the heart and circulatory system.

Surgery, Colon and Rectal—a subspecialty of surgery that deals only with the colon and rectum.

Surgery, General

Surgery, Hand—a subspecialty of surgery that deals with the hands.

Surgery, Head and Neck—a subspecialty of surgery that deals only with the head and neck (but not the brain).

Surgery, Neurological—a subspecialty of surgery that deals with the brain and nervous system.

Surgery, Orthopedic—a subspecialty of surgery that deals with bones and joints.

Surgery, Pediatric—a subspecialty of surgery that focuses on children.

Surgery, Plastic—a subspecialty of surgery that specializes in the repair of defects.

Surgery, Thoracic—a subspecialty of surgery that deals only with the chest cavity.

Surgery, Traumatic—a subspecialty of surgery that deals with the surgical repair of physical trauma (like automobile accidents, wounds, etc.).

Surgery, Urological—a subspecialty of surgery that deals with the genito-urinary tract.

Appendix F

AMERICAN
SPECIALTY BOARDS

According to the AMA's *American Medical Directory*, "The primary purposes of Specialty Boards are to: (1) conduct investigations and examinations to determine the competence of voluntary candidates; (2) grant and issue certificates of qualification to candidates successful in demonstrating their proficiency; (3) stimulate the development of adequate training facilities; (4) aid the Council on Medical Education of the American Medical Association in evaluating residencies; and (5) advise physicians desiring certification as to the course of study and training to be pursued." Certificates are granted in twenty-two specialty areas and eighteen subspecialties:

Specialty Board	Subspecialty (If Any)
American Board of Allergy and Immunology (a conjoint board of the American Board of Internal Medicine and the American Board of Pediatrics)	
American Board of Anesthesiology	
American Board of Colon and Rectal Surgery	
American Board of Dermatology	
American Board of Family Practice	
American Board of Internal Medicine	Cardiovascular Disease
	Endocrinology and Metabolism
	Gastroenterology
	Hematology
	Infectious Disease
	Medical Oncology
	Nephrology
	Pulmonary Disease
	Rheumatology
American Board of Neurological Surgery	
American Board of Nuclear Medicine (a conjoint board of the American Boards of Internal Medicine, Pathology and Radiology)	
American Board of Obstetrics and Gynecology	
American Board of Ophthalmology	
American Board of Orthopædic Surgery	
American Board of Pathology	
American Board of Pediatrics	Cardiology
	Endocrinology
	Hematology-Oncology
	Neonatal-Perinatal Medicine
	Nephrology
American Board of Physical Medicine and Rehabilitation	
American Board of Plastic Surgery	
American Board of Preventive Medicine	
American Board of Psychiatry and Neurology	Psychiatry
	Neurology
	Child Neurology
	Psychiatry and Neurology
	Child Psychiatry
American Board of Radiology	
American Board of Surgery	
American Board of Thoracic Surgery	
American Board of Urology	

329

Appendix G

TREATMENT INFORMATION AND RESOURCES

In chapter 6, "How to Find Help," we referred to a number of resources available for finding the best and nearest places to be diagnosed and/or treated. What follows is a list, organized alphabetically by state, of five of those resources:

1. Cancer Information Service.
2. American Cancer Society. We have listed the address and phone of the state chapter; local chapters can be found by calling the state chapter or by looking up "American Cancer Society" in the white pages of your phone book.
3. Comprehensive Cancer Center. The cancer centers we have listed are not the only ones qualified to diagnose and treat patients, but the ones designated by the National Cancer Institute. We have included them primarily for patients who have a cancer that is rare or hard to diagnose or treat, and who thus need highly qualified and experienced cancer specialists. If your state does not have a Comprehensive Cancer Center, we have listed the one closest to you.
4. Children's Hospitals. The list of children's hospitals or large departments of pediatrics was not meant to be complete. We have tried

to list all those facilities that have programs associated with NCI cooperative groups. In certain areas that have a concentration of major medical centers (New York, Boston, California, etc.), we have only listed a sampling of what is available.

5. Regional Medical Libraries. These are the medical libraries that have a direct computer hookup with the National Library of Medicine in Bethesda, Maryland.

If you are interested in experimental programs, information on the clinical cooperative groups listed in each site discussion can be found in Appendix H.

Canadian readers should note that the Canadian and American cancer programs work very closely with each other. There are Canadian hospitals and doctors who participate in the clinical cooperative groups; by calling the appropriate groups, you can find out where they are located. For general information on cancer diagnosis and treatment in Canada, call the National Cancer Institute of Canada and the Canadian Cancer Society. Both are located at 77 Bloor Street West, Suite 401, Toronto, Ontario, Canada M582 V7; phone (416) 961-7223.

Alabama

Cancer Information Service

(800) 638-6694

American Cancer Society

(205) 897-2242
2926 Central Avenue
Birmingham, Alabama 35209

Comprehensive Cancer Center

(205) 943-5077
University of Alabama Hospitals
and Clinics
619 South 19th Street
Birmingham, Alabama 35233

Children's Hospitals

The Children's Hospital
(205) 933-4167
1601 6th Avenue South
Birmingham, Alabama 35233

Regional Medical Library

See also GEORGIA.

Alaska

Cancer Information Service

1 (800) 638-6070

American Cancer Society

(907) 277-8696
1343 G Street
Anchorage, Alaska 99501

Comprehensive Cancer Center

See WASHINGTON.

Children's Hospitals

See WASHINGTON.

Nearest pediatric oncology department is located at:
University of British Columbia
Department of Pediatrics
715 West 12th Avenue
Vancouver, British Columbia,
Canada
Phone: (604) 873-5441 Ext. 2682

Regional Medical Library

See WASHINGTON.

331

Arizona

Cancer Information Service

(800) 638-6694

American Cancer Society

(602) 264-5861
634 West Indian School Road
P.O. Box 33187
Phoenix, Arizona 85067

Comprehensive Cancer Center

See CALIFORNIA.

Children's Hospitals

(602) 626-6300
University of Arizona Medical
School
Department of Pediatrics
Tucson, Arizona 85724

Regional Medical Library

See CALIFORNIA.

Arkansas

Cancer Information Service

(800) 638-6694

American Cancer Society

(501) 664-3480/1/2
P.O. Box 3822
Little Rock, Arkansas 72203

Comprehensive Cancer Center

See ALABAMA.

Children's Hospitals

Arkansas Children's Hospital
(501) 372-5622
804 Wolfe Street
Pediatric Division
Little Rock, Arkansas 72201

Regional Medical Library

See TEXAS.

California

Cancer Information Service

Southern California (213,714,805)
1 (800) 252-9066

Northern California
(213) 226-2374

American Cancer Society

(415) 777-1800
731 Market Street
San Francisco, California 94103

Comprehensive Cancer Center

Los Angeles County, University
of Southern California
(213) 226-2008
Comprehensive Cancer Center
2025 Zonal Avenue
Los Angeles, California 20033
G. Denman Hammond, M.D.,
Director

UCLA-Jonsson Comprehensive
Cancer Center
(213) 825-5268
UCLA School of Medicine
924 Westwood Boulevard,
Suite 940
Los Angeles, California 90024
Richard E. Steckel, M.D., Director

Children's Hospitals

Memorial Hospital Medical Center
of Long Beach
(213) 595-2311
Children's Medical Center
2801 Atlantic Avenue
Long Beach, California 90801

Harbor General Hospital
(213) 595-2311
1000 West Carson Street, E-6
Torrance, California 90509

Children's Hospital of Los Angeles
(213) 660-2450 Ext. 2656
P.O. Box 54700 Terminal Annex
Los Angeles, California 90054

UCLA Medical Center
(213) 825-7786
Department of Pediatric Oncology
Los Angeles, California 90024

Children's Hospital & Medical
Center of Northern California
(415) 654-5600
51st and Grove Street
Oakland, California 94609

Children's Hospital at Stanford
(415) 327-3800
520 Willow Road
Palo Alto, California 94304

Children's Hospital and Health
Center, San Diego
(714) 563-3186
8001 Frost Street
San Diego, California 92123

University of California Medical
Center (714) 294-6767
Pediatric Division
225 West Dickinson Street
San Diego, California 92103

Children's Hospital of San
Francisco (415) 981-4590
3700 California Street
San Francisco, California 94118

Regional Medical Library

Center for the Health Sciences
University of California
Los Angeles, California 90024

Colorado

Cancer Information Service

1 (800) 332-1850

American Cancer Society

(303) 321-2464
1809 East 18th Avenue
P.O. Box 18266
Denver, Colorado 80218

Comprehensive Cancer Center

(303) 320-5921
Colorado Regional Cancer Center
165 Cook Street
Denver, Colorado 80206

Children's Hospitals

(303) 861-6777
Children's Hospital of Denver
1056 East 19th Avenue
Denver, Colorado 80218

Regional Medical Library

See NEBRASKA.

Connecticut

Cancer Information Service

1 (800) 922-0824

American Cancer Society

(203) 265-7161
Barnes Park South
14 Village Lane
Wallingford, Connecticut 06492

Comprehensive Cancer Center

(203) 432-4122
Yale University Comprehensive
Cancer Center
333 Cedar Street
New Haven, Connecticut 06510

Children's Hospitals

Yale–New Haven Medical Center
(203) 436-4668
Department of Pediatrics
333 Cedar Street
New Haven, Connecticut 06510

Regional Medical Library

See MASSACHUSETTS.

Delaware

Cancer Information Service

1 (800) 523-3586

American Cancer Society

(302) 654-6267
Academy of Medicine Building
1925 Lovering Avenue
Wilmington, Delaware 19806

Comprehensive Cancer Center

See DISTRICT OF COLUMBIA.

Children's Hospitals

See DISTRICT OF COLUMBIA.

Regional Medical Library

See MARYLAND.

District of Columbia (Washington, D.C.)

Cancer Information Service

(202) 232-3833

American Cancer Society

(202) 483-2600
Universal Building, South
1825 Connecticut Avenue, N.W.
Washington, D.C. 20009

Comprehensive Cancer Center

Vincent T. Lombardi Cancer
   Research Center (202) 625-7066
Georgetown University
3800 Reservoir Road, N.W.
Washington, D.C. 20007

Howard University Cancer
   Research Center (202) 745-1406
Department of Oncology
2041 Georgia Avenue, N.W.
Washington, D.C. 20060

Children's Hospitals

Children's Hospital National
   Medical Center (202) 745-2140
111 Michigan Avenue, N.W.
Washington, D.C. 20010

Regional Medical Library

See MARYLAND.

Florida

Cancer Information Service

English: 1 (800) 432-5953
Spanish: 1 (800) 432-5955

Dade County:
   English: (305) 547-6920
Dade County:
   Spanish: (305) 547-6960

American Cancer Society

(813) 253-0541
1001 South MacDill Avenue
Tampa, Florida 33609

Comprehensive Cancer Center

(305) 547-6758/6678
C. Gordon Zubrod, M.D., Director
Comprehensive Cancer Center for
   the State of Florida
University of Miami School of
   Medicine
Jackson Memorial Medical Center
Centre House, Roof Garden
1400 N.W. 10th Avenue
Miami, Florida 33136

Children's Hospitals

Department of Pediatrics
   (305) 324-1180
University of Miami
P.O. Box 520875
Biscayne Annex
Miami, Florida 33152

University of South Florida
   (813) 974-2839
Pediatric Division
12901 North 30th Street
Tampa, Florida 33612

University of Florida/Gainesville
   (904) 392-3301
College of Medicine
Department of Pediatrics
Gainesville, Florida 32601

Regional Medical Library

See GEORGIA.

Georgia

Cancer Information Service

(800) 638-6694

American Cancer Society

(404) 351-3650/1/2
2025 Peachtree Road, N.E.
Suite 14
Atlanta, Georgia 30309

Comprehensive Cancer Center

See FLORIDA.

(Although not designated a comprehensive cancer center, you
may wish to contact Dr. Charles

H. Huguley, Jr., Director Emory
University Cancer Center
Rm. 606 F, Emory University
Hospital
Atlanta, Georgia 30322
(404) 329-7016)

Children's Hospitals

Emory University School of
Medicine (404) 588-3815
Pediatric Oncology
69 Butler Street, S.E.
Atlanta, Georgia 30303

Regional Medical Library

A. W. Calhoun Medical Library
Emory University
Atlanta, Georgia 30322

Hawaii

Cancer Information Service

Oahu: 524-1234

Other islands: Enterprise 6702

American Cancer Society

(808) 531-1662/3/4/5
Community Services Center Bldg.
200 North Vineyard Boulevard
Honolulu, Hawaii 96817

Comprehensive Cancer Center

See CALIFORNIA.

(Although not designated a
comprehensive cancer center,
you may wish to contact:
Cancer Center of Hawaii
University of Hawaii
1236 Lauhala Street
Honolulu, Hawaii 98613
(808) 538-9011)

Children's Hospitals

See CALIFORNIA.

Regional Medical Library

See CALIFORNIA.

Idaho

Cancer Information Service

(800) 638-6694

American Cancer Society

(208) 343-4609
1609 Abbs Street
P.O. Box 5386
Boise, Idaho 83705

Comprehensive Cancer Center

See COLORADO or WASHINGTON.

Children's Hospitals

See COLORADO or WASHINGTON.

Regional Medical Library

See WASHINGTON.

Illinois

Cancer Information Service

(800) 972-0586

American Cancer Society

(312) 372-0472
37 South Wabash Avenue
Chicago, Illinois 60603

Comprehensive Cancer Center

(312) 346-9813
Illinois Cancer Council
37 South Wabash Avenue
Chicago, Illinois 60603

Children's Hospitals

Wyler Children's Hospital
University of Chicago
950 East 59th Street
Box 97
Chicago, Illinois 60637

Children's Memorial Hospital
(312) 649-4584
2300 North Children's Plaza
Fullterton at Lincoln
Chicago, Illinois 60614

Regional Medical Library

John Crerar Library
35 West 33rd Street
Chicago, Illinois 60616

Indiana

Cancer Information Service

(800) 638-6694

American Cancer Society

(317) 257-5326
2702 East 55th Place
Indianapolis, Indiana 46220

Comprehensive Cancer Center

See ILLINOIS.

Children's Hospitals

James Whitcomb Riley Hospital
for Children
(317) 264-8784
Indiana University Medical Center
1100 West Michigan Street
Indianapolis, Indiana 46202

Regional Medical Library

See ILLINOIS.

Iowa

Cancer Information Service

(800) 638-6694

American Cancer Society

(515) 423-0712
Highway No. 18 West
P.O. Box 980
Mason City, Iowa 50401

Comprehensive Cancer Center

See ILLINOIS.

Children's Hospitals

Department of Pediatrics
(319) 356-3584
University of Iowa Hospitals and
Clinics
Iowa City, Iowa 52242

Regional Medical Library

See ILLINOIS.

Kansas

Cancer Information Service

(800) 638-6694

American Cancer Society

(913) 267-0131
3003 Van Buren Street
Topeka, Kansas 66611

Comprehensive Cancer Center

See COLORADO or ILLINOIS.

Children's Hospitals

University of Kansas Medical
Center, Pediatric Division
(913) 424-3341
Rainbow Boulevard at 39th Street
Kansas City, Kansas 66103

Regional Medical Library

See NEBRASKA.

Kentucky

Cancer Information Service

(800) 432-9321

American Cancer Society

(502) 459-1867
Medical Arts Building
1169 Eastern Parkway
Louisville, Kentucky 40217

Comprehensive Cancer Center

See OHIO.

Children's Hospitals

Department of Pediatrics
(606) 233-5694
Albert T. Chandler Medical Center
University of Kentucky
800 Rose Street
Lexington, Kentucky 40506

Children's Hospital of Louisville
(502) 589-8292
200 East Chestnut Street
Louisville, Kentucky 40202

Regional Medical Library

See MICHIGAN.

Louisiana

Cancer Information Service

(800) 638-6694

American Cancer Society

(504) 523-2029
Masonic Temple Building, Rm. 810
333 St. Charles Avenue
New Orleans, Louisiana 70130

Comprehensive Cancer Center

See ALABAMA.

(Although not comprehensive
cancer centers, there are major
cancer programs at:
Tulane University Medical Center
1430 Tulane Avenue
New Orleans, Louisiana 70112
(504) 588-5272
and
Louisiana State University
Medical Center
1542 Tulane Avenue
New Orleans, Louisiana 70112
(504) 568-4750)

Children's Hospitals

Pediatric Divisions, Tulane
University Medical Center
and Louisiana State University
Medical Center (see above)

Regional Medical Library

See TEXAS.

Maine

Cancer Information Service

(800) 225-7034

American Cancer Society

(207) 729-3339
Federal and Green Streets
Brunswick, Maine 04011

Comprehensive Cancer Center

See MASSACHUSETTS.

Children's Hospitals

See MASSACHUSETTS.

Regional Medical Library

See MASSACHUSETTS.

Maryland

Cancer Information Service

(800) 492-1444

American Cancer Society

(301) 828-8890
200 East Joppa Road
Towson, Maryland 21204

Comprehensive Cancer Center

(301) 955-3636
Johns Hopkins Comprehensive
Cancer Center
600 North Wolfe Street
Baltimore, Maryland 21205

Children's Hospitals

Johns Hopkins University
Pediatric Division
(301) 955-8816
600 North Wolfe Street
Baltimore, Maryland 21205

Regional Medical Library

National Library of Medicine
8600 Rockville Pike
Bethesda, Maryland 20014

Massachusetts

Cancer Information Service

1 (800) 952-7420

American Cancer Society

(617) 267-2650
247 Commonwealth Avenue
Boston, Massachusetts 02116

Comprehensive Cancer Center

(617) 732-3555/3150
Sidney Farber Cancer Institute
44 Binney Street
Boston, Massachusetts 02115

Children's Hospitals

Department of Pediatrics
(617) 726-8695
Massachusetts General Hospital
Boston, Massachusetts 02114

Tufts New England Medical
Center (617) 956-5000
Pediatric Division
171 Harrison Avenue
Boston, Massachusetts 02111

Regional Medical Library

Francis A. Countway Library of
Medicine
10 Shattuck Street
Boston, Massachusetts 02115

Michigan
Cancer Information Service

(800) 638-6694

American Cancer Society

(517) 371-2920

Comprehensive Cancer Center

(313) 833-0710
Comprehensive Cancer Center
of Metropolitan Detroit
110 East Warren Street
Detroit, Michigan 48201

Children's Hospitals

Mott Children's Hospital
(313) 764-7126
1405 East Ann Street
Ann Arbor, Michigan 48109

338

Children's Hospital of Michigan
(313) 494-5520
Wayne State University
3901 Beaubien Boulevard
Detroit, Michigan 48201

Regional Medical Library

Wayne State University Medical
Library
4325 Brush Street
Detroit, Michigan 48201

Minnesota
Cancer Information Service

1 (800) 582-5262

American Cancer Society

(612) 871-2111
2750 Park Avenue
Minneapolis, Minnesota 55407

Comprehensive Cancer Center

(507) 282-3261
Mayo Comprehensive Cancer
Center
200 First Street, S.W.
Rochester, Minnesota 55901

Children's Hospitals

Department of Pediatrics
(612) 373-4303
University of Minnesota Medical
School
University of Minnesota Hospitals
Minneapolis, Minnesota 55455

Pediatric Division
(507) 284-2511
Mayo Clinic
200 First Street, S.W.
Rochester, Minnesota 55901

St. Paul's Children's Hospital
(612) 227-6521
311 Pleasant Avenue
St. Paul, Minnesota 55102

Regional Medical Library

See ILLINOIS.

Mississippi

Cancer Information Service

(800) 638-6694

American Cancer Society

(601) 362-8874
345 North Mart Plaza
Jackson, Mississippi 39206

Comprehensive Cancer Center

See ALABAMA.

Children's Hospitals

University of Mississippi Medical
Center, Pediatric Division
(601) 987-4699
2500 North State Street
Jackson, Mississippi 39216

Regional Medical Library

See GEORGIA.

Missouri

Cancer Information Service

(800) 638-6694

American Cancer Society

(314) 636-3195
715 Jefferson Street
P.O. Box 1066
Jefferson City, Missouri 65101

Comprehensive Cancer Center

See ILLINOIS.

Children's Hospitals

St. Louis Children's Hospital
(314) 454-3306
Washington University
500 South Kingshighway Boulevard
St. Louis, Missouri 63178

Department of Pediatrics
(314) 882-3996
University of Missouri
Columbia, Missouri 65212

Regional Medical Library

See NEBRASKA.

Montana

Cancer Information Service

1 (800) 525-0231

American Cancer Society

(406) 252-7111
2820 First Avenue South
Billings, Montana 59101

Comprehensive Cancer Center

See WASHINGTON.

Children's Hospitals

See WASHINGTON.

Regional Medical Library

See WASHINGTON.

Nebraska

Cancer Information Service

(800) 638-6694

American Cancer Society

(402) 551-2422
Overland Wolfe Centre
6910 Pacific Street, Suite 210
Omaha, Nebraska

Comprehensive Cancer Center

See COLORADO.

Children's Hospitals

Pediatric Division
(402) 541-4802
University of Nebraska Medical
Center
42nd and Dewey Avenue
Omaha, Nebraska 68105

Regional Medical Library

University of Nebraska Medical
Center
42nd Street & Dewey Avenue
Omaha, Nebraska 68105

Nevada

Cancer Information Service

(800) 638-6694

American Cancer Society

(702) 733-7272
953-35B East Sahara
Suite 101 S. T. & P. Bldg.
Las Vegas, Nevada 89104

Comprehensive Cancer Center

See CALIFORNIA.

Children's Hospitals

See CALIFORNIA.

Regional Medical Library

See CALIFORNIA.

New Hampshire

Cancer Information Service

1 (800) 225-7034

American Cancer Society

(603) 669-3270
22 Bridge Street
Manchester, New Hampshire 03101

Comprehensive Cancer Center

See MASSACHUSETTS.

(Although not a comprehensive cancer center, you may wish to contact:
Norris Cotton Cancer Center
Dartmouth Medical School
Hanover, New Hampshire 03755
(603) 643-4000)

Children's Hospitals

Pediatric Division
(603) 643-4000 Ext. 2271
Dartmouth Medical School
Hanover, New Hampshire 03755

Regional Medical Library

See MASSACHUSETTS.

New Jersey

Cancer Information Service

(800) 523-3586

American Cancer Society

(201) 687-2100
2700 Route 22, P.O. Box 1220
Union, New Jersey 07083

Comprehensive Cancer Center

See NEW YORK and
PENNSYLVANIA.

Children's Hospitals

Pediatric Department
(201) 456-4481
College of Medicine and Dentistry
of New Jersey
Martland Hospital Unit
65 Bergen Street
Newark, New Jersey 07107

Regional Medical Library

See NEW YORK and
PENNSYLVANIA.

New Mexico

Cancer Information Service

1 (800) 525-0231

American Cancer Society

(505) 262-1727
525 San Pedro, N.E.
Albuquerque, New Mexico 87108

Comprehensive Cancer Center

See TEXAS.

(Although not a comprehensive cancer center, you may wish to contact:
University of New Mexico
Cancer Research and Treatment
Center
900 Camino De Saluo, N.E.
Albuquerque, New Mexico 87106
(505) 277-6337

Children's Hospitals

Pediatric Division, University of
New Mexico Cancer Research
and Treatment Center
(see above)

Regional Medical Library

See TEXAS.

New York

Cancer Information Service

New York State
1 (800) 462-7255
New York City (212) 794-7982

American Cancer Society

New York State Division
(315) 437-7025
6725 Lyons Street
P.O. Box 7
East Syracuse, New York 13057

New York City Division
(212) 586-8700
19 West 56th Street
New York, New York 10019

Long Island Division
(516) 420-1111
535 Broad Hollow Road
(Route 110)
Melville, New York 11746

Queens Division
(212) 263-2224
111-15 Queens Boulevard
Forest Hills, New York 11375

Westchester Division
(914) 949-4800
246 North Central Avenue
Hartsdale, New York 10530

Comprehensive Cancer Centers

Columbia University Cancer Center
(212) 694-4161/3807
Institute of Cancer Research
Hammer Health Sciences Center
701 West 168th Street
New York, New York 10032

Memorial Sloan-Kettering Cancer
Center
(212) 794-7646/7982/5957
1275 York Avenue
New York, New York 10021

Roswell Park Memorial Institute
(716) 845-2300
666 Elm Street
Buffalo, New York 14203

Children's Hospitals

Babies Hospital (212) 694-5882
3959 Broadway
New York, New York 10032

Department of Pediatrics
(516) 562-0100
Northshore University Hospital
300 Community Drive
Manhasset, New York 11030

Department of Pediatrics
(212) 470-2426
Long Island Jewish Medical Center
270-05 76th Avenue
New Hyde Park, New York 11040

Department of Pediatrics
(212) 472-6322
New York Hospital
Cornell Medical Center
525 East 68th Street
New York, New York 10021

Department of Pediatrics
(716) 275-3186
Strong Memorial Hospital
601 Elmwood Avenue
Rochester, New York 14642

Department of Pediatrics
(315) 473-4354
Upstate Medical Center
750 East Adams Street
Syracuse, New York 13210

Regional Medical Library

New York Academy of Medicine
Library
2 East 103rd Street
New York, New York 10029

North Carolina

Cancer Information Service

1 (800) 672-0943

American Cancer Society

(919) 834-8463
222 North Person Street
P.O. Box 27624
Raleigh, North Carolina 27611

Comprehensive Cancer Center

Duke University Comprehensive
  Cancer Center
  (919) 684-3765/2282
P.O. Box 3814
Durham, North Carolina 27710

Children's Hospitals

Department of Pediatrics
  (919) 966-1196
University of North Carolina
  School of Medicine
Chapel Hill, North Carolina 27514

Department of Pediatrics
  (919) 684-3765
Duke University Medical Center
Durham, North Carolina 27710

Department of Pediatrics
  (919) 727-4337
Bowman Gray School of Medicine
300 South Hawthorne Road
Winston-Salem, North Carolina
  27103

Regional Medical Library

See MARYLAND.

North Dakota

Cancer Information Service

(800) 638-6694

American Cancer Society

(701) 232-1385
Hotel Graver Annex Bldg.
115 Roberts Street
P.O. Box 426
Fargo, North Dakota 58102

Comprehensive Cancer Center

See MINNESOTA.

Children's Hospitals

See MINNESOTA.

Regional Medical Library

See ILLINOIS.

Ohio

Cancer Information Service

(800) 282-6522

American Cancer Society

(216) 771-6700
453 Lincoln Bldg.
1367 East Sixth Street
Cleveland, Ohio 44114

Comprehensive Cancer Center

(614) 422-5022
The Ohio State University
  Comprehensive Cancer Center
410 West 10th Avenue
Columbus, Ohio 43210

Children's Hospitals

Children's Hospital
  (513) 559-4266
Elland & Bethesda Ave.
Cincinnati, Ohio 45229

Cleveland Clinic
  (216) 444-5516
Pediatric Division
9500 Euclid Avenue
Cleveland, Ohio 44106

Rainbow Babies and Children's
  Hospital (216) 444-3345
2101 Adelbert Road
Cleveland, Ohio 44106

Children's Hospital of Columbus
  (614) 461-2310/2060
700 Children's Drive
Columbus, Ohio 43205

Regional Medical Library

See MICHIGAN.

342

Oklahoma

Cancer Information Service

(800) 638-6694

American Cancer Society

(504) 525-3515
1312 N.W. 24th Street
Oklahoma City, Oklahoma 73106

Comprehensive Cancer Center

See TEXAS and COLORADO.

Children's Hospitals

University of Oklahoma Health
  Sciences Center
  (405) 271-4485
Pediatric Division
P.O. Box 26901
Oklahoma City, Oklahoma 73190

Children's Memorial Hospital
  (405) 271-5311
P.O. Box 26307
Oklahoma City, Oklahoma 73190

Regional Medical Library

See TEXAS.

Oregon

Cancer Information Service

(800) 638-6694

American Cancer Society

(503) 231-5100
910 N.E. Union Avenue
Portland, Oregon 97232

Comprehensive Cancer Center

See WASHINGTON.

Children's Hospitals

Doernbecher Memorial Hospital
  for Children (503) 225-8194
University of Oregon Health
  Sciences Center
Portland, Oregon 97201

Regional Medical Library

See WASHINGTON.

Pennsylvania

Cancer Information Service

1 (800) 822-3963

American Cancer Society

(717) 545-4215
3309 Spring Street
P.O. Box 4175
Harrisburg, Pennsylvania 17111

Comprehensive Cancer Center

Fox Chase/University of
  Pennsylvania Cancer Center
  (215) 722-1900
7701 Burholme Avenue
Philadelphia, Pennsylvania 19111

Children's Hospitals

Children's Hospital of Philadelphia
  (215) 387-6000
34th and Civic Center Boulevard
Philadelphia, Pennsylvania 19104

Children's Hospital of Pittsburgh
  (412) 647-5055
125 DeSoto Street
Pittsburgh, Pennsylvania 15213

Regional Medical Library

Library of the College of Physicians
19 South 22nd Street
Philadelphia, Pennsylvania 19103

Puerto Rico/Virgin Islands

Cancer Information Service

1 (800) 638-6070

American Cancer Society

(809) 764-2295
Avenue Domenech 273
Hato Rey
GPO Box 6004
San Juan, Puerto Rico 00936

343

Comprehensive Cancer Center

See FLORIDA.

Children's Hospitals

See FLORIDA.

Regional Medical Library

See GEORGIA.

Rhode Island

Cancer Information Service

(800) 638-6694

American Cancer Society

(401) 831-6970
345 Blackstone Boulevard
Providence, Rhode Island 02906

Comprehensive Cancer Center

See MASSACHUSETTS.

Children's Hospitals

Rhode Island Hospital
(401) 277-4000
Pediatric Division
593 Eddy Street
Providence, Rhode Island 02902

Regional Medical Library

See MASSACHUSETTS.

South Carolina

Cancer Information Service

(800) 638-6694

American Cancer Society

(803) 787-5623
2442 Devine Street
Columbia, South Carolina 29205

Comprehensive Cancer Center

See NORTH CAROLINA.

Children's Hospitals

Department of Pediatrics
(803) 792-3271
Medical University of South
Carolina
171 Ashley Avenue
Charleston, South Carolina 29403

Regional Medical Library

See GEORGIA.

South Dakota

Cancer Information Service

(800) 638-6694

American Cancer Society

(605) 336-0897
700 South 4th Avenue
Sioux Falls, South Dakota 57104

Comprehensive Cancer Center

See MINNESOTA.

Children's Hospitals

See MINNESOTA.

Regional Medical Library

See NEBRASKA.

Tennessee

Cancer Information Service

(800) 638-6694

American Cancer Society

(615) 383-1710
2519 White Avenue
Nashville, Tennessee 37204

Comprehensive Cancer Center

See ALABAMA and NORTH
CAROLINA.

Children's Hospitals

St. Jude Children's Research
Hospital (901) 525-8381
332 North Lauderdale
Memphis, Tennessee 38101

344

Department of Pediatrics
(615) 322-7475
Vanderbilt University
Nashville, Tennessee 37203

Regional Medical Library

See GEORGIA.

Texas

Cancer Information Service

1 (800) 392-2040

American Cancer Society

(512) 345-4560
3834 Spicewood Springs Road
P.O. Box 9863
Austin, Texas 78766

Comprehensive Cancer Center

The University of Texas System
Cancer Center
(713) 792-2121/3000
M. D. Anderson Hospital and
Tumor Institute
6723 Bertner Drive
Houston, Texas 77025

Children's Hospitals

University of Texas Southwestern
Medical School
(214) 637-3820
Children's Medical Center
1935 Amelia Street
Dallas, Texas 75235

Baylor College of Medicine
(713) 521-4122
Pediatric Division
6621 Fannin Street
Houston, Texas 77030

University of Texas–San Antonio
(512) 691-6151
Department of Pediatrics
Health Science Center
7703 Floyd Curl Drive
San Antonio, Texas 78284

Regional Medical Library

University of Texas Southwestern
Medical School at Dallas
5323 Harry Hines Boulevard
Dallas, Texas 75235

Utah

Cancer Information Service

(800) 638-6694

American Cancer Society

(801) 322-0431
610 East South Temple
Salt Lake City, Utah 84102

Comprehensive Cancer Center

See COLORADO and CALIFORNIA.

Children's Hospitals

University of Utah Medical Center
(801) 581-7200
Department of Pediatrics
50 North Medical Drive
Salt Lake City, Utah 84132

Regional Medical Library

See NEBRASKA.

Vermont

Cancer Information Service

1 (800) 225-7034

American Cancer Society

(802) 223-2348
13 Loomis Street, Drawer C
Montpelier, Vermont 05602

Comprehensive Cancer Center

See MASSACHUSETTS and
NEW YORK.

Children's Hospitals

Pediatric Division
(802) 656-2296
University of Vermont
College of Medicine
Burlington, Vermont 05405

Regional Medical Library

See MASSACHUSETTS.

Virginia

Cancer Information Service

(800) 638-6694

American Cancer Society

(804) 359-0208
3218 West Cary Street
P.O. Box 7288
Richmond, Virginia 23221

Comprehensive Cancer Center

See DISTRICT OF COLUMBIA.

Children's Hospitals

Department of Pediatrics
(804) 924-5105
University of Virginia School of
Medicine
Charlottesville, Virginia 22901

Department of Pediatrics
(804) 786-9602
Medical College of Virginia
Virginia Commonwealth University
Richmond, Virginia 23298

Regional Medical Library

See MARYLAND.

Virgin Islands

See PUERTO RICO.

Washington, D.C.

See DISTRICT OF COLUMBIA.

Washington State

Cancer Information Service

1 (800) 552-7212

American Cancer Society

(206) 284-8390
323 First Avenue West
Seattle, Washington 98119

Comprehensive Cancer Center

Fred Hutchinson Cancer Center
(206) 292-2931
1102 Columbia Street
Seattle, Washington 98104

Children's Hospitals

Children's Orthopedic Hospital
and Medical Center
(206) 634-5000
4800 Sand Point Way, N.E.
Seattle, Washington 98105

Regional Medical Library

University of Washington
Health Sciences Library
Seattle, Washington 98105

West Virginia

Cancer Information Service

(800) 638-6694

American Cancer Society

(304) 344-3611
Suite 100
240 Capitol Street
Charleston, West Virginia 25301

Comprehensive Cancer Center

See OHIO, MARYLAND, DISTRICT
OF COLUMBIA, or PENNSYLVANIA.

Children's Hospitals

Charleston Area Medical Center
(304) 342-6179
3200 MacCorkle Avenue, S.E.
Charleston, West Virginia 25304

Department of Pediatrics
(304) 293-4451
West Virginia University Medical
Center
Morgantown, West Virginia 26505

Regional Medical Library

See MARYLAND.

Wisconsin

Cancer Information Service

(800) 362-8038

American Cancer Society

(608) 249-0487
611 North Sherman Avenue
P.O. Box 1626
Madison, Wisconsin 53701

Comprehensive Cancer Center

The University of Wisconsin
  Clinical Cancer Center
  (608) 263-8600
600 Highland Avenue
Madison, Wisconsin 53792

Children's Hospitals

Department of Pediatrics
  (608) 263-3188
University of Wisconsin Medical
  Center
1300 University Avenue
Madison, Wisconsin 53706

Children's Hospital of Milwaukee
  (414) 344-1944
1700 West Wisconsin Avenue
Milwaukee, Wisconsin 53233

Regional Medical Library

See ILLINOIS.

Wyoming

Cancer Information Service

1 (800) 525-0231

American Cancer Society

(307) 638-3331
Indian Hills Center
506 Shoshoni
Cheyenne, Wyoming 82001

Comprehensive Cancer Center

See COLORADO.

Children's Hospitals

See COLORADO.

Regional Medical Library

See NEBRASKA.

Canadian Resources

Treatment and research programs in Canada are coordinated by:

National Cancer Institute of Canada
77 Bloor Street West, Suite 401
Toronto, Ontario, Canada M582 V7
Phone: (416) 961-7223

The Canadian Cancer Society can be contacted at the same address and phone number.

Many Canadian cancer centers and hospitals are involved with the programs described in Appendix H. They are listed alphabetically by city below.

Calgary

Southern Alberta Cancer Centre
  NSABP
2104 2nd Street, S.W.
Calgary, Alberta T5S 1S5
Phone: (403) 263-0770

Edmonton

Cross Cancer Institute   RTOG,
  NSABP
11560 University Avenue
Edmonton, Alberta T6G 1Z2
Phone: (403) 432-8771

Halifax

Izaak Walton Killam Hospital for
   Children   CCG, NWTG
5850 University Avenue
Halifax, Nova Scotia B3J 3G9
Phone: (902) 424-6048

Hamilton

McMaster University   NSABP
50 Charlton Avenue East
Hamilton, Ontario L8N 1Y4
Phone: (416) 528-5403

Ontario Cancer Foundation
   NSABP
Hamilton Clinic
711 Concession Street
Hamilton, Ontario L8V 1C3
Phone: (416) 389-1371

Kingston

Kingston General Hospital   EST
Victory 4
Kingston, Ontario   K7L 2V7
Phone: (613) 546-3710

Queen's University   EST
Department of Medicine and
   Hematology/Oncology Services
2037 Etherington Hall
Stuart Street
Kingston, Ontario   K71 3N6
Phone: (613) 544-4536

London

University of Western Ontario and
   Ontario Cancer Foundation
   EST
London Clinic, Victoria Hospital
London, Ontario
Phone: (519) 432-5241

University Hospital   EST
London, Ontario
Phone: (519) 432-5261

Montreal

Hospital Saint-Luc   EST, NSABP
1058 Rue Saint-Denis
Montreal, Quebec H2X 3J4
Phone: (514) 285-1525 Ext. 263-
   309 (EST)
   (514) 254-8341 (NSABP)

Hospital L'Hotel-Dieu de Quebec
   NSABP
11 Cote du Palais
Montreal, Quebec G1R 2J6
Phone: (418) 694-5352

Hote-Dieu de Montreal   CLB
3840 Saint Urbain Street
Montreal, Quebec
Phone: (514) 844-0161

Jewish General Hospital   NSABP,
   PVSG, CLB
3755 Cote Saint Catherine Road
Montreal 26, Quebec
Phone: (514) 242-3111

McGill University Hospitals   CLB
Montreal General Hospital
1650 Cedar Avenue
Montreal, Quebec H3G 1A4
Phone: (514) 937-6011

Montreal Children's Hospital
   NWTG, SWOG
Pediatric Division
2300 Tupper Street
Montreal 25, Quebec H3H 1P3
Phone: (514) 937-8511

Montreal General Hospital
   NSABP
1650 Cedar Avenue
Montreal, Quebec H3G 1A4
Phone: (514) 937-7813

Royal Victoria Hospital   NSABP,
   CLB
687 Pine Avenue West
Montreal, Quebec H3A 1A1
Phone: (514) 842-1251

Ottawa

Ontario Cancer Foundation   EST,
   NSABP
Civic Hospital Division
Ottawa Civic Hospital Clinic
1053 Carling Avenue
Ottawa, Ontario K1Y 4E9
Phone: (613) 725-4361 (EST)
   (613) 728-2745 (NSABP)

Saskatoon

Saskatoon Cancer Center   NWTG
University Hospital
Saskatoon, Saskatchewan
Phone: (306) 652-3850

348

Toronto

Hospital for Sick Children   CCG
555 University Avenue
Toronto, Ontario L1A 1A1
Phone: (416) 597-1500

Mount Sinai Hospital   LCSG
600 University Avenue, Suite 441
Toronto, Ontario M5G 1X5
Phone: (416) 595-4380

Ontario Cancer Institute   TPN
500 Sherbourne Street
Toronto, Ontario
Phone: (416) 978-5588

Princess Margaret Hospital
   RHDG, LCSG
500 Sherbourne Street
Toronto, Ontario
Phone: (416) 924-0671

Saint Michael's Hospital   NSABP
30 Bond Street
Toronto, Ontario M5B 1WB
Phone: (416) 360-4245

Toronto General Hospital   LCSG
101 College Street
Toronto, Ontario M5G 1L7
Phone: (416) 595-3432

Toronto Western Hospital   LCSG
25 Leonard Avenue
Toronto, Ontario M5T 2R2
Phone: (406) 868-0555

Wellesley Hospital   LCSG
160 Wellesley Street East
Toronto, Ontario M4Y 1J3
Phone: (416) 966-6656

Vancouver

Saint Paul's Hospital   LCSG
Vancouver, B.C. V6Z 1Y6
Phone: (604) 682-2344

University of British Columbia
   CCG, NWTG
Department of Pediatrics
715 West 12th Avenue
Vancouver, B.C. V5Z 1M9
Phone: (604) 873-5441

Terry Fox Research Laboratory
B.C. Cancer Research Center
601 West 10th Avenue
Vancouver, B.C. V5Z123
Phone: (604) 873-8401

Winnipeg

Manitoba Cancer Foundation
   NSABP, NWTG
700 Bannatyne Avenue
Winnipeg, Manitoba R3E 0V9
Phone: (204) 787-2197

Appendix H

NATIONAL CANCER INSTITUTE PROGRAMS/ CLINICAL COOPERATIVE GROUPS*

National Cancer Institute (NCI)

NCI was established by the National Cancer Institute Act of 1937. It is one of the National Institutes of Health (NIH) of the Public Health Service, operating under the Department of Health and Human Services. The Institute was originally mandated to "investigate the

---

* Descriptions of the National Cancer Institute and its various departments have been taken from *National Cancer Institute: 1979 NCI FACT BOOK*, U.S. Department of Health and Human Services, Public Health Service, National Institutes of Health, National Cancer Program, Revised December 1979, NIH Publication No. 80–512, April 1980.

cause, diagnosis and treatment of cancer; assist and foster similar research activities by other public and private agencies; and promote the coordination of these activities.

"Thirty-four years later the National Cancer Act of 1979 (P. L. 92-218), and then the Amendments of 1974 (P. L. 93-352) and the Biomedical Research Extension Act of 1977 (P. L. 95-83), extended and expanded the activities of the National Cancer Institute and authorized a National Cancer Program to advance the national effort against cancer."* *

The National Cancer Institute is composed of five divisions and an office of the director.

The Office of the Director plans, develops, directs, and coordinates the activities and programs of the Institute and of the National Cancer Program and provides overall administrative guidance and services. It includes the Office of Program Planning and Analysis—which manages the development of the National Cancer Program Plan, the annual five-year plan, individual program plans, and the evaluation plan; analyzes programs of the Institute, evaluates resource needs for the National Cancer Program, and develops and provides support for management and scientific information systems.

The Office of Cancer Communications prepares and disseminates reports and other information to the professional community and the public.

The Office of International Affairs plans, coordinates, and manages cooperative international cancer-research activities, and provides leadership within the National Cancer Institute for the development of international programs and activities.

The Office of Administrative Management takes care of personnel, budgets, etc.

The Division of Cancer Cause and Prevention plans and directs a program of laboratory, field, and demographic research on the cause, natural history, and prevention of cancer through direct in-house research and through research contracts; evaluates mechanisms of cancer induction by viruses and by environmental carcinogenic hazards; serves as the focal point for the federal government on the synthesis of clinical, epidemiologic, and experimental data relating to the cause of cancer; and participates in the evaluation of and advises the Institute director on program-related aspects of cancer control activities and of grants and grant applications as they relate to cancer cause and prevention.

---

* * *National Cancer Program: Report of the Director 1978, Submitted to the President of the United States for Transmittal to the Congress.* U.S. Department of Health, Education and Welfare, Public Health Service, National Institutes of Health, NIH Publication No. 80–1986, November 1979, p. 3.

Within this division there are four programs: (1) the Field Studies and Statistics Program, which plans, conducts, and evaluates demographic research activities of the National Cancer Program and provides statistical services for all NCP research programs; (2) the Carcinogenesis Research Program, which plans, directs, and conducts basic and applied research programs on the role of chemical and physical causative factors and the prevention of cancer and conducts programs in the areas of carcinogenesis and related toxicology, metabolism, chemistry, cell biology, and experimental tumor pathology; (3) the Carcinogenesis Testing Program, which plans, directs, and conducts tests of chemical and physical agents in the environment for carcinogenic and cocarcinogenic effects; and conducts programs in the development and evaluation of standardized methods, designs, and models for carcinogenesis testing, related toxicology, and tumor pathology; and (4) the Viral Oncology Program, which plans and conducts the research and development programs dealing with viruses as causative agents of cancer.

The Division of Cancer Biology and Diagnosis plans and directs the Institute's general laboratory and clinical research activities; plans and manages collaborative programs in immunology, diagnosis, and breast cancer; and serves as the national focal point for programs to improve the detection and diagnosis of human cancers.

The Division of Cancer Treatment plans, directs, and coordinates an integrated program of cancer-treatment activities with the objective of curing or controlling cancer by utilizing combination modalities, including chemical, surgical, radiological, and certain immunological techniques. This division also administers a total drug-development program and serves as the national focal point for information and data on cancer-treatment studies. The division has four general programs: (1) the Cancer Therapy and Evaluation Program, which plans and directs the clinical contract and grant programs; tests combined-modality therapy approaches and new agents; and directs the evaluation of specific types and methods of cancer therapy; (2) the Clinical Oncology Program, which plans and directs the clinical research aspects of the programs of the division; (3) the Developmental Therapeutics Program, which plans, directs, conducts, and evaluates programs within and without the Institute, especially those related to chemotherapy; and (4) the Baltimore Cancer Research Program, which conducts an integrated program of laboratory and clinical research on the therapy and management of cancer patients, including pharmacologic investigations of how anticancer drugs work (this program will be described in more detail in the next section).

The Division of Cancer Research Resources and Centers plans and directs the Institute's grant-supported activities; recommends Institute policies relating to the administration of grant programs; develops, reviews, and coordinates plans and criteria for the implementation of NCI grants; and evaluates the effectiveness of grant-supported activities in achieving the Institute's missions. It also advises the Institute director, the National Cancer Advisory Board, and other advisory bodies of grant activities and developments. Within the division are three programs: (1) the Biological Research Program, which deals with biomedical and clinical research grant programs; (2) the Training and Education Program, which oversees professional training programs for researchers and clinical practitioners; and (3) the Centers and Treatment Program, which plans and directs the Cancer Centers Program, the Research Facilities Construction Program, and the Diagnosis and Treatment Program.

The Division of Cancer Control and Rehabilitation plans, directs, and coordinates an integrated program of cancer control and rehabilitation activities with the goal of identifying, testing, evaluating, demonstrating, communicating, and promoting the widespread application of available and new methods for reducing the incidence, morbidity, and mortality from cancer; serves as the focal point of a coordinated national effort to control cancer; in collaboration with the research divisions of NCI, identifies candidate-control techniques and methods for inclusion in the field-test and demonstration activities of the division; and advises the Institute director on program-related aspects of grants and contracts. This division has two programs: (1) the Intervention Programs, which focus on specific ways to control cancer and its effects; and (2) the Community Programs, which are involved in the development and direction of demonstration and education programs.

NCI Treatment Programs Available to Qualified Cancer Patients

NCI oversees and coordinates two sets of experimental treatment programs. One set of programs is conducted directly by NCI itself: These will be discussed in this section. The other set of programs is handled by Clinical Cooperative Groups, and will be discussed in the next section.

The Division of Cancer Treatment is divided into four programs. Two are of direct interest to patients: the Clinical Oncology Program and the Baltimore Cancer Research Program. Both treat patients directly. The Clinical Oncology Program is carried out at the Clinical Center, Building 10, National Institutes of Health, Bethesda, Maryland,

353

and at the Veterans Administration Hospital, 50 Irving Street, N.W., Washington, D.C. The Baltimore Cancer Research Center is located at 22 South Greene Street, Baltimore, Maryland.

We will try to give you a general idea of the experimental programs each facility is conducting. It should be noted, however, that specific protocols (treatment plans) close when they have all the patients they need, and new ones start up quite frequently. It is best to have your doctor check with the Patient Referral Service (301-496-4891) for up-to-date information on current programs and whom to contact for admission. Also, each branch chief can be contacted directly by calling (301) 496-4000. If for any reason your doctor cannot do this for you, you can get the information and refer yourself.

It should be emphasized again that NCI does not provide diagnostic services. Admissions can only be made on the basis of a confirmed diagnosis, although they will want to see your slides and all the clinical diagnostic information that has been gathered. If you need a confirmed diagnosis, contact a Comprehensive Cancer Center listed in Appendix G.

Medicine Branch: Robert D. Young, M.D., Chief.
Breast, endometrial carcinoma, Hodgkin's disease, lymphomas, melanomas, ovary, osteogenic sarcoma, and testicular cancer.

Pediatric Oncology Branch: Arthur S. Levine, M.D., Chief.
Acute leukemia, Ewing's sarcoma, neuroblastoma, non-Hodgkin's lymphomas, osteogenic sarcoma, rhabdomyosarcoma, and undifferentiated sarcomas.

NCI-VA Medical Oncology Branch: John D. Minna, M.D., Chief.
Lung, prostate, stomach, myeloma, macroglobulinemia, mycosis fungoides, Sézary syndrome, hepatocellular carcinoma. Also interested in patients with a strong family history of cancer.

Surgery Branch: Steven A. Rosenberg, M.D., Chief.
Breast, colon/rectum, melanoma, pancreas, urinary-tract tumors, and sarcomas of bone and soft tissue.

Radiation Oncology Branch: Eli J. Glatstein, M.D., Chief.
Esophagus, Hodgkin's disease, lung, lymphomas, unresectable chronosarcoma, and osteogenic sarcoma.

Dermatology Branch: Marvin A. Lutzer, M.D., Chief.
Ataxia telangiectasia, basal cell nevus syndrome, benign mucosal pemphigoid, cystic acne, Darier's disease, dermatitis herpetiformis, epidermodysplasia verruciformis, erythema elevatum diutinum, Fanconi's anemia, ichthyosis, keratosis palmaris et plantaris, multiple basal cell carcinoma, multiple warts, pemphigus vulgaris, pityriasis rubra pilaris, progeria, Rothmund-Thomson syndrome, Sézary syn-

drome, toxic epidermal necrolysis, Werner's syndrome, xeroderma pigmentosum.

Immunology Branch: William D. Terry, M.D., Chief.

Stage I and II melanoma patients.

Metabolism Branch: Thomas A. Waldmann, M.D., Chief.

Agammaglobulinemia, ataxia telangiectasia, calcium disorders, Di George syndrome, gastrointestinal disorders, growth-hormone deficiency, isolated IgA deficiency, serum-protein abnormalities, severe combined immunodeficiency, Sézary syndrome, Wiskott-Aldrich syndrome.

Clinical Oncology Branch/Baltimore Cancer Research Program: Peter H. Wiernik, M.D., Chief.

Breast, colon, lung (oat cell), acute and chronic leukemia, lymphomas, testicular carcinoma, and metastatic sarcoma.

Clinical Cooperative Programs*

Most experimental treatment programs funded and/or coordinated by NCI go on in other medical facilities throughout the world. In each site discussion in part II we have indicated which cooperative groups and projects are doing work on that type of cancer. What follows is a list of those groups located in the United States, organized alphabetically by acronym.

The groups and projects have several notable characteristics. First, the groups have been formed around several different types of criteria. Some have geographic names (although these can be misleading—the Southwest Oncology Group has members in New York, Washington State, and Cairo, Egypt), and these generally deal with many types of cancer. Other groups are organized around a single type of cancer, or the various cancers that affect one organ or system. Second, many groups may be involved with any one type of cancer. This should be clear from the number of cooperative groups listed in any one site discussion. Third, not all members of one group will offer all the protocols being conducted by the group as a whole.

---

* Information on clinical cooperative groups and experimental programs has been taken from *Membership Roster Cancer Clinical Trials Groups and Projects,* Cancer Therapy Evaluation Program, Division of Cancer Treatment, National Cancer Institute, September 1980, and *Compilation of Cancer Therapy Protocol Summaries,* April 1980, Fourth Edition, NIH Publication No. 80–1116. Both are published by the U.S. Department of Health and Human Services, Public Health Service, National Institutes of Health, Bethesda, Maryland 20205.

Fourth, despite the name of the group or the location of the chairman for each group, members may be found throughout the United States, Canada, and the world. For example, the Wilms's tumor Study Group deals only with experimental treatments for Wilms's tumor. It is comprised of 500 individual doctors associated with 107 hospitals; the group tests seven protocols. The Southwest Oncology Group includes over 600 doctors associated with 85 hospitals in 29 states and 4 foreign countries, and tests 267 protocols involving most types of cancers.

Because of the large number of doctors and hospitals involved, we have listed only the chairman for each group. A call to him will give your doctor or you the information about which protocol best suits your type of cancer and is located nearest to your home.

Cancer Clinical Trials Groups and Projects

BCRC   Baltimore Cancer Research Center
22 South Greene Street
Baltimore, Maryland 21201
Phone: (301) 528-7912   Dr. Peter Wiernik

BTRC   Brain Tumor Research Center
University of California, San Francisco Campus
551 Parnassus Avenue
San Francisco, California 94122
Phone: (415) 666-9000   Dr. V. A. Levin

BTSG   Brain Tumor Chemotherapy Study Group
David A. Pistenna, M.D., Chairman
Landow Building, Rm. 422A
National Cancer Institute, NIH
Bethesda, Maryland 20205
Phone: (301) 496-9361

CBCG   Cooperative Breast Cancer Group
1514 Jefferson Highway
New Orleans, Louisiana 70121
Phone: (504) 837-3000 Ext. 5834   Dr. A. Segaloff

CCG   Children's Cancer Study Group
Denman Hammond, M.D., Chairman
University of Southern California
2025 Zonal Avenue
Keith Administration Building, Rm. 509
Los Angeles, California 90033
Phone: (213) 226-2008

CCSF   Comprehensive Cancer Center for the State of Florida
c/o University of Miami
School of Medicine
Miami, Florida 33152
Phone: (305) 547-6090

CHOC   Children's Hospital Oncology Center
1056 East 19th Avenue
Denver, Colorado 80218
Phone: (303) 861-8888   Dr. David G. Tubergen

CHOP   Children's Hospital of Philadelphia
34th Street and Civic Center Boulevard
Philadelphia, Pennsylvania 19104
Phone: (215) 387-6000   Dr. Audrey E. Evans

CLB   Cancer and Leukemia Cooperative Group B
James F. Holland, M.D., Chairman
Department of Neoplastic Disease
Mt. Sinai School of Medicine
100th Street and Fifth Avenue
New York, New York 10029
Phone: (212) 650-6316

COG   Central Oncology Group
1120 West Johnson Street
Madison, Wisconsin 53706
Phone: (608) 263-2938   Dr. Fletcher

EORTC   European Organization for Research on the Treatment of
Cancer
c/o Inst. Jules Bordet
1000 Brussels, Belgium
Phone: (02) 538.65.33

EST   Eastern Cooperative Oncology Group
Paul Carbone, M.D., Chairman
Wisconsin Clinical Cancer Center, Rm. K4-614
600 Highland Avenue
Madison, Wisconsin 53792
Phone: (608) 263-8610

GOG   Gynecological Oncology Group
George C. Lewis, Jr., M.D., Chairman
Gynecologic Group Headquarters
1234 Market Street, Suite 430
Philadelphia, Pennsylvania 19107
Phone: (215) 854-0770

GTSG   Gastrointestinal Tumor Study Group
Douglas Holyoke, M.D., Chairman
Roswell Park Memorial Institute
666 Elm Street
Buffalo, New York 14263
Phone: (716) 854-2300
Philip Schein, M.D., Cochairman
Georgetown University Medical Center
Rm. 2230
3800 Reservoir Road, N.W.
Washington, D.C. 20007
Phone: (202) 652-7081

GUMO   Georgetown University Hospital
Division of Medical Oncology
3800 Reservoir Road, N.W.
Washington, D.C. 20007
Phone: (202) 625-7081   Dr. M. Slavik

357

HNCP	Head and Neck Contracts Program
	William DeWys, M.D., Project Officer
	Landow Building, Rm. 414A
	National Cancer Institute, NIII
	Bethesda, Maryland 20205
	Phone: (301) 496-2522
ITS	Intergroup Testicular Studies
	William DeWys, M.D., Project Officer
	Landow Building, Rm. 414A
	National Cancer Institute, NIH
	Bethesda, Maryland 20205
	Phone: (301) 496-2522
LCSG	Lung Cancer Study Group
	John Y. Killen, Jr., M.D., Project Officer
	Landow Building, Rm. 433B
	National Cancer Institute, NIH
	Bethesda, Maryland 20205
	Phone: (301) 496-2522
MAYO	Mayo Clinic
	200 1st Street, S.W.
	Rochester, Minnesota
	Phone: (507) 282-2511
MDA	M. D. Anderson Hospital and Tumor Institute
	University of Texas Health Science Center at Houston
	6723 Bertner Drive
	Houston, Texas 77025
	Phone: (713) 792-2121
MSKCC	Memorial Sloan-Kettering Cancer Center
	1275 York Avenue
	New York, New York, 10021
	Phone: (212) 794-5957
MTS	Mt. Sinai Hospital
	Fifth Avenue and 100th Street
	New York, New York 10029
	Phone: (212) 650-6361
NBCCGA	National Bladder Cancer Collaborative Group A
	c/o Massachusetts General Hospital
	Boston, Massachusetts 02114
	Phone: (617) 726-3009 Dr. G. R. Prout
NBCP	National Bladder Cancer Project
	Dr. Gilbert Friedell, Project Director
	St. Vincent Hospital
	25 Winthrop Avenue
	Worcester, Massachusetts 01610
	Phone: (617) 798-1234
NCCTG	North Central Cancer Treatment Group
	James M. Ingle, M.D., Chairman
	Department of Medical Oncology
	Mayo Clinic
	200 First Street, S.W.
	Rochester, Minnesota 55901
	Phone: (507) 284-8227

NCIC	National Cancer Institute of Canada
	77 Bloor Street West, Suite 401
	Toronto, Ontario, Canada M582 V7
	Phone: (416) 961-7223 Dr. Peter Scholefield
NCOG	Northern California Oncology Group
	Stephen K. Carter, M.D., Chairman
	1801 Page Mill Road
	Building B., Suite 200
	Palo Alto, California 14304
	Phone: (415) 497-7431
NPCP	National Prostatic Cancer Project (prostate)
	Dr. Gerald P. Murphy, Project Director
	Roswell Park Memorial Institute
	666 Elm Street
	Buffalo, New York 14203
	Phone: (716) 854-2300
NSABP	National Surgical Adjuvant Project for Breast and Bowel Cancers
	Bernard Fisher, M.D., Chairman
	914 Scaife Hall
	3550 Terrace Street
	Pittsburgh, Pennsylvania 15261
	Phone: (412) 624-2671
NWTS	National Wilms' Tumor Study Group
	Giulio D'Angio, M.D., Chairman
	Children's Cancer Research Center
	34th and Civic Center Boulevard
	Philadelphia, Pennsylvania 19104
	Phone: (215) 596-9614
OCSG	Ovarian Cancer Study Group
	Building 37, Rm. 6d28
	National Cancer Institute, NIH
	Bethesda, Maryland 20014
	Phone: (301) 496-1774
PhI/II	Phase I/II Studies of New Anticancer Drugs
	Vincent Bono, M.D., Project Officer
	Cancer Therapy Evaluation Program
	Landow Building, Rm. 409C
	National Cancer Institute, NIH
	Bethesda, Maryland 20205
	Phone: (301) 496-5223
PhII/III	Phase II/III Studies in Patients with Disseminated Solid Tumors
	Raymond B. Weiss, M.D., Coordinator
	Landow Building, Rm. 404A
	National Cancer Institute, NIH
	Bethesda, Maryland 20205
	Phone: (301) 496-6056
PhIIGC	Phase II Trials in Gastrointestinal Carcinoma
	Gary Witman, M.D., Project Officer
	Landow Building, Rm. 433C
	National Cancer Institute, NIH
	Bethesda, Maryland 20205
	Phone: (301) 496-2522

359

PVSG   Polycythemia Vera Study Group
        Louis R. Wasserman, M.D., Chairman
        Mt. Sinai Hospital
        19 East 98th Street
        New York, New York 10029
        Phone: (212) 876-2734

RHDG   Radiotherapy Hodgkin's Disease Group
        George B. Hutchison, M.D., Chairman
        Harvard University
        School of Public Health
        Department of Epidemiology
        677 Huntington Avenue
        Boston, Massachusetts 02115
        Phone: (617) 732-1050

RPMI   Roswell Park Memorial Institute
        666 Elm Street
        Buffalo, New York 14203
        Phone: (716) 854-2300

RTOG   Radiation Therapy Oncology Group
        Simon Kramer, M.D., Chairman
        Thomas Jefferson University Hospital
        1025 Walnut Street
        Philadelphia, Pennsylvania 19107
        Phone: (215) 574-3176

SEG   Southeastern Cancer Study Group
        John R. Durant, M.D., Chairman
        Comprehensive Cancer Center
        University of Alabama
        Tumor Institute, Rm. 214
        Birmingham, Alabama 35294
        Phone: (205) 934-5270

SFCC   Sidney Farber Cancer Center
        35 Binney Street
        Boston, Massachusetts 02115
        Phone: (617) 732-3470

SVH   St. Vincent's Hospital and Medical Center
        36 Seventh Avenue
        New York, New York 10011
        Phone: (212) 790-7000

SWOG   Southwest Oncology Group
        Barth Hoogstraten, M.D., Chairman
        Carol Fabian, M.D., Special Asst. to Chairman
        University of Kansas Medical Center
        Kansas City, Kansas 66103
        Phone: (913) 588-5966

TPN   Total Parenteral Nutrition Studies
        William DeWys, M.D., Project Officer
        Landow Building, Rm. 406B
        National Cancer Institute, NIH
        Bethesda, Maryland 20205
        Phone: (301) 496-4844

SJCRH	St. Jude's Children's Research Hospital
	332 North Lauderdale
	P.O. Box 318
	Memphis, Tennessee 38101
	Phone: (901) 525-8381 Dr. Charles Pratt
UARIZ	University of Arizona
	School of Medicine
	Department of Internal Medicine
	1501 North Campbell Avenue
	Tucson, Arizona 85721
	Phone: (602) 882-6372
UCLA	University of California at Los Angeles
	School of Medicine
	2025 Zonal Avenue
	Los Angeles, California 90033
	Phone: (213) 825-7786
UORG	Uro-Oncology Research Group
	David F. Paulson, M.D., Chairman
	P.O. Box 2977
	Duke University Medical Center
	Durham, North Carolina 27710
	Phone: (919) 684-5057
VALG	Veterans Administration Lung Cancer Study Group
	U.S. Veterans Administration
	Department of Medicine & Surgery
	Lung Cancer Study Group
	130 West Kingsbridge Road
	Bronx, New York 10468
	Phone: (212) 584-9000 Ext. 604 Dr. J. Wolf
VASAG & VASOG	Veterans Administration Surgical Adjuvant Cancer Chemotherapy Study Group
	Veterans Administration Surgical Oncology Group
	George A. Higgins, M.D., Chairman
	Chief, Surgical Service
	Veterans Administration Hospital
	50 Irving Street, N.W.
	Washington, D.C. 20422
	Phone: (202) 389-7266
WCCC	Wisconsin Clinical Cancer Center
	University of Wisconsin
	Department of Human Oncology
	1300 University Avenue
	Madison, Wisconsin 53706
	Phone: (608) 263-8600 Dr. D. C. Tormey
WCG	Western Cancer Study Group
	2825 South Hope Street
	Los Angeles, California 90007
	Phone: (213) 748-3111 Ext. 331 Dr. J. R. Bateman

361

WFU   Wake Forest University
Bowman Gray School of Medicine
Department of Medicine
300 South Hawthorne Road
Winston-Salem, North Carolina 27103
Phone: (919) 727-4397   Dr. H. B. Muss

WPL   Working Party for Therapy of Lung Cancer
666 Elm Street
Buffalo, New York 12403
Phone: (716) 845-2333   Dr. R. Vincent

WSU   Wayne State University
Adult Division
   Wayne State University Medical Center
   Detroit, Michigan 48201
   Phone: (313) 494-6433   Dr. Laurence Baker
Pediatric Division
   Children's Hospital of Michigan
   3901 Beaubien Boulevard
   Detroit, Michigan 48201
   Phone: (313) 494-5520   Dr. Barbara Cushing

YALE   Yale University
Yale School of Medicine
Section of Medical Oncology
LSOG 444
333 Cedar Street
New Haven, Connecticut 06510
Phone: (203) 436-8860   Dr. David P. Purpora

Appendix I

MAJOR ANTICANCER DRUGS BY GROUP*

Drugs useful in four or more types of cancer	Drugs useful in three or fewer types of cancer
Alkylating Agents	
Cyclophosphamide	Busulfan
Chlorambucil	Streptozotocin
Melphalan	Mechlorethamine
Dacarbazine	Thio-TEPA
Semustine	
Carmustine	
Lomustine	
Antimetabolites	
Methotrexate	Cytarabine
Fluorouracil	Thioguanine
	Azaribine
	Mercaptopurine
Antibiotics	
Dactinomycin	Daunorubicin
Mitomycin C	Mithramycin
Adriamycin	
Bleomycin	

Drugs useful in four or more types of cancer	Drugs useful in three or fewer types of cancer
Vinca Alkaloids	
Vincristine Vinblastine	
Hormones	
Glucocorticoids	Androgens Estrogens Progestogens
Miscellaneous	
cis-Platinum	L-Asparaginase Hydroxyurea Procarbazine Mitotane Nafoxidine Radioisotopes

* Adapted from William B. Pratt and Raymond W. Ruddon, *The Anticancer Drugs* (New York: Oxford University Press, 1979), p. 44.

364

Appendix J

TOXICITY OF ANTICANCER DRUGS IN VARIOUS ORGAN SYSTEMS*

Bone Marrow:

Antitumor antibiotics
(except bleomycin)
Busulfan
Cytarabine
Dacarbazine
Fluorouracil
Hydroxyurea
Mercaptopurine
Methotrexate
Nitrogen mustards
Nitrosoureas

Procarbazine
Thioguanine
Thio-TEPA

Central Nervous System:

Fluorouracil
L-Asparaginase
Methotrexate (intrathecal)
Mithramycin
Mitotane
Procarbazine
Vincristine

---

* Adapted from William B. Pratt and Raymond W. Ruddon, *The Anticancer Drugs* (New York: Oxford University Press, 1979), p. 53.

Heart:

Adriamycin
Daunomycin

Gastrointestinal Tract:

Cytarabine
Fluorouracil
Mercaptopurine
Methotrexate

Kidney:

cis-Platinum
Methotrexate
Mitomycin D
Streptozotocin

Liver:

Cytarabine
Mercaptopurine
Methotrexate
Mithramycin
Thioguanine

Lung:

Bleomycin
Busulfan
Methotrexate

Oral Mucosa:

Adriamycin
Azacytidine
Bleomycin
Cytarabine
Dactinomycin
Daunorubicin
Fluorouracil
Hydroxyurea
Methotrexate
Procarbazine

Skin:

Adriamycin
Bleomycin
Dactinomycin
Fluorouracil
Methotrexate
Nafoxidine
Procarbazine

Appendix K

DRUGS USED IN STANDARD AND EXPERIMENTAL CHEMOTHERAPY, HORMONE THERAPY, AND IMMUNOTHERAPY*

The organization of this section is that used by the National Cancer Institute. All drugs have been listed in alphabetical order, arranged by site. Italicized drugs are those which are commonly used for that type of cancer, and which appear in many treatment protocols.

---

* Adapted from *Compilation of Cancer Therapy Protocol Summaries*, April 1980, fourth edition, NIH publication no. 80–1116.

Although alphabetical, sites are generally grouped by system: For example, "Ovary" is listed under "Gynecological Tumors: Ovary." Also, you will notice that in addition to listing specific cancers, two other classifications are used: "general" and "other." "General" refers to drugs used to combat all types of cancer that affect that site or system, usually in advanced stages. "Other" refers to treatments for other specified types of cancer affecting that site. For example, there are three listings for lung cancers: Under "Lung Tumors: Oat Cell" are those drugs currently used against oat-cell tumors of the lungs; under "Lung Tumors: general" are those drugs currently used against all types of lung cancers, regardless of specific cell type; under "Lung Tumors: other" are drugs used in protocols aimed at specific types of non–oat cell tumors. This broad classification is used because there is not enough of any one type of protocol to create separate classifications.

Adrenal Gland (see ENDOCRINE TUMORS)

Bladder (see GENITOURINARY TUMORS)

Brain and other CNS Tumors

Adriamycin, Anguidine, Baker's Antifol, *BCNU*, Broxuridine, *CCNU*, Citrovorum Factor, Cycloleucine, Cyclophosphamide, DDMP, *Dexamethasone*, Dianhydrogalactitol, Dibromodulcitol, DTIC, 5-Fluorouracil, Ftorafur, Galactitol, Hydroxyurea, Imidazole mustard, 6-Mercaptopurine, *Methotrexate*, Methyl-CCNU, Methylprednisolone, Metronidazole, *Misonidazole*, Nitrogen Mustard, cis-Platinum, *Prednisone, Procarbazine,* Streptozotocin, Thio-TEPA, *Vincristine, VM-26,* VP-16

Breast Cancer

Actinomycin-D, *Adriamycin,* Adriamycin–DNA Complex, Aminoglutethimide, Amphotericin-B, *AMSA,* Anguidine, Antibiotics, Asparaginase, Azacytidine, Azaserine, Baker's Antifol, BCG-Cell Wall Skeleton, *BCG-Connaught,* BCG-Pasteur, BCG-Tice, *BCG-Unspecified,* BCNU, Bleomycin, Bruceantin, Calusterone, CCNU, Chlorambucil, Chlorozotocin, Chromomycin, Cisclomiphene, *Citrovorum Factor,* Colchicine, Cortisone, *Corynebacterium Parvum-Burroughs,* Corynebacterium parvum-Merieux, Cyclocytidine, *Cyclophosphamide,* Cytosine arabinoside, Dexamethasone, DHEA Mustard, Dibromodulcitol, Dichloromethotrexate, Diethylstilbestrol, Dromostanolone, DTIC, Estradiol, Floxuridine, *5-Fluorouracil,* Fluoxymesterone, Ftorafur, Galactitol, Gallium nitrate, Hexamethylmelamine, Hycanthone mesylate, Hydrocortisone, Hydroxyurea, ICRF, Interferon, Isophosphamide, *Levamisole,* Maytansine, Medroxyprogesterone acetate, Megestrol acetate, *Melphalan,* MER-BCG, *Methotrexate,* Methyl-GAG, Misonidazole, Mithramycin, *Mitomycin-C,* Nafoxidine, Neocarzinostatin, Norethisterone acetate, PALA, PCNU, Peptichemio, Piperazinedione, *cis-Platinum,* Prednisolone, *Prednisone,* Procarbazine, Progesterone, Pyrazofurin, Rubidazone, Shionogi, Streptonigrin, *Tamoxifen,* Testosterone, Thio-TEPA, Thioguanine, Thymidine, Triiodothyronine, *Vinblastine, Vincristine,* Vindesine, Vitamin A, Vitamin D, VP-16

Carcinoid Tumors

Adriamycin, Cyclophosphamide, 5-Fluorouracil, Methotrexate, Mitomycin-C, Streptozotocin

Cervix (see GYNECOLOGIC TUMORS)

Colon (See GASTROINTESTINAL TUMORS)

Endocrine Tumors: Adrenal

Adriamycin, Cortisone, Mitotane, cis-Platinum

Endocrine Tumors: Endocrine Pancreas

Chlorozotocin, Streptozotocin

Endocrine Tumors: Thyroid

Adriamycin, Bleomycin, PALA, cis-Platinum

Esophagus (see GASTROINTESTINAL TUMORS)

Ewing's Sarcoma (see PEDIATRIC SOLID TUMORS)

Gastrointestinal Tumors: Colon and Rectum

Actinomycin-D, *Adriamycin,* AMSA, Anguidine, Azacytidine, Azaserine, *Baker's Antifol,* BCG-Connaught, BCG-Glaxo, BCG-Pasteur, BCG-Tice, BCG-Unspecified, BCNU, Bleomycin, CCNU, Chlorozotocin, Chromomycin A-3, Citrovorum Factor, Corynebacterium parvum-Burroughs, Cycloleucine, *Cyclophosphamide,* Cytosine arabinoside, Dibromodulcitol, Dichlorometho-trexate, Diglycoaldehyde, DTIC, Floxuridine, *5-Fluorouracil, Ftorafur,* Galactitol, Hycanthone, Hycanthone mesylate, *Hydroxyurea,* ICRF, Indicine (N-oxide), Levamisole, Lithium carbonate, Melphalan, MER-BCG, *Methotrexate, Methyl-CCNU, Mitomycin-C,* Neocarzinostatin, PALA, Piperazinedione, cis-Platinum, Prednisone, Rubidazone, Streptonigrin, Streptozotocin, Tamoxifen, beta-TGdR, Thio-TEPA, Thioguanine, Thymidine, Vinblastine, *Vincristine,* Vindesine, VM-26, VP-16, Warfarin, Yoshi-864

Gastrointestinal Tumors: Esophagus

Adriamycin, *Bleomycin,* Citrovorum Factor, Cyclophosphamide, DDMP, Dibromodulcitol, 5-Fluorouracil, Hydroxyurea, MER-BCG, *Methotrexate,* Methyl-CCNU, Methyl-GAG, Misonidazole, Mitomycin-C, *cis-Platinum,* Vindesine

Gastrointestinal Tumors: Liver

Actinomycin-D, *Adriamycin,* AMSA, Aspirin, Bleomycin, Chlorambucil, Chlorozotocin, Citrovorum Factor, Corynebacterium parvum-Burroughs, Cyclophosphamide, DTIC, Floxuridine, *5-Fluorouracil,* Methotrexate, Methyl-CCNU, Misonidazole, Mitomycin-C, Neocarzinostatin, Streptozotocin, Vincristine, VP-16

369

Gastrointestinal Tumors: Pancreas

Actinomycin-D, Adriamycin, BCG-Glaxo, CCNU, Chlorozotocin, Citrovorum Factor, Cyclophosphamide, Cytosine arabinoside, *5-Fluorouracil*, Galactitol, Hexamethylmelamine, ICRF-159, Melphalan, Methotrexate, Methyl-CCNU, Methyl-GAG, Misonidazole, *Mitomycin-C*, Rubidazone, Spironolactone, *Streptozotocin*, Testolactone, beta-TGdR, Tubercidin, Vincristine, VP-16

Gastrointestinal Tumors: Stomach

AAFC, *Adriamycin*, AMSA, Anguidine, Baker's Antifol, BCG-Connaught, BCG-Unspecified, BCNU, Camptothecin, Chlorambucil, Chlorozotocin, Citrovorum Factor, Corynebacterium parvum-Burroughs, *Cyclophosphamide*, Cytosine arabinoside, Dibromodulcitol, Dichloromethotrexate, Floxuridine, *5-Fluorouracil*, Ftorafur, Galactitol, Hydroxyurea, ICRF, Melphalan, MER-BCG, *Methotrexate*, *Methyl-CCNU*, Misonidazole, *Mitomycin-C*, Neocarzinostatin, OK-432, cis-Platinum, Testolactone, Vinblastine, Vincristine, Vindesine, VP-16

Gastrointestinal Tumors: general

AAFC, Adriamycin, AMSA, Azacytidine, Baker's Antifol, BCG-Glaxo, BCG-Unspecified, BCNU, Bleomycin, Chlorozotocin, Citrovorum Factor, Corynebacterium parvum-Burroughs, *5-Fluorouracil*, Ftorafur, Galactitol, MER-BCG, Methotrexate, Methyl-CCNU, Misonidazole, Mitomycin-C, cis-Platinum, Streptozotocin, Vincristine, Vindesine, VP-16

Genitourinary Tumors: Bladder

Adriamycin, AMSA, Anguidine, Bleomycin, Chlorambucil, Cyclophosphamide, Dibromodulcitol, *5-Fluorouracil*, Gallium nitrate, Hexamethylmelamine, Levamisole, *Misonidazole*, Mitomycin-C, Neocarzinostatin, *cis-Platinum*, Poly IC, Thio-TEPA, Vincristine, VM-26, VP-16

Genitourinary Tumors: Kidney

Actinomycin-D, *Adriamycin*, AMSA, Anguidine, Azacytidine, Baker's Antifol, Bleomycin, CCNU, Chlorambucil, Citrovorum Factor, Cyclophosphamide, Cytosine arabinoside, DDMP, Dibromodulcitol, Estracyt, 5-Fluorouracil, Galactitol, Gallium nitrate, Hydrocortisone, Hydroxyurea, Indicine (N-oxide), Medroxyprogesterone acetate, Megestrol acetate, 6-Mercaptopurine, Methotrexate, Methyl-GAG, Methylprednisolone, Neocarzinostatin, PALA, *cis-Platinum*, Prednisone, Progesterone, Pyrazofurin, Rubidazone, Tamoxifen, Vinblastine, *Vincristine*, Vindesine, VP-16

Genitourinary Tumors: Prostate

Adriamycin, AMSA, Anguidine, *Cyclophosphamide*, Cyproterone acetate, Dibromodulcitol, *Diethylstilbestrol*, DTIC, Emetine, *Estracyt*, *5-Fluorouracil*, Gallium nitrate, Hydroxyurea, ICRF-159, Levamisole, Medroxyprogesterone acetate, Melphalan, MER-BCG, Methotrexate, Methyl CCNU, Misonidazole, cis-Platinum, Procarbazine, Stilphostrol, Streptozotocin, Tamoxifen, Testosterone, Vincristine, VP-16

Genitourinary Tumors: Testis

Actinomycin-D, Adriamycin, Anguidine, BCG-Unspecified, *Bleomycin,* CCNU, Chlorambucil, Citrovorum Factor, Cyclophosphamide, Cytosine arabinoside, Daunomycin, Dibromodulcitol, 5-Fluorouracil, Gallium nitrate, Hydrocortisone, Isophosphamide, MER-BCG, 6-Mercaptopurine, Methotrexate, Mithramycin, Piperazinedione, *cis-Platinum,* Prednisone, *Vinblastine, Vincristine,* Vindesine, VP-16

Genitourinary Tumors: general

Adriamycin, Anguidine, Cyclophosphamide, Galactitol, Peptichemio, cis-Platinum

Genitourinary Tumors: other

Adriamycin, BCG-Unspecified, Bleomycin, cis-Platinum, VP-16

Gynecologic Tumors: Cervix

Adriamycin, AMSA, BCG-Unspecified, *Bleomycin,* Citrovorum Factor, *Corynebacterium parvum-Burroughs, Cyclophosphamide,* DDMP, *5-Fluorouracil,* Hexamethylmelamine, Hydroxyurea, ICRF-159, Levamisole, Megestrol acetate, Melphalan, Methotrexate, Misonidazole, Mitomycin-C, *cis-Platinum, Vincristine,* Yoshi-864

Gynecologic Tumors: Ovary

Actinomycin-D, Adriamycin, AMSA, BCG-Connaught, BCG-Pasteur, BCG-Tice, BCG-Unspecified, BCNU, Bleomycin, Chlorambucil, Citrovorum Factor, Corynebacterium parvum-Burroughs, Cycloleucine, *Cyclophosphamide,* Cytembena, Dibromodulcitol, *5-Fluorouracil, Hexamethylmelamine,* ICRF, Isoniazid, Maytansine, Medroxyprogesterone acetate, Megestrol acetate, *Melphalan,* MER-BCG, *Methotrexate,* Misonidazole, Mitomycin-C, Phosphorus-32, *cis-Platinum,* Pyrazofurin, Thio-TEPA, Vinblastine, *Vincristine,* VM-26, VP-16, Yoshi-864

Gynecologic Tumors: Uterus

Adriamycin, AMSA, BCG-Pasteur, Chlorambucil, Corynebacterium parvum-Burroughs, *Cyclophosphamide,* Dibromodulcitol, DTIC, 5-Fluorouracil, *Medroxyprogesterone acetate,* Melphalan, Methotrexate, Misonidazole, Neocarzinostatin, cis-Platinum, Progesterone, Tamoxifen, Vincristine, Yoshi-864

Gynecologic Tumors: Vagina

Adriamycin, AMSA, BCG-Pasteur, Cyclophosphamide

Gynecologic Tumors: Vulva

Adriamycin, AMSA, BCG-Pasteur, Bleomycin, Cyclophosphamide, Yoshi-864

Gynecologic Tumors: general

AMSA, Baker's Antifol, Bleomycin, CCNU, Chlorozotocin, Dianhydrogalactitol, ICRF-159, Maytansine, Methyl CCNU, Piperazinedione, cis-Platinum, VP-16, Yoshi-864

Head and Neck Tumors

Adriamycin, Allopurinol, Aminopterin, AMSA, BCG-Connaught, BCG-Glaxo, BCG-Pasteur, BCG-Tice, BCG-Unspecified, *Bleomycin,* Citrovorum Factor, Corynebacterium parvum-Burroughs, Corynebacterium parvum-Merieux, *Cyclophosphamide,* DDMP, Dibromodulcitol, Dinitrofluorobenzene, 5-*Fluorouracil,* Ftorafur, Galactitol, Gallium nitrate, Hydroxyurea, Interferon, Levamisole, Maytasine, MER-BCG, 6-Mercaptopurine, *Methotrexate,* Methyl CCNU, Methyl-GAG, *Misonidazole,* Mitomycin-C, PALA, Peptichemio, *cis-Platinum,* Thymosin, Vinblastine, *Vincristine,* Vindesine

Hematologic Malignancies: general

Aspirin, Cyclophosphamide, Dipyridamole, Melphalan, Nitrogen Mustard, Oxymetholone, Phosphorus-32, Testosterone enanthate, Vitamin C

Histiocytosis

Chlorambucil, Cyclophosphamide, 6-Mercaptopurine, Methotrexate, Nitrogen Mustard, Prednisolone, Prednisone, Procarbazine, Vinblastine, Vincristine

Hodgkin's Disease (see LYMPHOMA)

Kidney (see GENITOURINARY TUMORS)

Larynx (see HEAD AND NECK TUMORS)

Leukemia: Acute Leukemia (general)

Adriamycin, Allopurinol, *AMSA,* L-Asparaginase, Azacytidine, Baker's Antifol, Benadryl, Chlorambucil, Chromomycin A-3, Citrovorum Factor, *Cyclophosphamide, Cytosine arabinoside,* Daunomycin, Dianhydrogalactitol, Diglycoaldehyde, DTIC, 5-Fluorouracil, Hydrocortisone, Isophosphamide, Levamisole, Lithium carbonate, Maytansine, 6-Mercaptopurine, *Methotrexate,* Neocarzinostatin, Piperazinedione, cis-Platinum, Prednimustine, *Prednisone,* Pyrazofurin, Rubidazone, beta-TGdR, Thioguanine, *Vincristine,* Vindesine, VM-26, VP-16

Leukemia: Acute Lymphocytic Leukemia

Acetaminophen, Actinomycin-D, *Adriamycin,* Anguidine, Asaley, *L-Asparaginase,* Azacytidine, BCG-Unspecified, *BCNU,* Benadryl, Bleomycin, CCNU, *Citrovorum Factor,* Corynebacterium parvum-Burroughs, Cyclocytidine, *Cyclophosphamide, Cytosine arabinoside, Daunomycin,* Deazauridine, Dexamethasone, Dibromodulcitol, Diglycoaldehyde, Hydrocortisone, ICRF-159, Interferon, Isophosphamide, Levamisole, MER-BCG, 6-*Mercaptopurine, Methotrexate,* Methylprednisolone, Neocarzinostatin, cis-Platinum, Poly-IC, *Prednisolone, Prednisone,* Rubidazone, Streptozotocin, beta-TGdR, *Thioguanine,* Trofosfamid, Vinblastine, *Vincristine,* Vitamin C, VM-26, VP-16

Leukemia: Acute Nonlymphocytic Leukemia

AAFC, Acetaminophen, *Adriamycin,* AMSA, Antibiotics, L-Asparaginase, *Azacytidine,* BCG-Tice, BCG-Unspecified, *BCNU,* Benadryl, CCNU, Chlorambucil, Chlorozotocin, Citrovorum Factor, Corynebacterium parvum-

Burroughs, Cyclocytidine, *Cyclophosphamide, Cytosine arabinoside, Dauno-mycin,* Deazauridine, Dexamethasone, Diglycoaldehyde, Hydrocortisone, Hydroxyurea, ICRF, Interferon, Lithium carbonate, MER-BCG, *6-Mercapto-purine, Methotrexate,* Methyl-GAG, Neocarzinostatin, Nitrogen Mustard, cis-Platinum, Poly-IC, Prednisolone, *Prednisone,* Pyrazofurin, Rubidazone, Stanozolol, beta-TGdR, *Thioguanine,* Trofosfamid, Vinblastine, *Vincristine,* Vindesine, VM-26, VP-16

Leukemia: Chronic Lymphocytic Leukemia

Adriamycin, BCNU, Chlorambucil, Chlorozotocin, Colchicine, Cyclophos-phamide, Cytosine arabinoside, Gallium nitrate, Hexamethylmelamine, Melphalan, Phosphorus-32, Prednisone, Thymosin, Vincristine

Leukemia: Chronic Nonlymphocytic Leukemia

Adriamycin, AMSA, Azacytidine, BCG-Unspecified, Busulfan, CCNU, Cyclophosphamide, *Cytosine arabinoside, Daunomycin,* Dexamethasone, 5-Fluorouracil, Hydroxyurea, Levamisole, MER-BCG, 6-Mercaptopurine, Methotrexate, Piperazinedione, Poly-IC, *Prednisone,* Pyrazofurin, Rubida-zone, Tetrahydrouridine, beta-TGdR, Thioguanine, Vinblastine, *Vincristine,* Vindesine, Vitamin A, VP-16, Yoshi-864

Leukemia: Extramedullary Leukemia

Adriamycin, L-Asparaginase, Azacytidine, BCG-Unspecified, BCNU, Citro-vorum Factor, Cyclophosphamide, *Cytosine arabinoside,* Daunomycin, Hydrocortisone, Hydroxyurea, MER-BCG, *6-Mercaptopurine, Methotrexate,* Methyl CCNU, Piperazinedione, Prednisolone, *Prednisone,* Thioguanine, *Vincristine*

Leukemia: general

Adriamycin, Adriamycin–DNA Complex, Anguidine, Bleomycin, Citrovorum Factor, Cyclophosphamide, Cytosine arabinoside, Deazauridine, Digly-coaldehyde, Galactitol, Hydrocortisone, Maytansine, 6-Mercaptopurine, Methotrexate, Neocarzinostatin, Peptichemio, Prednisone, Rubidazone, Thali-carpine, Thioguanine, Trifluridine, Vincristine, Vindesine, Yoshi-864

Liver (see GASTROINTESTINAL TUMORS)

Lung Tumors: Oat Cell

Adriamycin, ASMA, Antibiotics, Baker's Antifol, BCG-Pasteur, BCG-Tice, BCG-Unspecified, BCNU, *Bleomycin, CCNU,* Citrovorum Factor, Coryne-bacterium parvum-Burroughs, Corynebacterium parvum-Merieux, *Cyclo-phosphamide,* Dehydroemetine, Dexamethasone, Dibromodulcitol, DTIC, 5-Fluorouracil, Ftorafur, *Hexamethylmelamine,* Hydroxyurea, Isophospha-mide, Levamisole, MER-BCG, *Methotrexate,* Methyl CCNU, Mitomycin-C, PALA, Piperazinedione, *cis-Platinum,* Prednisone, *Procarbazine,* Thymosin, Vinblastine, *Vincristine, VP-16.*

Lung Tumors: general

Adriamycin, AMSA, Baker's Antifol, BCG-Connaught, BCG-Unspecified, Bleomycin, *CCNU,* Chlorozotocin, Citrovorum Factor, Colchicine, Corynebacterium parvum-Burroughs, *Cyclophosphamide*, Daunomycin, DDMP, Dexamethasone, Dibromodulcitol, Dichloromethotrexate, 5-Fluorouracil, Freund's Complete Adjuvant, Gallium nitrate, Guanazole, Hexamethylmelamine, Hydroxyurea, Levamisole, Maytansine, MER-BCG, *Methotrexate*, Methyl CCNU, Methyl-GAG, Misonidazole, PALA, cis-Platinum, Procarbazine, Rubidazone, Thio-TEPA, Thymidine, *Vincristine*, Vindesine, VP-16

Lung tumors: other

ACTH, Actinomycin-D, *Adriamycin*, Amphotericin-B, AMSA, Azacytidine, *Baker's Antifol*, BCG-Connaught, BCG-Glaxo, BCG-Pasteur, BCG-Tice, BCG-Unspecified, BCNU, *Bleomycin*, Bruceantin, *CCNU*, Chlorambucil, Chlorozotocin, Citrovorum Factor, *Corynebacterium parvum-Burroughs*, Corynebacterium parvum-Merieux, *Cyclophosphamide*, Dehydroemetine, Dianhydrogalactitol, DTIC, *5-Fluorouracil*, Ftorafur, Galactitol, *Hexamethylmelamine*, Hydrocortisone, ICRF-159, Isoniazid, Isophosphamide, *Levamisole*, Maytansine, Melphalan, MER-BCG, *Methotrexate*, Methyl CCNU, Methyl-GAG, Misonidazole, Mitomycin-C, Neocarzinostatin, Nitrogen Mustard, *cis-Platinum*, Prednisone, *Procarbazine*, Pyrazofurin, Streptozotocin, Thiabendazole, Thymosin, Vinblastine, *Vincristine*, Vindesine, Vitamin C, VM-26, *VP-16*

Lymphoma: Hodgkin's Disease

Adriamycin, AMSA, BCG-Tice, BCG-Unspecified, *BCNU*, Benadryl, *Bleomycin*, Camptothecin, *CCNU*, *Chlorambucil*, Chlorozotocin, Chromomycin A-3, Colchicine, *Cyclophosphamide*, *DTIC*, Gallium nitrate, Hexamethylmelamine, ICRF-159, Levamisole, Maytansine, MER-BCG, Methyl CCNU, *Nitrogen Mustard*, Piperazinedione, cis-Platinum, Prednisolone, *Prednisone*, *Procarbazine*, Rubidazone, Streptozotocin, Thio-TEPA, *Vinblastine*, *Vincristine*, Vindesine, VM-26, VP-16

Lymphoma: Lymphosarcoma

Adriamycin, L-Asparaginase, Chlorozotocin, Citrovorum Factor, Cyclophosphamide, Cytosine arabinoside, Daunomycin, 6-Mercaptopurine, Methotrexate, Methylprednisolone, Prednisolone, Prednisone, Streptonigrin, Vincristine

Lymphoma: Reticulum Cell Sarcoma

Adriamycin, AMSA, Antibiotics, BCG-Unspecified, BCNU, Bleomycin, CCNU, Citrovorum Factor, *Cyclophosphamide*, Cytosine arabinoside, Daunomycin, Dexamethasone, Hydroxyurea, ICRF-159, Imidazole mustard, Methotrexate, Methyl CCNU, *Prednisone*, Procarbazine, Streptonigrin, Thioguanine, Vinblastine, *Vincristine*, VM-26, VP-16

Lymphoma: general

Actinomycin-D, *Adriamycin*, Adriamycin–DNA Complex, Aminopterin, AMSA, Azaserine, BCG-Pasteur, BCG-Unspecified, *BCNU*, Benadryl, *Bleomycin*, Camptothecin, *CCNU*, Chlorambucil, Chlorozotocin, Citrovorum Factor, Corynebacterium parvum-Burroughs, *Cyclophosphamide*, *Cytosine arabinoside*, Daunomycin, Dexamethasone, DTIC, Gallium nitrate, Hexamethylmelamine, Hydrocortisone, Hydroxyurea, ICRF-159, Isophosphamide,

Levamisole, Maytansine, Melphalan, MER-BCG, *6-Mercaptopurine, Methotrexate*, Methyl CCNU, Methyl-GAG, Neocarzinostatin, Nitrogen Mustard, Piperazinedione, *cis-Platinum*, Prednisolone, *Prednisone, Procarbazine*, Pyrazofurin, Rubidazone, Streptonigrin, Streptozotocin, Thio-TEPA, *Thioguanine*, Vinblastine, *Vincristine*, Vindesine, VM-26, VP-16

Melanoma (see SKIN TUMORS)

Mesothelioma

Adriamycin, Bleomycin, Chlorozotocin, Dibromodulcitol, ICRF-159, Maytansine, cis-Platinum

Mycosis Fungoides

Adriamycin, Bleomycin, Cyclophosphamide, Cytosine arabinoside, ICRF-159, Levamisole, Methotrexate, cis-Platinum, Prednisone, Pyrazofurin, Vincristine

Myeloma

Adriamycin, Allopurinal, AMSA, Aniline Mustard, Azathioprine, BCG-Pasteur, BCG-Unspecified, *BCNU*, Calcium gluconate, CCNU, Chlorozotocin, Chromomycin A-3, *Cyclophosphamide*, Cytosine arabinoside, Daunomycin, Fluoxymesterone, Hexamethylmelamine, Levamisole, *Melphalan*, Methotrexate, Methyl CCNU, Methyl-GAG, Piperazinedione, cis-Platinum, *Prednisone*, Pyrazofurin, Sodium fluoride, Stanozolol, Testosterone enenthate, Thioguanine, *Vincristine*, Vitamin D

Neuroblastoma (see PEDIATRIC SOLID TUMORS)

Oat Cell Carcinoma (see LUNG TUMORS)

Ovary (see GYNECOLOGIC TUMORS)

Pancreas (see GASTROINTESTINAL TUMORS and ENDOCRINE TUMORS)

Pediatric Solid Tumors: Ewing's Sarcoma

Actinomycin-D, Adriamycin, CCNU, *Cyclophosphamide*, DTIC, 5-Fluorouracil, Methotrexate, Nitrogen Mustard, Rubidazone, *Vincristine*

Pediatric Solid Tumors: Neuroblastoma

Actinomycin-D, *Adriamycin*, Allopurinol, BCG-Connaught, BCG-Glaxo, BCNU, Bleomycin, CCNU, Citrovorum Factor, *Cyclophosphamide*, Cytosine arabinoside, Daunomycin, *DTIC*, Levamisole, MER-BCG, Methotrexate, Methyl CCNU, Nitrogen Mustard, cis-Platinum, Prednisone, Procarbazine, Sodium butyrate, Trifluorodeoxyuridine, *Vincristine*, VM-26, VP-16

Pediatric Solid Tumors: Retinoblastoma

Adriamycin, Citrovorum Factor, Cyclocytidine, Cyclophosphamide, Methotrexate, cis-Platinum, Vincristine, VM-26

Pediatric Solid Tumors: Rhabdomyosarcoma

Actinomycin-D, Adriamycin, Azapicyl, Bleomycin, CCNU, Chlorozotocin, Corynebacterium parvum-Burroughs, Cyclocytidine, Cycloleucine, *Cyclophosphamide,* Cytosine arabinoside, DTIC, ICRF-159, Melphalan, Methotrexate, cis-Platinum, *Vincristine,* VM-26

Pediatric Solid Tumors: Wilms's Embryoma

Actinomycin-D, Adriamycin, Bleomycin, Cyclocytidine, Cyclophosphamide, 5-Fluorouracil, ICRF-159, cis-Platinum, Vinblastine, *Vincristine,* Vindesine, VM-26, VP-16

Pediatric Solid Tumors: general

Actinomycin-D, Adriamycin, Baker's Antifol, Bleomycin, CCNU, Chromomycin A-3, Cyclocytidine, Cyclophosphamide, Dianhydrogalactitol, Diglycoaldehyde, DTIC, 5-Fluorouracil, Nitrogen Mustard, Piperazinedione, cis-Platinum, Prednisone, Procarbazine, Vinblastine, Vincristine, Vindesine, VM-26, VP-16, Yoshi-864

Pediatric Solid Tumors: other

Actinomycin-D, Bleomycin, Cyclophosphamide, 5-Fluorouracil, Galactitol, Methyl-GAG, cis-Platinum, Vincristine, Vindesine

Pharynx (see HEAD AND NECK TUMORS)

Polycythemia Vera

Adriamycin, Azaribine, Busulfan, Chlorambucil, Cytosine arabinoside, Hydroxyurea, Phosphorus, Prednisone, Thioguanine, Vincristine

Prostate (see GENITOURINARY TUMORS)

Rectum (see GASTROINTESTINAL TUMORS)

Reticulum Cell Sarcoma (see LYMPHOMA)

Retinoblastoma (see PEDIATRIC SOLID TUMORS)

Rhabdomyosarcoma (see PEDIATRIC SOLID TUMORS)

Sarcoma: Osteogenic Sarcoma

Actinomycin-D, Adriamycin, Allopurinol, Amphotericin-B, AMSA, Anguidine, L-Asparaginase, Baker's Antifol, BCG-Unspecified, Bleomycin, Chlorambucil, Chlorozotocin, *Citrovorum Factor,* Corynebacterium parvum-Burroughs, Cyclocytidine, Cycloleucine, *Cyclophosphamide,* Dibromodulcitol, *DTIC,* Galactitol, Gallium nitrate, ICRF-159, Maytansine, *Melphalan,* MER-BCG, *Methotrexate,* Methyl CCNU, Misonidazole, Piperazinedione, *cis-Platinum,* Pyrazofurin, Rubidazone, Vinblastine, *Vincristine,* Vindesine, VM-26, VP-16

376

Sarcoma: Soft Tissue Sarcoma

Actinomycin-D, Adriamycin, Allopurinol, Amphotericin-B, AMSA, Anguidine, Asparaginase, Azapicyl, Baker's Antifol, BCG-Unspecified, BCNU, Bleomycin, CCNU, Chlorambucil, Chlorozotocin, Citrovorum Factor, Cornyebacterium parvum-Burroughs, Cyclocytidine, Cycloleucine, *Cyclophosphamide,* Cytosine arabinoside, Daunomycin, DDMP, Dibromodulcitol, *DTIC,* 5-Fluorouracil, Galactitol, Gallium nitrate, Hydroxyurea, ICRF-159, Imidazole mustard, Maytansine, Melphalan, MER-BCG, *Methotrexate,* Methyl CCNU, Misonidazole, Piperazinedione, *cis-Platinum, Prednisone,* Procarbazine, Pyrazofurin, Rubidazone, Streptonigrin, Thioguanine, Vinblastine, *Vincristine,* Vindesine, VM-26, VP-16

Skin Tumors: Melanoma

Actinomycin-D, Adriamycin, *AMSA,* Azacytidine, Azaserine, Baker's Antifol, BCG-Cell Wall Skeleton, BCG-Connaught, BCG-Glaxo, BCG-Pasteur, BCG-Tice, *BCG-Unspecified, BCNU,* Bleomycin, CCNU, Chlorambucil, Chlorozotocin, Citrovorum Factor, *Corynebacterium parvum-Burroughs,* Corynebacterium parvum-Merieux, Cyclocytidine, Cycloleucine, *Cyclophosphamide,* DDMP, Dexamethasone, Dibromodulcitol, Diglocoaldehyde, *DTIC,* Duborimycin, 5-Fluorouracil, Galactitol, *Hydroxyurea,* ICRF-159, Interferon, Isophosphamide, Levamisole, Maytansine, Melphalan, *MER-BCG,* Methotrexate, Methyl CCNU, Misonidazole, Neocarzinostatin, PALA, Papaverine, Peptichemio, Piperazinedione, *cis-Platinum,* Procarbazine, Pyrazofurin, Streptonigrin, Streptozotocin, Tamoxifen, Thio-TEPA, Thymidine, Vinblastine, *Vincristine,* Vindesine, Vitamin C, VP-16

Skin Tumors: other

BCG-Pasteur, BCG-Unspecified, BCNU, Citrovorum Factor, DDMP, DTIC, Hydroxyurea, Misonidazole, Vincristine

Solid Tumors: general

Actinomycin-D, *Adriamycin,* Adriamycin–DNA Complex, AMSA, Anguidine, Azacytidine, Azaserine, Baker's Antifol, BCG-Pasteur, BCNU, Bleomycin, Camptothecin, CCNU, Chlorambucil, Chlorozotocin, Chromomycin A-3, Citrovorum Factor, Corynebacterium parvum-Burroughs, Cycloleucine, *Cyclosphosphamide,* Cytosine arabinoside, Daunomycin, Deazauridine, Dexamethasone, DHEA Mustard, Dianhydrogalactitol, Dibromodulcitol, Diglycoaldehyde, DTIC, *5-Fluorouracil,* Ftorafur, Galactitol, Gallium nitrate, Guanazole, Hexamethylmelamine, ICRF-159, Isophosphamide, Maytansine, *Methotrexate,* Methyl CCNU, Methyl-GAG, Misonidazole, Mithramycin, Mitomycin-C, Neocarzinostatin, Nitrogen Mustard, Peptichemio, Piperazinedione, cis-Platinum, Prednisone, Pyrazofurin, Rubidazone, Streptozotocin, Thalicarpine, Thio-TEPA, Trifluridine, Vinblastine, *Vincristine,* Vindesine, Vitamin C, VP-16, Yoshi-864

Stomach (see GASTROINTESTINAL TUMORS)

Testis (see GENITOURINARY TUMORS)

Thyroid (see ENDOCRINE TUMORS and
HEAD AND NECK TUMORS)

Uterus (see GYNECOLOGIC TUMORS)

Vagina (see GYNECOLOGIC TUMORS)

Vulva (see GYNECOLOGIC TUMORS)

Wilms's Embryoma (see PEDIATRIC SOLID TUMORS)